Innovation Leadership

Creating the Landscape of Health Care

Edited by

Tim Porter-O'Grady, DM, EdD, APRN, FAAN

Senior Partner and Registered Mediator, Tim Porter-O'Grady Associates, Inc., Atlanta, Georgia
Associate Professor, Leadership Scholar
Arizona State University College of Nursing & Health Innovation, Phoenix, Arizona

Kathy Malloch, PhD, MBA, RN, FAAN

Clinical Professor, Arizona State University College of Nursing & Health Innovation, Phoenix, Arizona
Clinical Consultant, API Healthcare, Inc., Hartford, Wisconsin

JONES AND BARTLETT PUBLISHERS
Sudbury, Massachusetts
BOSTON   TORONTO   LONDON   SINGAPORE

World Headquarters
Jones and Bartlett Publishers
40 Tall Pine Drive
Sudbury, MA 01776
978-443-5000
info@jbpub.com
www.jbpub.com

Jones and Bartlett Publishers
Canada
6339 Ormindale Way
Mississauga, Ontario L5V 1J2
Canada

Jones and Bartlett Publishers
International
Barb House, Barb Mews
London W6 7PA
United Kingdom

Jones and Bartlett's books and products are available through most bookstores and online booksellers. To contact Jones and Bartlett Publishers directly, call 800-832-0034, fax 978-443-8000, or visit our website, www.jbpub.com.

Substantial discounts on bulk quantities of Jones and Bartlett's publications are available to corporations, professional associations, and other qualified organizations. For details and specific discount information, contact the special sales department at Jones and Bartlett via the above contact information or send an email to specialsales@jbpub.com.

The authors, editor, and publisher have made every effort to provide accurate information. However, they are not responsible for errors, omissions, or for any outcomes related to the use of the contents of this book and take no responsibility for the use of the products and procedures described. Treatments and side effects described in this book may not be applicable to all people; likewise, some people may require a dose or experience a side effect that is not described herein. Drugs and medical devices are discussed that may have limited availability controlled by the Food and Drug Administration (FDA) for use only in a research study or clinical trial. Research, clinical practice, and government regulations often change the accepted standard in this field. When consideration is being given to use of any drug in the clinical setting, the health care provider or reader is responsible for determining FDA status of the drug, reading the package insert, and reviewing prescribing information for the most up-to-date recommendations on dose, precautions, and contraindications, and determining the appropriate usage for the product. This is especially important in the case of drugs that are new or seldom used.

Production Credits
Publisher: Kevin Sullivan
Acquisitions Editor: Emily Ekle
Acquisitions Editor: Amy Sibley
Associate Editor: Patricia Donnelly
Editorial Assistant: Rachel Shuster
Associate Production Editor: Lisa Cerrone
Marketing Manager: Rebecca Wasley
V.P., Manufacturing and Inventory Control: Therese Connell
Composition: Circle Graphics
Cover Design: Kate Ternullo
Cover Image: © Petr Vaciavek/Dreamstime.com
Printing and Binding: Malloy, Inc.
Cover Printing: Malloy, Inc.

Library of Congress Cataloging-in-Publication Data
Innovation leadership : creating the landscape of health care / [edited by] Tim Porter-O'Grady, Kathy Malloch.
    p. ; cm.
Includes bibliographical references and index.
ISBN 978-0-7637-6543-9 (pbk.)
1. Health services administration. 2. Leadership. I. Porter-O'Grady, Timothy. II. Malloch, Kathy.
[DNLM: 1. Health Services Administration. 2. Organizational Innovation. 3. Leadership. W 84.1 I572 2010]
RA971.I475 2010
362.1068—dc22
                                                                    2009024781

6048
Printed in the United States of America
13 12 11 10 09   10 9 8 7 6 5 4 3 2 1

Table of Contents

Preface

It has been said that this is the "Age of Innovation." Contemporary challenges with social, political, economic, and environmental arenas affecting human life have forever altered our individual and social priorities. In this time of challenge, the requisite contemporary prevailing realities and the need to suggest more sustainable options for addressing them have become primary. This primacy now requires leaders to more fully engage innovation as a way of life and to provide the kind of leadership necessary to inculcate innovation into every organization's way of doing business.

The globe is rife with innovators and innovations. There is no paucity of change agents and creative individuals in any enterprise or work capacity. The issue is not capacity to innovate; it is instead a need for the requisite skills to coordinate, integrate, and facilitate the innovation dynamic within a social and organizational context. Here the challenge is more precise and far more difficult to address. The leadership of innovation is a particular skill set requiring both an understanding of the innovation dynamic and a broader capacity to understand and manage the context within which sustainable innovation unfolds. Yes, understanding the skills and capacity for the leadership of constant change and creativity is in its infancy. Old industrial models of leadership application in relatively linear and stable organizations still abound and predominate the leadership literature and learning for contemporary readers. Nothing could be more devastating than this mismatch between the creative process unfolding in a complex framework and the management and leadership skills inadequate to address it.

It is in attempting to confront this prevailing reality that this text emerges. It reflects the robbed range of beginning thinking related to both a deeper understanding of the foundations of the innovation process and some of its applications matched with an elementary attempt to more clearly define and refine the requisites of leadership for innovation. Like any text of its kind, it cannot be considered as a complete reference but can be used in partnership with other vehicles of understanding for the true student of innovation. In this text we attempt to lay some relatively well-validated foundations for successful innovation processes and work to establish some leadership corollaries that best fit the dynamics of innovation. We've also tried to introduce some new thinking that projects emerging insights with regard to personal and collective skills that help to better guide the leader of innovation along the development and refinement of the innovation process.

Of course, this is a work in progress. Texts of this kind simply represent a moment in time, such that as soon as they are completed they dance around the edges of irrelevance. Our commitment is to continue to develop the concepts found in this text, expand on them, and reflect the prevailing reality of change and innovation that is more journey than point of arrival. Still, the foundations laid in this work by well-established thinkers and doers in the innovation process will surely withstand the test of time and establish the ground on which new ideas related to innovation and its leadership can be safely built. In addition, we hope that some challenges to contemporary thinking have been broached that will stimulate the dialogue out of which comes new thinking and approaches that might have otherwise lain dormant. These new modes of thinking are essential to the health and vitality of the leadership discourse. By raising these challenges, the contributors to this text do not seek merely to provide answers to prevailing questions concerning innovation and its leadership, but also to raise the level of dialogue and discernment.

Although the primary focus and exemplars in this text come out of the healthcare experience, their implications are not limited to health care. The concepts and practices outlined have drawn liberally from the business experience and reflections on the business of innovation. In a highly integrated world experience, compartmentalized thinking and acting are no longer appropriate. Elements and applications found in this text have major significance for the healthcare experience. At the same time, there are implications for the broader service and business environment. A review of the contributors of this text clearly demonstrates both the breadth and depth of interdisciplinary thinking and relationships woven throughout the content of this book. This has been purposeful, reflecting the necessary interdisciplinary conversation and collaboration essential to the future of leadership and innovation. We hope it demonstrates more clearly the value gained and the net increased aggregate value of broad interdisciplinary communication and relationship.

We look forward to continuing the development and dialogue necessary to advance the leadership of innovation. It is hoped that our readers will guide and inform future developments of this text through their communication with the publisher, editors, and contributors. Innovation is a reflection of the application of collective wisdom and discipline of the process. In that spirit, the editors wish to continue the dialogue and development that will refine learning and application of the innovation process and be further reflected in future editions. Finally, we hope and anticipate that the value of this text will be found in its usefulness, and that it will be one of a number of meaningful resources that will continue to inform and advance real and sustainable innovation in health care and throughout the world.

TIM PORTER-O'GRADY AND KATHY MALLOCH

Acknowledgments

I thank all the contributors to this text who generously shared their wisdom and insight in participating collectively to advance the dynamic and the leadership of innovation. A personal thanks goes to my writing and editing partner, Kathy Malloch, for her wonderful friendship, great insight, and continuous lifelong quest for knowledge and personal growth. I also thank Mark Ponder, partner and corporate administrator, whose commitments, generosity, and love are a constant source of renewal and encouragement. Finally, I thank my professional colleagues who in untold ways have influenced and guided my thinking throughout my career and who continually serve as a source of inspiration and encouragement in my professional and personal life journey.

Tim Porter-O'Grady

To be sure, no man or woman is an island, and in writing this book reminders of our interconnectedness with colleagues, friends, and family abound. I, too, am grateful to be blessed with Tim's friendship and colleagueship, which are now inexorably linked. The synergy of our collaboration and sharing of new ideas and approaches for our colleagues are a source of daily renewal and energy. A very special thank you goes to Bryan Malloch, my husband and best friend, who never sways in his support. He is my biggest supporter and the best partner anyone could ask for.

Kathy Malloch

Editors

Tim Porter-O'Grady, DM, EdD, APRN, FAAN
Senior Partner and Registered Mediator
Tim Porter-O'Grady Associates, Inc.
Atlanta, Georgia
Associate Professor and Leadership Scholar
Arizona State University College of Nursing & Health Innovation
Phoenix, Arizona

Kathy Malloch, PhD, MBA, RN, FAAN
President
Kathy Malloch Leadership Systems, LLC
Glendale, Arizona
Clinical Professor
Arizona State University College of Nursing & Health Innovation
Phoenix, Arizona
Clinical Consultant
API Healthcare, Inc.
Hartford, Wisconsin

Contributors

Jamil AlShraiky, MArch, MS
Director, Healthcare Design Initiative
Assistant Professor, Department of Interior Design
Arizona State University Herberger Institute for Design and the Arts
Tempe, Arizona

Sharon C. Ballard
President and CEO
EnableVentures, Inc.
Scottsdale, Arizona

Prasad Boradkar
Codirector and Project Leader
InnovationSpace
Associate Professor
Arizona State University Herberger Institute for Design and the Arts
Tempe, Arizona

Gregory Crow, EdD, RN
Professor Emeritus
Sonoma State University Department of Nursing
Rohnert Park, California
Senior Consultant
Tim Porter-O'Grady Associates, Inc.
Atlanta, Georgia

Sandra Davidson, MSN, RN, PhD(c), CNE
Director, Master of Healthcare Innovation Program
Clinical Associate Professor
Arizona State University College of Nursing & Health Innovation
Phoenix, Arizona

Gregory A. DeBourgh, EdD, RN, ANEF
Associate Professor and Chair, Adult Health Department
University of San Francisco School of Nursing
San Francisco, California

Scott Endsley, MD, MSc
Vice President, System Design
Health Services Advisory Group
Phoenix, Arizona

Ellen Fineout-Overholt, PhD, RN, FNAP, FAAN
Director
Center for the Advancement of Evidence-Based Practice
Arizona State University College of Nursing & Health Innovation
Phoenix, Arizona

Dr. Jonathan Levie
Reader
Hunter Centre for Entrepreneurship
University of Strathclyde
Glasgow, Scotland, United Kingdom

Bernadette Mazurek Melnyk, PhD, RN, CPNP/NPP, FAAN, FNAP
Dean and Distinguished Foundation Professor in Nursing
Arizona State University College of Nursing & Health Innovation
Associate Editor, *Worldviews on Evidence-Based Nursing*
Phoenix, Arizona

Gerald D. O'Neill, Jr.
Director
Entrepreneurship and Research Initiatives
Arizona State University
Tempe, Arizona

Paul Plsek
Consultant
Paul E. Plsek & Associates, Inc.
Roswell, Georgia
Mark Hutcheson Chair of Innovation
Virginia Mason Medical Center

Seattle, Washington
Director
Academy for Large-Scale Change
NHS Institute for Innovation & Improvement
United Kingdom

Jaynelle F. Stichler, DNSc, RN, FACHE, FAAN
Associate Professor
San Diego State University School of Nursing
Professional Development and Research Consultant
Sharp Memorial Hospital and Sharp Mary Birch Hospital for Women
San Diego, California
Faculty Associate
Arizona State University College of Nursing & Health Innovation
Phoenix, Arizona
Founding Co-Editor
Health Environments Research & Design (HERD) Journal

Susan B. Stillwell, MSN, RN, CNE
Clinical Associate Professor
Center for the Advancement of Evidence-Based Practice
Arizona State University College of Nursing & Health Innovation
Phoenix, Arizona

Dominique Surel, DM, MBA
President
CSA Group
Evergreen, Colorado

Kathleen Williamson, PhD, RN
Associate Director
Center for Advancement of Evidence-Based Practice
Arizona State University College of Nursing & Health Innovation
Phoenix, Arizona

CHAPTER 1

Leadership for Innovation: From Knowledge Creation to Transforming Health Care

Tim Porter-O'Grady

In the history of human enterprise, leadership has been a requisite for advancing the human condition. Regardless of the time in history or the human endeavors undertaken, leaders have emerged consistently at the right time to act out the roles necessary to coordinate, integrate, and facilitate human change (Hesselbein, 2002). Times and methods of leading the human enterprise have changed dramatically over the eons; the need for leadership has not.

The long history of leadership expression has been accompanied by an equally long history of the study of leadership (Bass, 1990). From the earliest times in recorded history in the Western World, through Greek and Roman epochs, the Middle Ages, the Age of Enlightenment, the Industrial Age, to our present Socio-Technical Age, detailed analysis of leadership and its impact has been consistently recorded. This focused study of leadership in the Western World has a corollary in Eastern writings, where the study of leadership followed a different trajectory but represented as much emphasis and interest.

Interest in leadership in democratic societies accelerated in the early Industrial Age and has advanced continuously ever since (Schein, 2004). This increased interest during the 20th century resulted in the development of specific leadership theories. These theories first focused on the characteristics and qualities that distinguished leaders from others, then moved through subsequent theories that more often focused on natural ability, skills, and contextual and situational factors, and finally settled in contemporary relational and quantum scientific theories that articulate integration and synthesis.

Although a number of broad-ranging theoretical constructs for leadership emerged over the past century, most of them fall within the context or are related to eight major theoretical frames that codified leadership during the course of the 20th century. These theoretical "frames" are the great man theories (leaders are born, not made), trait theories (inherent leadership qualities), contingency theories (environmental factors influence particular styles of leadership), situational theories (leaders choosing the best course of action based on the situation in which they find themselves), behavioral theories (focusing on the learned action of leaders obtained through teaching and observation), participative theories (ideal leadership is that which takes the input and

---

Box 1-1 Eight Major Leadership Theories

- Great man theories
- Trait theories
- Contingency theories
- Situational theories

- Behavioral theories
- Participative theories
- Management theories
- Relational theories

---

participation of others into consideration), management theories (transactional; focusing on the role of supervision, structure, and performance), and relational theories (transformational; emphasizing the relations and interactions between leaders and followers and focusing on motivating individuals and groups to perform at their highest potential) (Hersey & Blanchard, 1999) (Box 1-1).

An intensive, broad array of related research and theories reflecting one or the other of these eight major theories has regularly emerged over the course of concentrated study of leadership during the entirety of the Industrial Age (Bass, 1990). However, at the end of the Industrial Age, the influence of complex thinking and quantum science changed much of the foundation of the consideration of human action and leadership behavior. Furthermore, advances in psycho-neurobiology have had a tremendous impact on the understanding of human thought, motivation, and action. All these contemporary forces are merging to create newer foundations for thinking about leadership in a way that challenges many of the theoretical constructs developed during the 20th century (Hazy, Goldstein, & Lichtenstein, 2007).

LEADERSHIP AND THE HEALTHCARE PROFESSIONS

In addition to generalized thinking and challenges with regard to leadership, there are clearly unique considerations regarding the foundations and action of leadership within health care (Porter-O'Grady & Malloch, 2007). Recent focus on healthcare systems and the translation of current understanding about the needs of knowledge workers and the professions within which they hold membership leads to the consideration of unique and particular approaches to both structuring and expressing leadership. The contextual conditions and considerations for professional workers and the needs of knowledge workers create unique circumstances for the expression of leadership.

Each of the professions in health care has a unique body of knowledge and particular professional affiliations for applying it. Over the course of the 20th century, increased specialization has resulted from the expansion of the knowledge foundation for particular clinical practices (Stewart, 2002). This radical expansion of the knowledge base for clinical practice has created a whole range of knowledge-based practices in ways not previously conceived in earlier ages. In addition to physician practices, entire new areas of clinical focus have emerged from nursing and pharmacy to diagnostics, technology, and clinical therapeutics. Although the traditional medical model locus of control has maintained generalized control over much of healthcare decision making, in recent years that control has been less relevant and continuing legal protection of it has been more broadly questioned. As control for practice decisions has become more generally shared between specialty knowledge workers, hierarchical and unilateral locus of control leadership and decision-making models have become less viable (Coombs & Ersser, 2004). The independence of areas of specialty practice and the interdependence of all clinical decision making have created significant challenges within the healthcare disciplines. Linking and intersecting decision making across the health service spectrum has become a serious concern over the past two decades. Issues of evidence-based decision making, patient safety, decisional contradictions, lack of integration of decisions, and a structure that lacks synthesis have resulted in many contemporary problems and issues affecting the appropriate delivery of high-quality care.

In addition to thinking about the need to support, integrate, and facilitate the complex array of health professions, new thinking about leadership and complex systems has emerged. This newer thinking around complex adaptive systems challenges some of the basic concepts of leadership long held to be foundational to the exercise of leadership roles. Notions of power and authority, directing work, "buck stopping," being "captain of the ship," management, and imposing mandates as traditionally conceived are being severely challenged. In a time marked by the explosion of innovations and the need for radical reconfiguration and change, these traditional long-held notions of leadership are no longer viable (Gratton & Erickson, 2007).

It is a time of overwhelming and unpredictable transformation, with the sudden emergence of new knowledge, universal information access, global economic and social change, broad-based technological innovations, and the explosion of new scientific concepts and principles challenging long-held understanding of the universe and the very essence of life itself (Stone & Maxwell, 2005). In the midst of this drama lies the constant challenge to fundamental beliefs, theories, practices, and processes. Almost universally, people feel overwhelmed, challenged at the very core, uncertain about meaning and value, and unclear about how these challenges affect how they think and what they do.

At the same time, it is this emergence of the new science and the unpredictability of the emergence that so clearly represent the thinking that drives the age. Emergence and self-organizing complex systems are intriguing arenas of current research exploring the unpredictable and unanticipated complex system patterns, networks, and structures that function according to an entirely different set of rules and composed of newly discovered properties (Martin & Ernst, 2005). This pattern of networked emergent phenomena operates all around us at multiple levels, affecting us consciously and unconsciously and influencing our behavior, relationships, and organizations. The more historically "fixed" bureaucratic and hierarchical organizations and operating structures actually serve to prevent us from observing the full extent of the action of complexity and constant emergence. The need to constantly exercise control and provide a high level of order often serves to mask the chaos and serendipity so necessary to creativity, growth, and innovation.

The value of informal leadership and its role in influencing and directing systems are becoming clear. The more formal officially sanctioned leadership positions as described in bureaucratic or structured hierarchies often act counter to the requisites of informal leadership, which is located in the system and better reflects the needs and requisites of relationship, goodness-of-fit, and in response to the spontaneous demand for decision and action frequently required for successful innovation and change (Foti & Hauenstein, 2007). Box 1-2 highlights the differences between formal and informal leaders.

The divergence between concepts of formal leadership and emergent leadership brings uncertainty and confusion throughout healthcare systems. The traditionally well-defined and clearly structured hierarchical and tightly controlled structural approaches to managing the healthcare environment well served those who controlled it. Assumptions regarding the legitimacy of control over decisions, the medical decisional hierarchy, rigidity, and employer-directed roles for specific disciplines (most notably nursing) clearly articulated the locus of control and power legitimacy in healthcare organizations. In complex adaptive systems, on the other hand, these roles and relationships are less inflexible and require a different set of relational applications that represents both the value and the contribution of all roles, actions, and interactions in light of specifically defined and sustainable outcomes. Notions of mutuality, intersection, and synthesis redescribe and reconfigure decisions and actions. This then leads to the need for a different understanding and a change in the structures that support a more dynamic, interactive, and fluid set of relationships, decisions, and actions (Barrow, Davies, & Harper, 2004).

Box 1-2 Formal and Informal Leaders

Formal Leaders:
- Positional
- Hierarchical
- Controlling
- Directing
- Responsible
- Role-defined

Informal Leaders:
- Emergent
- Networked
- Locational
- Situational
- Relational
- Issue-defined

LEADERSHIP AND THE ELEMENTS OF COMPLEXITY

The historical metaphor for human organizations has been more mechanistic, suggesting that organizations are great machines (Freeman, Werhane, & Hogue, 2004). Over the long history of leadership, people and groups at any level of complexity have often been characterized and explained using military metaphors. Rigidly hierarchical and compartmentalized, control-driven military references have traditionally and historically often formed the structural frame for governing human relationships, especially at work. Almost all those substructures, policies, rules and regulations, and work processes reflect, in some way, this mechanistic, military metaphor for organizing people, decisions, and work.

Within the broader application of quantum mechanics, the emergence of complex adaptive systems demonstrates a singularly different understanding of the interaction among many elements and agents in human systems. The use of tightly controlled and rigidly hierarchical role, decisional, and process mechanics actually rails against the normative dynamics of system complexity. The assumption that all circumstances that affect human dynamics can be rigidly controlled and managed has no legitimacy in contemporary science. This is not to suggest that there is no role for military applications. It does suggest, however, that military applications and operations apply to a very narrow and specific set of variables in extremely particular situations and do not generalize well to the broader, more normative dynamics of human behavior.

Behavior in systems is fundamentally unpredictable. Therefore all linear, vertical, directed, and structured responses to action and change do little to actually manage or influence it. The complexity theory that undergirds complex adaptive systems is based on an understanding of relationships and interactions. In every aspect of the universe, multiple systems act in an interdependent way internally and with each other. Furthermore, these complex systems constantly adapt, shift, and change in relationship to their environment, forming the frame for complex adaptive systems.

The components of a system are the agents of the system. Flora and fauna act as the agents of an ecosystem, water molecules and air are the agents of the weather system, and so on. Like all systems, these agents are constantly relating and interacting with each other in a way that cannot be predicted or planned. Still, out of them come patterns of interaction that continually relate and feed back on each other, constantly informing these agents in creating the conditions of adjustment and adaptation. During this process extended periods of chaos and uncertainty emerge, moving inexorably to a new and different balance that, for a period, reflects a different set of circumstances or conditions. Complex adaptive systems have a number of characteristics and elements that define them (Figure 1-1). Those most significant affecting leadership are as follows:

- *Emergence:* Randomness appears to be the foundation of interaction between agents in the system. Out of these interactions particular patterns emerge that

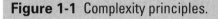

Figure 1-1 Complexity principles.

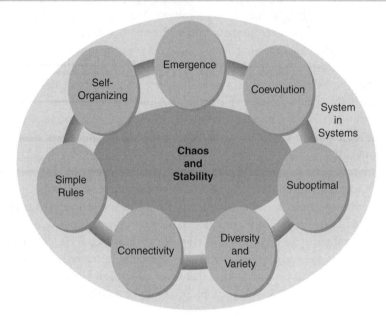

result in new configurations but also inform the agents of change in the system about the system and the rules in place that will sustain and change it.

- *Coevolution:* All systems interact internally and externally. These systems have their own internal environment but, at the same time, interact with an equally influencing external environment. The goodness-of-fit between internal and external environments recognizes that each influences the other; internal changes affect the external environment, and external changes influence the internal environment. This dynamic is continuous and unending, a sort of constant dynamic dance between external and internal forces. The latest thinking suggests that these systems continually learn from this interaction and evolve in ways that enable them to directly influence their environment and predict more precisely the implications and impact of future change.

- *Suboptimal:* Systems do not have to be perfect to successfully adapt and thrive. Over the course of evolving or emerging systems, or changes in old systems, they need only be slightly better than other existing systems. This notion of "good enough" in a complex adaptive system suggests that the system will often sacrifice efficiency for effectiveness. Sometimes this means the consumption of significant resources in the effort to obtain a more desirable outcome.

Important to the c cognition. This type of cognit of each team member with the & Bell, 2004). Important to this struc-ture within a team depend struc-

- *Variety:* The more variable a system is, or the more variety existing within, the stronger the system becomes. Ambiguity, uncertainty, paradox, and chaos are always present in these systems. The confluence of these forces and the challenges they create lead to the initiation of new concepts, processes, and products. Complex adaptive systems require variety and diversity to maintain viability and sustain over the long term.

- *Connectivity:* In complexity all things intersect and interact with each other. These interactions and feedback mechanisms provide the framework for the dynamic and life of the system. It is within these nodes and networks of connectivity that patterns and relationships are formed that intersect and interact with each other in a way that informs and forms the foundation for change. In complexity, it is these intersections in the energy and relationships that generate from them that are important to the life of a system.

- *Simple rules:* The rules governing complexity are not themselves unnecessarily complex. The mosaic of patterns in a system may appear exceptionally complex, but these patterns are often guided by rules that are profoundly simple. The principles that guide complex action are easily generalizable and, more frequently than not, influence the particular operation of complexity in all its circumstances. If one seeks to understand complexity, one need only understand the simplicity that drives it.

- *Butterfly effect (iteration):* Small changes generating from inside the system can be quite significant as they move through their emergence–feedback loop a particular number of times. Much like a snowball grows more quickly as it gets larger, these small initial changes can have large significant impacts on a system as they grow or aggregate.

- *Self-organizing:* Hierarchy has little meaning in complex adaptive systems. Formal structured vertical strategic planning or management processes are not viable here. Systems are continuously self-organizing, adapting to the continuous change of interactions, intersections, and relationships going on within. As external and internal forces continually change and adapt, these relationships between forces adjust and accommodate along a continuum operating through the dynamic processes of emergence and feedback.

- *Tightrope of chaos:* Organizations or systems that live in absolute stability are non-adaptive and quickly die. Systems that live constantly in the midst of chaos die just as quickly. Organizations that balance between the energy of chaos and the equilibrium of stability are more likely to adapt and thrive. Leaders constantly monitor this delicate "tightrope," drawing from the energy of chaos, which enables the system to maximize its variety and creativity without descending into either permanent chaos or absolute stability.

- *Nodes and networks:* All systems are smaller systems of larger systems or larger systems of smaller systems. This view of systems as a network of intersections and interactions between larger and smaller systems helps establish a framework for conceptualizing self-organizing and adaptation. In health care, a patient is a part of the local system (the care unit), which is a part of a larger system (the hospital), which relates to an even larger system (a community or region), intersecting with even larger communities (payment, regulatory, accreditation, partnership, etc.). Each single system is a part of a network of a number of larger systems whose life and direction are determined by the nature of the relationship, intersections, and interactions between all these various related systems.

These principles form the core that most notably defines the elements or principles of complex adaptive systems. Leaders operating at every level of systems need to fully understand how these principles operate to coordinate, integrate, and facilitate decisions and actions within systems (http://www.trojanmice.com/articles/complexadaptive systems.htm).

EMERGENCE AND LEADERSHIP IN COMPLEX SYSTEMS

In complex systems emergence is an important construct. Emergence occurs during a systems process of self-organization. The activities of self-organization occur at every level of life in the universe and are a part of the complex theoretical framework of all quantum systems. Although this relationship is still subject to further debate and discussion (e.g., whether emergent states result from self-organization or self-organization is itself an emergent phenomenon and can even exist without self-organization) (Wolf & Holvoet, 2005), emergence generally refers to new or emergent patterns of behavior, coherent structures, or states produced by the interaction between individual agents within a system, patterns that cannot be predicted from the characteristics of the individual agents alone, and from the rules that generate from their interactions (Goldstein, 2000). For leaders, the suggested implications are that emergent states are epiphenomena that result from the social interactions among members of the human group. Emergent states are defined as constructs that evidence properties and characteristics of the team that are usually dynamic in nature. Emergent properties can often differentiate or vary in the characteristics of the team's context, input, processes, and outcomes (Marks, Mathieu, & Zaccaro, 2001).

Important to the concept of emergence and leadership is the notion of team cognition. This type of cognition emerges from the interplay of the individual cognition of each team member with the process behaviors of the team as a whole (Cook, Kiekel, & Bell, 2004). Important to this concept is the understanding that individual knowledge structure within a team depends on team members sharing different types of knowledge structures. To remember particular knowledge structures in use during group interactions, group members have to share as much task-related information as possible. Shared cognition approaches focus on what team members share and how the integration of that shared information affects each member and the team as a whole. Theoretical approaches enumerate information processing as the interaction between members at three levels: selection, memory, and communication. Teams select a part of the available information and, by communicating their understanding of it, unfold representations that are contained in the long-term memory of the team. This representation simply means a particular way in which a team understands the body of knowledge, called the team frame of reference, collective cognitive representation, or team cognition (Gottlieb, 2003).

Because of these inherent relationships and operational processes, the appointed or formal leader of a given group may be considered the official leader, but this person is not often the operational leader of the group. This "operational" leader can be classified as "emergent" leader. This emergent leader often unfolds in roles that the official leader has not or does not fulfill. This emergent leader essentially "fills the gap" that results from unplayed (or emergent) or inadequate functions of the formal leader.

In many organizations, if not most, much of the description of leadership is an outflow of the understanding of leader as a formalized role. However, much current understanding of the dynamics and interactions of teams or groups suggests that this frame of reference for leadership description and characteristics is incomplete. Based on the understanding of emergence shared in this chapter, individuals frequently emerge into leadership roles in an informal construct because that individual is perceived by team members to possess skills both in group affiliation and in particular leadership skills. In this scenario the individual identifies or asserts particular leader skills; or the group identifies and acknowledges particular skills or talents of an individual member; or a task, function, or priority of the group aligns well with a specific leader talent of an individual member and is recognized by the member and the group. In this set of circumstances, the leader with these particular talents "emerges" based on the needs, characteristics, and/or dynamics of team interaction or process. In this context, the individual most likely to "emerge" and to be accepted as leader in the group is one who possesses high ingroup prototypicality and demonstrates the group's cognition and agreement regarding characteristics, mannerisms, and behaviors that they idealized as valuable to their leader conception. Although there are certainly well-researched modifiers influencing group perceptive dynamics such as gender, gender roles, and gender-specific tasks; skill value; social, physical, and personality characteristics; dominance; and verbal and expressive acuity, leader emergence (distributive leadership) is a common and important dynamic of team function, including innovation processes. The system's leader recognizes the essential centrality of emergence and group process and creates the constructs, structures, frames, and processes that reflect this value in group dialogue, decision making, and action (Rippin, 2007).

LEADERSHIP AND THE FOUR LEVELS OF EMERGENCE

In organizational systems a number of different configurations operate in conjunction in ways that continue to support the dynamic of the overall system from point of service or productivity and throughout the system. Essentially, four levels of emergence in complex systems exist where nodes and networks that link the system together converge to enable and sustain its life and future (Figure 1-2). The first level, *networks*, suggests looking at leadership and its role across the system. Here, the interface between formal and emergent leadership characteristics is more identified in the selection of network leadership than it is serendipitous or predominantly emergent. Reflected in this first level are the salient characteristics of a leader and his or her ability to understand life in complex adaptive systems and the fundamental characteristics of context, integration, intersection, and relationships as they ebb and flow throughout a dynamic system. It is important that leaders at this level of the system demonstrate their work leadership skills that address at least the following implications:

- Advance the ability to "see" networked systemness as a construct for the lived experience in organizations and a framework for the operation of leadership at every level of the system.
- Express the capacity to fully engage, involve, empower, and maximize the role of individuals and teams at every level of function in the system.
- Create conditions and circumstances where individuals and teams work to reach both separate and mutual goals and to renew goal processes in a continuous dynamic.
- Promote interaction and synthesis within and across the system, acting in the role of coordinating, integrating, and facilitating interaction between agents,

Figure 1-2 Four levels of emergence.

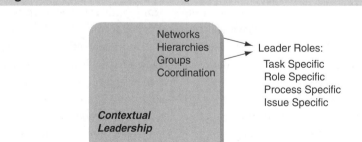

processes, groups, and network interfaces in a way that continually advances the integrity and viability of the system.

- Maintain and advance the connections, linkages, and interfaces of agents, groups, and components of the system in a way that continues the dynamic toward sustainability.
- Use the elements of knowledge creation and the structures of creative tension in a process that maintains the drama, energy, and accomplishments that inherently motivate and maintain levels of enthusiasm and excitement at every systems level.
- Operate successfully in the network exclusive role of contextual synthesis, continually advancing awareness and response to the changing internal and external interface that alters the contextual, strategic, and operational characteristics influencing action (Harmaakorpi & Niukkanen, 2007).

At the network level of leadership, the interaction across the network, between its nodes and points of intersection, is the critical perspective of the network leader. Furthermore, in this formalized role the network leader continually assesses, adjusts, and acts specifically to respond to the external and internal environmental interface, making decisions and drawing conclusions regarding the impact of that interface on structure, decisions, actions, and the trajectory of the system. In this role a highly developed skill set of predictive and adaptive capacity forms the foundation of performance expectations and of role application. Because these rules are formal and generally administrative, the preparation and capacity of the individuals filling these roles is a critical prerequisite to their appropriate exercise. In addition, because of the critical nature of the role and the confidence required to fulfill it, the necessary goodness-of-fit between individual and team at this level of the organization is vital to the efficacy of the performance expectations located within and between these leaders.

One of the main characteristics of leadership capacity in networks is the fundamental requisite that skills and behaviors successfully advance and impact the evolution and refinement of the network structure and the life of the organization. The constant interplay between external and internal forces creates the contextual framework within which the culture and life of the organization are directed. Because this interplay is constant and unrelenting, the network leader is ever vigilant to constantly maintain focus at this point and to successfully undertake the translational work necessary to accurately interpret and apply the forces interacting at this conjunction impacting the mission, purposes, strategy, direction, operation, priorities, and activities at every point in the system.

The primary role and focus of network leadership in dynamic and innovative organizations is on the three "i's": intersection, interface, and interaction. Also, confluence and synthesis of effort and action across the system drive the capacity and skill set of network leaders. From the perspective of innovation, the network leader's primary obligation is to ensure that the contextual and operational infrastructures necessary to support the dynamic of innovation as a way of doing business are operating effectively and are consistently and continuously supportive of the innovative processes. From the network perspective, structural, strategic, and operational infrastructures must operate relatively seamlessly to create both the context and the culture necessary to support the system/organization in its effort to maintain the dynamic tension/balance between the external and internal agents interacting to drive change and systems relevance (Figure 1-3).

For network leaders sources of innovation are both external and internal. Whereas the sources of innovation may originate in a variety of loci, the translation of innovation origination/generation into viable process and products positively affecting the organization involves the successful balancing and managing of the related and relevant external and internal dynamics in a way that drives the innovation toward value positively impacting the financial or operational viability of the system/organization. Where an innovation originates is not nearly as important to the network leader as its translation into application and value. As noted in other points in this text, the innovation process may originate in any number of ways and take form at any number of points along the trajectory of its flow. The system may address some innovations at the point of origin, others in the midst of translation and application, and still others as refinements or transformations of an existing innovation process or product. The network leader ensures that systems infrastructures can benefit and support the innovation and its related processes at any point in the continuum and at any place in the organization to which the innovation relates or that plays a role in successfully unfolding it.

Different from the innovators themselves, the network leader sees innovation and strategy as directly related. Although all successful innovations may have inherent value,

Figure 1-3 Network leadership roles in complex systems.

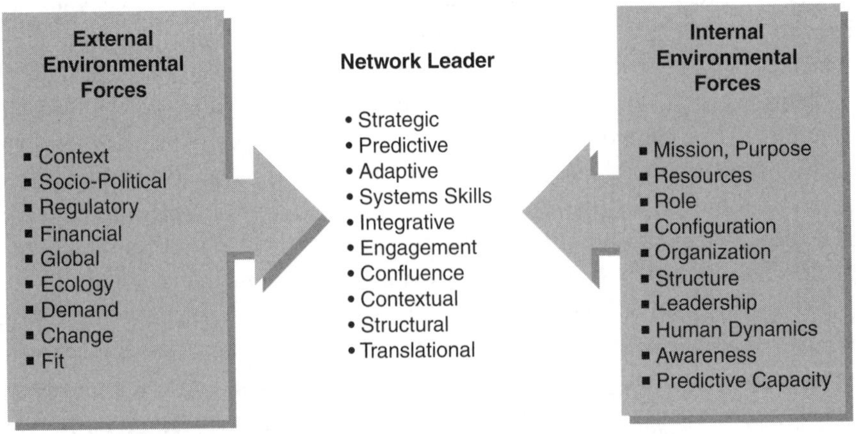

External Environmental Forces	Network Leader	Internal Environmental Forces
■ Context ■ Socio-Political ■ Regulatory ■ Financial ■ Global ■ Ecology ■ Demand ■ Change ■ Fit	• Strategic • Predictive • Adaptive • Systems Skills • Integrative • Engagement • Confluence • Contextual • Structural • Translational	■ Mission, Purpose ■ Resources ■ Role ■ Configuration ■ Organization ■ Structure ■ Leadership ■ Human Dynamics ■ Awareness ■ Predictive Capacity

for the network leader inherent value represents a direct line to strategic imperative. The mission, values, and purposes of the organization inform strategic priorities. These elements are influenced directly by the organization's goodness-of-fit with the external environment within which it lives. The network leader constantly scans this relationship for both opportunities and challenges because they both inform and impact the strategic requisites of the operating organization. Developing the appropriate management, strategic tools, and processes necessary to successfully anticipate, predict, and adapt to emerging or prevailing external shifts and using them effectively forms the critical skill set of the network leader. This leader is driven by relational realities at the macro level and their interface with the micro systems most frequently responsible for the innovation processes and applications. For the network leader innovation is a means, not an end. This leader sees innovation as a major dynamic, strongly linked to the strategic trajectory of the system, working to advance its relevance and viability. The network leader supports innovation not simply because it is a value (which it is) but rather because it underpins and ensures the continuing vitality and sustainability of the enterprise. All effort in this category of leadership is, thereby, focused on how well strategy and innovation interface, measured by indicators of continuing success of the mission and value of the organization within its broader context and constituency.

The network leader has specific competencies that are essential to the exercise of the role. As previously indicated, the competence of the network leader, primarily a positional role, needs to be ascertained before the individual assumes the role. It is primarily administrative (as opposed to situational or innovative) and lives predominantly in the contextual and relational domains. Skills in both arenas are a part of the essential foundation for the appropriate and successful exercise of the network leader role. Other major competencies related to the effective exercise of network leadership in the innovative organizations are as follows:

- An understanding of the key drivers of change within health care
- The ability to connect to the core work of the healthcare enterprise
- Scanning skills related to the confluence of forces in the external environment
- The talent to synthesize large aggregates of data as they relate to the strategic and core activities of the healthcare enterprise
- Highly leveraged translational skills in adapting external–internal integration challenges as they reconceptualize or redefine the character and content of health service
- A highly refined capacity for establishing a network of relationships throughout the external and internal networks having an impact on the viability and sustainability of the organization
- The structural insights necessary to ensure fluidity and mobility of the organizational infrastructure in a way that adjusts network configurations to more quickly adapt to changing circumstances and realities that affect the system's viability

- The ability to configure intersections and points of conjunction between and among the disciplines and constituencies from the system's internal and external environments with the power to quickly decide and act in the presence of change and innovation
- The capacity to inculcate the strategic imperative throughout the network such that it drives the lives and the work of all members of the system and informs decision and action at every level of the organization
- The ability to recognize and use both formal and informal nodes in the network and recognize the capacities and limitations of formal and emergent leadership, applying each rule to its fullest extent in maintaining the life of the organization and advancing its sustainability

As this discussion indicates, systems/organizations do not live in isolation. The confluence of forces and the dynamics of continuous change constantly intersect and interact within systems and between them. Because this is the dynamic, and therefore endless, the activity of the network leader related to this intense interaction is focused on it and fully invested in it. Indeed, network leaders are driven by the content of the interaction between elements of the network and the external and internal convergence that continuously affects the life and direction of the organization. Although fully aware of the content issues of the operation and actions of the system, the network leader sees these as a part of a larger aggregation of energy and forces. Because of this constant "dance" between these influencing and converging forces, the network leader acts both as agent and catalyst, giving form to response and ensuring that the outflow of the action between internal environments serves to positively inform and influence the decisions, actions, and outcomes of the work of the organization.

In complex adaptive systems, the network leader understands that directing specific activity and controlling the variables influencing them and the actions applying them to the realities of work are a local concern, not to be controlled from the top. Indeed, the network leader understands, in complex systems, exerting hierarchical control over the efforts and actions of the point of service or productivity in the system almost always guarantees a lack of goodness-of-fit between the exercise of control and the specific quality and efficacy of the local actions and creates a structural frame that quickly becomes rigid and nonresponsive. Engagement rather than direction is the key construct here, and the network leader is aware of how much engagement must be embedded in the very infrastructure of the system so that rather than a subset of behavioral empowerment, it is instead a construct applied as a structural imperative.

The network leader understands the power and value of the structure as system. It is important to acknowledge the fundamental characteristics of complex adaptive systems and recognize that, although structure is fluid and malleable, it is not formless or incongruent. The dynamic between structure and behavior is just as powerful as it is between behavior and action. The role and function of the network leader demonstrate a depth of understanding of the intensity of this interaction and recognize that building a congruent adaptive structure is as important in ensuring system effectiveness and vitality as is creating fluid, adaptive, and productive patterns of relationship and behavior at the point of service.

LEADERSHIP AND COMPLEX ADAPTIVE SYSTEMS HIERARCHY

The second level of emergence in complex adaptive systems/networks is *hierarchy*. In traditional management structures systems in health care can generally manage, structure, design, develop, practice, and service. At the same time health systems struggle more diligently to control external environmental issues such as health policy, health practices, competence, education, and individual users. The prerequisite of leaders in this scenario is attempting to manage the complex interaction of these forces through monitoring mechanisms and structural and process activities and adapting and changing them to shifts in reality. This means requiring leaders to focus critically on system structure and architecture.

Managing complex adaptive systems is especially challenging because, by definition, these systems operate within the continuous and unending dynamic of change. In traditional industrial models, management process focused on the management of costs and revenues. In complex adaptive systems, value becomes the driving force and management for value becomes the leadership process construct. Managing and leading to value means creating architecture (relational hierarchy) to support that effort, one that focuses on outcome rather than process and input. Another normative impact of this shift to value is refocusing the constructs and dynamics of the system toward clinical outcomes (health states) rather than toward provider rewards (Porter & Teisberg, 2006; Rouse, 2007a).

Leadership in complex adaptive systems, additionally, focuses on two significant issues: structuring for constant change and developing and ensuring highly responsive and adaptive human behaviors and dynamics within an organizational construct. Here, hierarchy refers to establishing relational priorities from the creation of an infrastructure that establishes the rules of engagement in a highly adaptive system to a set of rules and behaviors that represents the responsive and adaptive demands of systems and people with the changes affecting what they do. Even with a construct providing appropriate framework, it too must be adaptive and changing as the issues of goodness-of-fit between internal structure and response configure with the external–internal confluence with the forces of change (Figure 1-4).

Hierarchy in complex adaptive processes does not follow traditional linear notions of relationship. In a cyclical or systems view, there are locational realities that demand

Figure 1-4 Interacting network and organizational hierarchies.

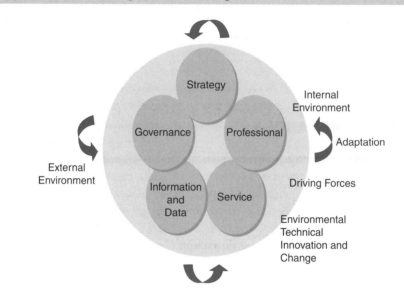

particular kinds of configuration to maximize appropriate response at the various loci of control. In this view expectations at the point of service require particular skill sets, competencies, and role performance. At the network location different skills, competencies, and performance expectations must be demonstrated. At the same time the level of support, integration, and synthesis between these points of performance, although unique to their location, must demonstrate a level of consistency, integration, and confluence to ensure the full needs of a responsive and effective system are in place (Rouse, 2007b).

Although hierarchies are inherent in complex adaptive systems, they are not absolutely vertical or linear in their design, structure, or relationships. In traditional industrial model approaches, hierarchies were ascendant, each subordinating element of the hierarchy directed and controlled by the ascendant hierarchical component. From a systems view hierarchy is more a locational device with specific performance and role assignments and expectations that ultimately intersect, influence, and interact with other hierarchy components or hierarchy locations. In this dynamic each position, role, or placement of hierarchy in the network has a direct impact on the relationship, fit, performance, and role of other places and people in the system. Much more interdependency and relational capacity is necessary to energize the relationship between hierarchies in the system. This level of intense interdependence demonstrates how important contribution and collaboration are between hierarchies in complex adaptive systems (Rouse, 2008).

Furthermore, complex adaptive systems require a stronger and more seamless commitment to consistent organizational behaviors across the system. In more traditional approaches organizational demands required more management behaviors instead of the more clearly described leadership behaviors required in complex adaptive systems. Hierarchies and structures as well as operational management processes historically required command and control approaches instead of more incentive and inhibition methods and processes. Also, complexity requires the measurement of outcomes rather than simply the review of processes and activities. The focus of complex adaptive systems is on patience and agility rather than simply measures of efficiency. Because complex systems are dynamic and highly relational, the development of intense personal relationships and interactions is more critical to their success than has historically been valued. Systems hierarchies in traditional organizations have been more linear and vertical in their orientation. In networked organizations, hierarchy represents more of a heterarchy (a system of organization), demonstrated by overlap, multiplicity, mixed ascendancy, and/or divergent but coexistent patterns of relation. Finally, organizational constructs represent a design that is less formal and linear and allows for more significant action of self-organization and reconfiguration, reflecting the organization's relevant response to changing internal/external demands, innovation, and change (Rouse, 2008).

In contemporary understanding of hierarchy, no permanent externally imposed structure can exist in a dynamic and responsive organizational context. Imposing external design operates against the action of complexity and adaptation. Formal structure is continually morphed by various stakeholders as they continue to learn and adapt and create ever-improving approaches that respond to the conjuncture of external and internal forces. For the leader, life occurs at the intersections of networks and hierarchies. This leader, therefore, spends a great deal of personal capital on this intersectional focus, ensuring that architecture, hierarchy, and systems constructs (Figure 1-5) both support and advance predictability, adaptation, creativity, innovation, and responsiveness (Basole & Rouse, 2008).

LEADERSHIP, GROUPS, AND INNOVATION

The third level of emergence in complex adaptive systems/networks is *groups*. In all human dynamics the network of social relationships and the quality of those relationships both predict and describe the level and value of community and social interaction. Leadership is vital to establishing and sustaining the structure and circumstances to support the level of intensity so necessary to the innovation process (Gratton & Erickson, 2007). In contemporary organizations especially, now reflecting a high level of complexity, distance, and role specificity, constructing social networks becomes critical to establishing identity, advancing strategy, and building the overarching

Figure 1-5 Life at the intersections.

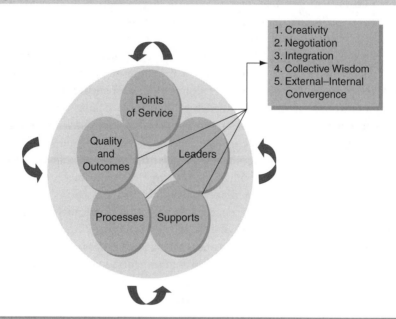

1. Creativity
2. Negotiation
3. Integration
4. Collective Wisdom
5. External–Internal Convergence

Points of Service

Quality and Outcomes

Leaders

Processes

Supports

connections and linkages necessary to ensure organizational integrity and competence related to the essential work of the organization.

In complex adaptive systems it is critical to recognize the fundamental interdependence of roles and processes, each acting in its own way to impact the strategic trajectory of the organization. However, sustainability within the system is built at the intersections of these various unilateral and compartmentalized processes and requires an infrastructure and the dynamic that maintains this connection. Translated into healthcare realities, no discipline or practice can ever act unilaterally or independently of its relationship with those on whom it depends and those who depend on it. This essential interdependence defines the nature of the social structure and requires from the highest levels of leadership the competence necessary to build the organizational infrastructure that has the capacity to create and use social networks and collaborative processes to address necessary changes and demands in the organization with a high level of creativity representing personal and collective engagement.

In innovative infrastructures it is necessary to look at teams as highly variable and temporary. The innovative process needs to be well served by those who have particular gifts and talents to offer it at the appropriate time within the innovation process flow. Here leadership understands that the core innovation team, charged with the responsibility for the innovation process itself, never has all the skills, talents, data, and resources necessary to accomplish its task. Therefore, although the core may be constant, membership in the group is not. A good portion of the leadership dynamics of an innovation team is to know and address what talent, resources, insights, and skills might be necessary at particular given times in the process with mechanisms constructed to make sure that that talent is accessed and used at the appropriate time and in the right way. Also, because the health system is predominantly a professional environment, every professional should expect to be accessed because of his or her unique skill capacities and to apply that talent at some point to the innovation process. Furthermore, in professional social networks each member must come to understand that he or she will play a role both at one's particular point of service and at points of intersection in the system at times when one's contribution may be required to undertake necessary systems change. Building this kind of infrastructure and incorporating these sets of expectations within the organizational construct is the fundamental obligation of executive leadership.

Group work is collaborative behavior. For collaboration to exist in systems as a way of relating and working, it must be a primary value embedded in the very fabric of the organization and exemplified by the constructs, models, and processes of leadership. Building this kind of culture and the infrastructure that represents it is an executive requisite in the contemporary organization that seeks to be available to successful innovation. Collaborative interaction, role sharing, collective problem solving, equity processes, and group decision making must be evident in the senior team's methods of leadership and doing business, such that this behavior becomes a prototype that represents the expected behaviors in leaders throughout the organization. Although it is not possible to know the whole business of delivering health-related services from every perspective, senior executives should be a familiar enough with the roles, decisions, and processes across departments and components of the system in a way that allows each of them to act for the other. This level of interaction must be clear and visible to all members of the system so that these behaviors seen at the executive level become the model for leadership behaviors that will unfold at any point in the health system. In systems where senior leaders represent these behaviors in their own practice, evidence of these behaviors also exists in other places in the system (Gratton & Erickson, 2007).

Group dialogue, decision making, and interaction should not be seen as exceptional or extracurricular work. So often in clinical environments professionals see their specific patient-related work to be the primary, if not the only, important focus of their professional obligation. In fact, these professionals often get so involved in the functional focus of their work activities that they see time spans and collective and collaborative processes as impeding or drawing them away from what they consider as their singularly most important activity: patient care. What these professionals fail to consider is that all activities related to deliberation and dialogue around the appropriateness, applicability, evidence, and viability of that action depend almost entirely on the quality, intensity, and veracity of the dialogue and agreement obtained on which the validity of clinical action is based. Time not spent in these activities condemns action to a level of relativity and uncertainty. Indeed, it is the strongest indictment of current clinical practices of many disciplines that their practice represents a failure of time not spent in the more critical clinical activity of collective dialogue and interaction related to practice that would help practitioners better discern appropriate practice and deliver it. In addition, complex adaptive systems pay a heavy price to the extent that their social networks and infrastructure are not congruent. The supporting infrastructure necessary to facilitate networked intersection and interaction requires a configuration that enables cross discipline and diverse dialogue and collective dynamics in order to sustain them. Management leadership, understanding this, ensures that the essential infrastructure coalesces around people and processes along with building the tools and skills necessary to ensure it lives and thrives.

A network infrastructure presupposes a highly collaborative frame for organizational decision making and action. Systems leaders know that the most effective decisions and resulting process actions occur as close to the point of productivity or service as can be obtained. As well, service leaders are aware that engagement demands ownership. This ownership is demonstrated in both the freedom and the capacity of those who do the work to fully participate in decisions that affect it. This is, however, not an accidental or chaotic set of circumstances. The discipline of network leadership is embedded both in structure and in the requisites of good process and interactional dynamics. Through use of good process tools, deliberation techniques, group dynamics, and emergence thinking and processing, an effective frame for the expression of worker ownership and participation can operate. Further, innovation and creative process at all levels of the system are disciplined by mission and strategic directives that give both form to the culture and direction to the organization.

Point-of-Service Leadership

Thus far, much of the focus on leadership in this chapter has related particularly to the formal and executive or network leadership capacity. However, in dynamic organizations decisions and actions taken here represent less than 10% of that demanded by the network. Although a critical 10%, it is limited to governance, strategic, structural, operational, and cultural concerns. The 90% majority decisions and actions are those that relate to the usual and ordinary daily obligations of work operating at the point of service where the vast majority of the life of a system is experienced. This holds especially true in healthcare systems/clinical organizations. The predominant "I–Thou" exchange occurs primarily at various intersections in various service sectors of the system. It is here where the changes and cultural reconfigurations necessary for networks to live and respond in complex adaptive systems must occur for adaptation and thriving to be sustained. And, of course, it is here where much of the action of innovation and creativity is embedded in highly adaptive and responsive systems.

Innovative culture is an expectation environment. The management frame of reference at the point of service is one that inculcates the expectation for creativity, adaptation, and change to occur. In highly adaptive systems change is not considered an external condition or circumstance; rather, it is considered the essential characteristic of the work itself. When change is the work, all the structural elements (performance expectations, role descriptions, goals, performance evaluations, outcomes) are configured to demonstrate the living application of those expectations. As this is inculcated into the infrastructure, expectation leads to a particular set of protocols and behaviors that articulate the values, roles, and functions of individual and collective performance.

For the innovative systems executive, creating a management team that articulates and demonstrates by their own behavior the living acceptance of change as the normative behavior becomes the seminal leadership development activity. Leaders at the point of service in the innovative organization are driven to create a culture within which change and adaptation is the foundational expectation and is seen by all players as the common characteristic element of every role. The group or service leader, in this set of circumstances, shows in his or her own role behavior the visual expression of the character of change and adaptation as expressed in the role. Holding themselves accountable for visual representation of change ownership, these leaders express, mentor, and motivate individuals and groups to inculcating and living that understanding within the context of their own roles. Service informal group leaders recognize that the only effective way of deciding and acting requires full engagement, participation, and ownership of deciders and actors. The imperative to decide and act in the innovative organization is not a requisite or demand of the policy and management of the organization. It is, instead, a requisite of membership, a rite of passage, and an experiential obligation of participation in action from each stakeholder to the extent of his or her capacity and potential for contribution. It is, quite simply, an expectation.

As this gets more clearly articulated and demonstrated in the role of leadership and the prevailing infrastructure makes such individual and collective engagement a part of the way of doing business, the convergence of structure and behavior creates the appropriate format for truly innovative action. It is within this framework that the dynamics and processes of innovation explored further in later chapters have life and take flight. Truly emergent leadership, common in innovation group process, cannot occur without the culture of expectation and engagement. All the characteristics of trust, investment, disclosure, expression, and open partnership simply cannot be generated or maintained in a culture that does not make it safe by making it real. In this case, obligation for full engagement does not come through discipline and order; instead, it arises as a function of the context, culture, and the life of the organization expressed through the concert of shared membership and the inherent peer obligations embedded in it.

The service or point-of-service leader respects the potential of emergent leadership in each member of the network's community. Emergent leadership arises out of a particular and specific need for a skill or contribution embedded in individuals and drawn on by the demand of the moment in the innovation process. Point-of-service and/or group leadership can often enumerate and select for the potential for leadership contribution in individuals in emergent circumstances. This leader can also alert the group to the potential and characteristics of emergence in group dynamics and to expect and respect its viability in group deliberation and decision making. Throughout the innovative scenario the point-of-service or group leader continually monitors the dynamics of deliberation and provides resource support and access, including other individuals who can contribute to the group's dynamics and to the successful movement of the innovation process. Inherent in all these performance characteristics is the point-of-service leader's continuing obligation to challenge, develop, expand, educate, and model knowledge, role, skill, and behavioral enhancements. The point-of-service leader can create the urge and the opportunity for successfully generating continuously relevant behaviors in the work group by informal mentoring and demonstrating and exemplifying the challenges and opportunities in learning, adapting, and experimenting (Gratton & Erickson, 2007).

A specific set of skills and behaviors is crucial to ensure a sustaining innovative environment. These skills and abilities are not accidental. The point-of-service leader recognizes the need to specifically delineate, clarify, train, and educate for the kinds of behaviors research has demonstrated are essential to building collaborative communities and to generating the innovations that can result from them. Human relations, conflict, interaction, and the dynamics of creative and innovation process must be reasonably clear with both structure and process well enumerated for those who will participate in it. Techniques and tools for stimulating critical and creative thinking, good group process, positive deviance, conflict generation, convergence, and synthesis are all a part of the basic cycle of learning and development necessary to spawning the outcomes of truly innovative relationships and processes.

Good leadership is intentional. Assessing both context and content helps the leader establish the environmental and behavioral circumstances of the work group. No leader initiates the innovative process without cause. It is the particular and unique complex of both talent and need that informs the leader with regard to the support, learning, and application trajectory unique to his or her human collective. Further, the leader searches the intersections between points of service and the other nodes of the network. In this, the leader looks for strong points of reference, facility, conflict, resonance, and "noise" between the obligations of his or her service and its goodness-of-fit with other components or with the whole of the greater system. This notion of "fit" is critical to the leader's understanding of synthesis between all work effort and all obligations of one service component, its impact on others, and the ultimate linkage in connection with the system as a whole. In a complex adaptive system, the point-of-service leader sees him- or herself not so much as the leader of a component of the system but as a systems leader operating from the perspective of a particular place in the system. The frame of reference for this leader is the whole system with "fit" of the component(s) he or she is responsible for within the system or the network. A strategic imperative that drives the point-of-service leader answers the question of how the mission and strategy of the system is advanced through the intention, deliberation, and action of the service component(s). The answer to this question disciplines the action to which the question relates.

Unique Leadership Needs of Innovation Groups/Teams

Team foundations for innovative groups and team action are fundamentally no different from any other collaborative group processes. Although many of the characteristics and actions of the innovative groups are unique to the innovation process, many of the structural considerations remain essentially the same. Creating a context for the dynamic group process is a major leadership activity and requires two foci: (1) a continuous human dynamic and relational framework embedded in the structure of the system, unit, or service and (2) good methods, techniques, and applications in managing the dynamics of the group process itself.

The major role of formal leaders in complex adaptive systems is to see to it that the systems remain adaptive and the context for decision, action, and work provides the appropriate frame (context) for the energetic and active coalescing of forces, agents, and activities in a continuous and dynamic confluence of interactions that sustain and advance the life of the system. The appropriate context for vibrant group process is one that meets the following conditions:

- An open and accessible relationship and interaction between management and staff that exemplify equity, respect, and understanding
- An open framework for communication and interaction that represents acceptance, trust, engagement, and an absence of fear
- A free sharing of relevant information impacting the decisions and actions of the work group that is particularly need-driven specific to the group
- The establishment and acceptance of conflict processes that incorporate normative conflict into the ordinary and usual activities of human interaction and work process
- An overall systems-generated expectation of openness and access to systems leaders and to information relevant to decisions and actions of groups
- An environment of continuous learning, growth, and development in both management and staff, exemplified in learning partnerships directed to developing individual and collective skills

- An environment that creates, implements, and supports an information-driven infrastructure that serves as the vehicle for knowledge creation, generation, management, application, and evaluation
- A human resource management system that reflects flexibility, adaptation, and specificity with regard to the encouragement, support, advancement, and rewarding of creative and innovative individuals, groups, and processes
- The continuous development and refinement of techniques and methodology in effective group process related to the specific purposes and action of the group yielding relevant and viable value and/or outcome

These contextual requisites are essential foundations for effecting a dynamic and adaptive pattern and system representing the interface of structure, process, and behavior (both management and participant) necessary to the creation and sustenance of an organization that is in any way creative, predictive, and adaptive. One can note the absence of emphasis on unilateral control, direction, discipline, and knowledge on the part of management. Instead, emphasis reflects what research suggests are the more communitarian needs in networks for competence, relationship, expectation, clarity, understanding, and good methodology for idea management and problem solving. Finally, the contextual imperative for personal and role accountability is an essential constituent for all participants, regardless of position or location, necessary to ensure the full investment and engagement of each person in the mission of the enterprise and the contribution of each person in advancing it (Box 1-3).

Skill and confidence in good group dynamics are critical to the effectiveness of collaborative groups, especially innovation groups. Innovation group process occurs at all levels and places in the network depending on the focus, issues, and intersections affected or invested. Stakeholders to the innovation process are not determined by location in the network so much as they are identified by contribution and impact. Good collaboration and group dynamics in the innovation process require access to whatever people and resources lead to effective decision making and action. Wherever the emergent need for

---

Box 1-3 Sample Innovation Process Techniques

- Nominal process
- Action lists
- Brainstorming
- Forced choice
- Jigsaw learning
- Delphi technique

- Strategy maps
- Social judgment analysis
- Cognitive maps
- Role defined
- Post-it boards

innovation process occurs in the network, informative needs for success can be enumerated as follows:

- Good predictive capacity that can use the tools of information management and evaluation to determine the need and timing for particular innovation group process
- Strong relationships between the mission and strategic requisites of the system and its responsive processes that can be quickly and easily generated in response to external challenges, threats, opportunities, or changes as they arise
- A well-inculcated and tightly-fitted relationship between the supportive and dynamic contextual infrastructure for engagement and the ability and willingness to engage stakeholders in creativity and innovation as an ordinary expectation of systems membership
- Good methodology, technique, and processes for managing innovation group dynamics (Box 1-3), which can both identify and apply state-of-the-art methods for relevant, applicable, and useful innovation process (see Chapter 3, which details effective innovation process)
- Effective methods of evaluating the success (and failure) of process and of outcome that provide the additional opportunity for learning, improving, and transforming group dynamics and process in a way that enhances the innovation process and increases its utility for future practice
- An opportunity to discover, identify, and use the particular talents of emergent leaders within the innovation process and to enumerate their unique skills and contributions in a way that can both access and reward emergent leadership capacity both situationally and systemwide

Recent research on group leadership suggests far more situational and emergent conditions and circumstances that create a high variation in the skill set of good leadership (Malloch & Porter-O'Grady, 2009). In complex adaptive systems, change drives the life of the organization and creates the circumstances that create the conditions for predictive and adaptive potential. Because the fit and interaction between external and internal forces are constantly in flux, the ability of the leader to assess the conditions and content of this constantly changing interaction and to determine the most appropriate immediate and long-term responses is critical to the system's ability to thrive. Engaging stakeholders at the right time in the right place for the right purpose becomes a centerpiece of the exercise of formal leadership in the system. Because leadership and management within a network relate more specifically to the management of "flow" and life at the various intersections in the network, it is essential for adaptive capacity to be highly refined in the role of leader. The innovation process is a response to the challenges and opportunities that emerge in this constant confluence between internal dynamics and external forces. The role of the formal leader in this process, whether it is network or point-of-service, is to bring a kind of discipline to the dynamic, allowing infrastructure, method, technique, and skill to interact in a way that best addresses those decisions and actions that lead to the most appropriate response in the system.

LEADERSHIP AND COORDINATION IN THE INNOVATIVE ORGANIZATION

The fourth and final level of emergence in complex adaptive systems/networks is *coordination*. This is perhaps one of the most significant components of the leadership role that supports both adaptation and innovation. In the network the constant ebb and flow of energy and activity in itself transforms the life and processes of the organization. In highly adaptive organizations, leadership practices are as variable as the demands and shifts that occur at the various intersections in the organizational network. Innovative adaptive organizations are able to vary their practice based on shifting knowledge, data, experience, outcomes, and circumstances. The life cycle of organizational networks constantly demands the creation of new configurations, approaches, processes, and relationships. The life of these organizations demands constant improvement and tighter goodness-of-fit between the demands of external forces and the configuration adaptation of internal operations.

In this set of circumstances the leader of innovation is rarely married to a particular method or style. However, the leader of innovation does reflect a specific set of values and demonstrates leadership skills and characteristics that conform expression to predictive and adaptive capacity. This leader understands the configurations, actions, and implications of complexity in the context of the networked system and is able to visualize the action of "flow" and the convergence of changing forces and necessary response in a way that positions the system to thrive. The leader of innovation is aware of the action of chaos and complexity. This leader understands that even seemingly inconsequential interactions and actions extrapolated over the course of time can have dramatic impact on the life of the system (strange attractors or the "butterfly effect"). The action of coordination relates directly to both understanding the action of this phenomenon and managing process in the face of it. Because, for this leader, it is impossible to know where the system/network is moving at each or any moment, it is necessary to see patterns in the life of the network as it interacts with itself and in the context of its external environment. The leader of innovation, constantly aware of this dynamic dance and continuous yet unforeseeable movement, looks for the themes, arrays, and relationships where form and future take shape, where trajectory originates, and where some level of prediction can lead to systemic and personal adaptation. This leader recognizes the tight relationship between chaos and order, knowing that one leads to the other in a dynamic process. Leaders and systems try not to avoid chaos but instead understand it and use the "attractors" within it to help the system self-organize. Because turbulent environments are the rule of existence, leaders try not to change the rules reflecting the essential chaos; instead, they develop an understanding of the characteristics of complexity and help manage its flow guided by clearly enumerated behavioral parameters (values). Therefore for leaders and organizations change is the reality, ever constant, ever present. To deal successfully with this complexity and chaos means, for the leader, to be constantly embroiled in the turbulence of movement. Through defining the strange attractors, a set of values is formed that enables the system to adapt and to live in this turbulence. The work of coordinating this dynamic involves the following conditions operating in the system/network (Dolan, Garcia, & Aurbach, 2003):

- Developing a shared set of principles, understanding of the mission, and strategic imperatives of the system and the ends to which they are directed
- Engendering trust and confidence, engagement, and ownership sufficient to deal with constant uncertainty
- Introducing infrastructure, structure, processes, and work dynamics that emphasize and value flexibility and fluidity and collective and individual work and action
- Working diligently to establish the patterns embedded in chaotic circumstances and situations looking for the creative and innovative challenge and opportunity embedded within
- Recognizing that self-organizing is an extant dynamic and can be positively influenced by creating the best goodness-of-fit between the prevailing environment and the internal operating dynamics of the system/network
- Establishing that ownership, investment, engagement, accountability, and collaboration are requisites of membership within the network and predescribe the roles essential to thriving there
- Recognizing the inherent relationship between the network and its external environment representing that relationship and a high level of social connection and responsibility that operates in a way to sustain the environment within which the life of the network/system is supported and sustained
- Acknowledging that the intensity of human relationships and their interactions are critical to the life of the organization and the goodness-of-fit between the action of each of its members and the integrity of the whole
- Remembering that esteem, ethics, and emotional intelligence lead to a state of high value and meaning, generating in all members a sense of well-being and recognition.

A common characteristic of the leader of innovation is the ability and high-level skill in the act of synchronicity. Real-time collaborative and synchronous coordination of the various operating characteristics, strategy, structure, processes, and human dynamics is a strong indicator of effectiveness in complex adaptive systems.

Box 1-4 Evidencing Synchronicity

- Interactions
- Relationships
- Partnerships
- Group process

- Agreement
- Collaboration
- Resonance

Synchronicity in a leadership role relates to the constant balancing and rebalancing of these interacting elements in a dynamic dance that represents the congruence, compatibility, and life of the organization. The higher the level of synchronicity, the more clearly it is demonstrated in the viability and sustainability of the organization and its sustenance.

Extreme collaboration and interdependence between all these network components are essential to ensure positive determinants for the organizations/system. Networks thrive on the effective confluence of interdependencies at the various intersections in the network: external–internal, mission–strategy, executive–service leader, network–node, service leader–team, discipline–discipline, group–individual, and point of service–network. Synchronicity is a sign that the confluence of interactions, relationships, collaborations, partnership, decisions, and processes is converging in a way that demonstrates resonance between them exemplified by the network's ability to adapt and thrive (Box 1-4). Truly effective and meaningful innovation relies, indeed depends, on this level of synchronicity. The leader of innovation focuses attention on the enterprise requiring constancy, awareness, and vigilance.

CONCLUSION

The leadership of innovation in complex adaptive systems requires a whole new leadership skill set in an emergent notion of leadership itself. Although it can be suggested by some that the role of leader in these complex organizations is diminished in its value, the real truth is that the need for leadership is advanced in complex adaptive systems. However, it is incumbent upon contemporary leadership to demonstrate the ability to transform the character and culture of systems and organizations to reflect emerging knowledge regarding the action and impact of chaos and complexity on human and organizational systems. Indeed, much innovation needs to be applied to the transforming role of leadership in 21st century systems/networks (Ben Saoud & Mark, 2006).

The innovative organization needs first to recognize what is necessary to thrive in an ever-changing, increasingly global community driven to a new level of understanding of complexity and the interconnectedness of everything. Building appropriate connections and linkages of major and small networks, internal and external environments, and relationships is the major construct of the leadership role for the perceivable future. Just as innovation is no longer an option for organizations, redescribing and represcribing the meaning, role, and function of leadership are major works of the time. In health care this is especially true. Increasingly, the external circumstances and environment exemplified in the sociopolitical, economic, and technological transformations unfolding in it now seek a different intersection, with healthcare delivery requiring newer configurations for addressing the health of individuals and communities in sustaining the future of a democratic society.

Leadership in the 21st century is also a work in progress. It is subject to the same dynamics of transformation in the context of chaos and complexity as the networks and systems within which its role unfolds. As more data related to emergence and complex adaptive systems are generated, the role of the leader will become clearer and more refined within them. The need for congruence and synchronicity in the ebb and flow of intersections, relationships, operating dynamics, adaptation, and innovation also requires strong insight and capacity in the leader to coordinate, integrate, and facilitate the necessary interactions effectively. Of one thing we can be sure: The need for effective leadership will not diminish. It will instead expand, requiring a deeper and richer competence. Leadership in the 21st century will now reflect a higher level of human understanding and will finally emerge out of the functional, militaristic, hierarchical, and rigidly controlling historical frame. Creating this kind of leader will be the seminal work of the time (Riney, 2008).

Innovation in healthcare organizations is simply no longer an option. Therefore creating the culture and infrastructure that make innovation a way of doing business is the critical role of healthcare leadership in all places in the system. This continues to require a reconceptualization of the content and development of leaders and the specific skill needs necessary to create and lead truly innovative healthcare environments. The premises and principles of complex adaptive systems form the frame for conceiving and thinking about the application of leadership within a healthcare context. Driven by the partnership between the disciplines and life at the point of service, innovation in health care now relates to building an evidentiary, information-driven foundation for healthcare practice: safer and better practices, better coordinated and integrated health outcomes, and, ultimately, impact on the social health of the nation. These ends simply cannot be achieved through the same mental model that brought health care to this point. At the same time, creating an innovation-driven organization requires an understanding of the application of concepts and principles of complex adaptive systems and the interactions and human dynamics that sustain them. This chapter merely serves as an introduction both to this understanding and to its implications for facilitating innovation in health systems/networks. Although this discussion on innovation leadership requires a much broader forum than this chapter can ever approach, the chapter does serve to introduce leaders of innovation to a beginning understanding of the need for new roles and behaviors. As subsequent chapters will more certainly and clearly show, time is of the essence. The leadership capacities necessary to facilitate, coordinate, and integrate comprehensive innovation in health care are now in major demand of the time.

REFERENCES

Barrow, J. D., Davies, P. C. W., & Harper, C. L. (2004). *Science and ultimate reality: Quantum theory, cosmology, and complexity.* Cambridge, UK: Cambridge University Press.

Basole, R., & Rouse, W. (2008). Complexity of service value networks: Conceptualization and empirical investigation. *IBM Systems Journal, 47*(1), 53–70.

Bass, B. (1990). *Bass & Stogdill's handbook of leadership: Theory, research, & managerial applications.* New York: Free Press.

Ben Saoud, N., & Mark, G. (2006). Complexity theory and collaboration: An agent-based simulator for a space mission design team. *Computational and Mathematical Organization Theory, 13*(2), 113–147.

Cook, N., Kiekel, P., & Bell, B. (2004). Advances in measuring team cognition. In E. Sales & S. Fiore (Eds.), *Team cognition: Understanding the factors that drive process and performance* (pp. 83–106). Washington, DC: American Psychological Association.

Coombs, M., & Ersser, S. (2004). Medical hegemony in decision-making—A barrier to interdisciplinary working in intensive care? *Journal of Advanced Nursing, 46*(3), 245–252.

Dolan, S., Garcia, S., & Aurbach, A. (2003). Understanding and managing chaos in organizations. *International Journal of Management, 20*(1), 23–35.

Foti, R., & Hauenstein, N. (2007). Pattern and variable approaches in leadership emergence and effectiveness. *Journal of Applied Psychology, 92*(2), 347–355.

Freeman, R., Werhane, E., & Hogue, P. (2004). *Business, science, and ethics.* Charlottesville, VA: Society for Business Ethics.

Goldstein, J. (2000). Emergence: A concept amid a thicket of conceptual snares. *Emergence, 2*(1), 5–22.

Gottlieb, M. (2003). *Managing group process* (p. 233). Westport, CT: Praeger.

Gratton, L., & Erickson, T. (2007). Eight ways to build collaborative teams. *Harvard Business Review, 85*(11), 100–111.

Harmaakorpi, V., & Niukkanen, H. (2007). Leadership in different kinds of regional development networks. *Baltic Journal of Management, 2*(1), 80–96.

Hazy, J., Goldstein, J., & Lichtenstein, B. (2007). *Complex systems leadership theory: New perspectives from complexity science on social and organizational effectiveness.* New York: Vintage Press.

Hersey, P., & Blanchard, K. (1999). *Management of organizational behavior* (6th ed.). Englewood Cliffs, NJ: Prentice-Hall.

Hesselbein, F. (2002). *Hesselbein on leadership* (1st ed.). San Francisco: Jossey-Bass.

Malloch, K., & Porter-O'Grady, T. (2009). *The quantum leader: Applications for the new world of work* (2nd ed.). Sudbury, MA: Jones and Bartlett.

Marks, M., Mathieu, J., & Zaccaro, S. (2001). A temporally based framework and taxonomy of team processes. *Academy of Management Review, 26*(3), 356–376.

Martin, A., & Ernst, C. (2005). Leadership, learning and human resource management: Exploring leadership in times of Paradox and complexity. *Corporate Governance, 5*(3), 82–94.

Porter, M., & Teisberg, E. (2006). *Redefining health care: Creating value-based competition on results.* Boston: Harvard Business School Press.

Porter-O'Grady, T., & Malloch, K. (2007). *Quantum leadership: A resource for health care innovation.* Sudbury, MA: Jones and Bartlett.

Riney, R. (2008). Healing leadership disorders. *H R Magazine, 53*(5), 62–66.

Rippin, A. (2007). Stitching up the leader: Empirically based reflections on leadership and gender. *Journal of Organizational Change Management, 20*(2), 209–226.

Rouse, W. (2007a). Complex engineered, organizational and natural systems: Issues underlying the complexity of systems and fundamental research needed to address these issues. *Systems Engineering, 10*(3), 260–271.

Rouse, W. (2007b). *People and organizations: Explorations of human-centered design.* New York: Wiley.

Rouse, W. (2008). Healthcare is a complex adaptive system: Implications for design and management. *The Bridge* [On-line], *38*, 1–2. Available: http://www.nae.edu/nae/bridgecom.nsf/weblinks/MKEZ-7CLKRV? OpenDocument

Schein, E. (2004). *Organizational culture and leadership.* San Francisco: Jossey-Bass.

Stewart, T. (2002). *The wealth of knowledge: Intellectual capital in the twenty-first century organization.* New York: Currency-Doubleday Books.

Stone, D., & Maxwell, S. (2005). *Global knowledge networks and international development bridges across boundaries.* New York: Routledge.

Wolf, D. T., & Holvoet. (2005). Emergence and self-organization: Different concepts but promising when combined. In S. Brueckner, G. di Marzo Seruguendo, A. Karageorgos, & R. Nagpal (Eds.), *Lecture notes in computer science* (pp. 1–15). New York: Springer.

CHAPTER 2

Creating the Organizational Context for Innovation

Kathy Malloch

"Were there none who were discontented with what they have, the world would never reach anything better."

—FLORENCE NIGHTINGALE

Traditional organizational infrastructures are effective for just that, traditional organizations created to function in the Industrial Age. As the transition from the Industrial Age to the age of technology and information availability accelerates, the processes of work, relationships between workers and customers, and the speed at which all of this occurs require a new emphasis for organizations. The contemporary organization requires an infrastructure that effectively supports both operations and innovations as well as the work of the organization and an openness to testing and implementing new ideas. At first glance this does not appear to be different from the work in which organizations are currently engaged. However, the speed and accelerated introduction of new ideas have increased dramatically, creating the need for a greater emphasis on innovation as well as an emphasis on the transition from innovation to operations.

Changes in communication modalities, new workflow processes, multivariate evaluation and measurement variables, innovative outcome expectations, and the quest for clear and visible value are undeniable for organizations. These evolutions reflect the new realities of space, time, structure, and substance. Effective organizational cultures must now support a more pronounced bimodal work model: effective operations and the continual creation, evaluation, and introduction of new and better ideas. According to Scharmer and Kaufer (2000) and Castells (1998), the changes occurring because of the Information Age are significant. There are now social structures based on networks, an economy tightly linked to information, and cultures steeped in virtual reality. These changes call for redefinitions of just about everything a leader does from visioning to planning to collaborating to implementing to evaluating and on and on.

In this chapter the transformations occurring because of the digital age, the new culture for a trimodal organization, and the emerging characteristics of innovation leaders are discussed. Readers are cautioned that the innovation leadership content and model are continually evolving and must necessarily adapt to new iterations and changes in the marketplace. The context in which an organization exists is always an essential consideration for the innovation leader—although there are common principles and behaviors associated with success, there is no one size that fits all.

I am a digital immigrant . . . my two young daughters are digital natives. They do not know a world without ubiquitous broadband Internet access. We may never become true digital natives, but we can and must begin to assimilate to their culture and way of thinking.

—RUPERT MURDOCH, 2005

A NEW LOOK AT THE ENVIRONMENT

The new world taking shape before us necessarily impacts the very nature of health care and the ways in which healthcare services are organized, packaged, delivered, and evaluated. Specifically, the availability and sharing of information, the media used for knowledge transfer, the range and types of relationships between and among providers and patients, and the time required to transfer and share information now require new structures, principles for communication, and outcome expectations for leaders. The changes in how information is communicated, who can access information, real-time availability of information on the Internet, and the availability of digitized media for nearly every bit of information are discussed in this next section. Table 2-1 provides an overview of traditional and Information Age characteristics as well as advantages and disadvantages for the four dimensions of structure, media, space, and time.

Redefining Structure

The first dimension that has changed dramatically is structure. Traditional organizational structure serves to define levels of authority, communication pathways, and span of control. The organizational chart at one time defined clear lines of accountability and role relationships believed appropriate for organizational effectiveness and efficiency. Now with the widespread use of the Internet and digital device real-time communication and

Table 2-1 Comparison of Traditional and Information Age Dimensions

Traditional vs. Information Age: Structure, Media, Space and Time Comparisons

	Traditional	Information Age	Advantages	Disadvantages
Structure for communication and authority designation Who is involved?	Organizational chart Vertical communication	Internet Social networks Open communication	Eliminates silos Increases integration of work products	Uncertainty with open communication Perceived loss of control and power
Media How is knowledge transferred?	Paper, books, Video, Audio	Digital	Consistency; quality of information	Lack of resources to implement
Space Where does it happen?	Physical buildings/offices Local	Virtual Nonlocal	Space available for open collaboration	Perceived loss of privacy
Time When does it occur?	Business hours	No limits 24 hours/day	Decreases lag time across time zones and between individuals	Blurs the boundaries between work and personal time

self-organizing networks, these boundaries have become blurred at best and nearly obsolete in many organizations.

The availability of text messaging, instant messaging, and social networks has contributed greatly to the new model for work. Communication with anyone at any time is now possible and occurs regularly. Power relationships are now dramatically reconfigured. Communications between executive, managers, and staff are now horizontal, vertical, diagonal, up-and-down historical lines of authority and chains of command. According to Bennis, Goleman, and Biederman (2008), the effectiveness of an organization depends on the flow of information. Further, the organization's capacity to compete, solve problems, innovate, meet challenges, and achieve goals requires all the organization's intelligence—and this is directly related to the healthy flow of information.

The structure for patient care also changes dramatically with the introduction of virtual patient care room and electronic oversight of patients. Not only does the leader need to ensure appropriate space for patient care but also effective virtual systems and the availability of staff to provide the virtual oversight from remote locations. Staffing and scheduling processes necessarily become more complex as needs increase and staff locations vary more widely. Creating staffing models that link clinicians with patients and supporting technology for the oversight requires new staffing and scheduling models.

Another example of evolving communication is the creation of blogs by most senior leaders, inviting members of the organization to share ideas and feedback. Rather than the traditional formal face-to-face meeting, leaders are now accessible to employees with Internet access 24 hours a day, 7 days a week. Based on these changes, new assumptions about the structure of organizations are needed. The new infrastructure is now based on openness and minimal lines of authority or divisions of work units. Behaviors and structures that support unconstrained communication and open relationships are redefining the roles and accountabilities of both leaders and staff.

Redefining Media

The second dimension that has changed significantly involves the media by which information is transmitted and shared. Communication media have evolved from physical to electronic and from isolated to interactive. The assumptions related to the media or vehicle for transfer of information, including written, oral, and video modalities as the primary vehicles, are challenged in nearly every venue. No matter how well text is written, it is not an interactive medium. Paper was once the most reliable form for communication; now digital files are becoming the norm. No longer is paper the most efficient and effective medium for communication. Audio-video media have also dramatically decreased the need for travel and physical presence. Physical presence has long been managed with the multiuser conference line. As global communication occurs quickly and efficiently with access to the Internet and a video camera, connections with multiple individuals in many locations are commonplace. With the introduction of affordable video conferencing, physical presence is less important. Heavy desktop computers have been replaced with flat-screen monitors and handheld devices. Data storage capacity is significant because sophisticated users have unlimited access to information on the Internet. Leadership roles have evolved to roles of accessing, filtering, and interpreting information for others.

The assumptions specific to media impact the expectations about workflow, the length of processing time, data storage, and hardware and software management. Further, although media have been more readily available to others, it is nearly impossible for workers to access, interpret, and manage the information as quickly as it is now available. Limitations are now human personnel rather than the timely movement of media.

Redefining Space

As structures and media evolve, the role of physical space and location is also changing. Communication modalities are more electronic, data are available virtually, and new assumptions about physical space are emerging. Gathering together at common sites is becoming the exception rather than the rule.

In the current context of large and complex facilities, the physical space between individuals, offices, and geographical locations that once resulted in a delay in communication between individuals, as well as a delay in the transmittal of paper documents, is now minimized and in some cases eliminated. The need for individual office space is now questioned regularly. The utility and purpose of individual private office space, and the affordability of spaces used less than 10% of the time, provide an opportunity for new configurations. Space for teamwork rather than individual workspace is preferred. What is not clear is the appropriate mix of face time on-site and off-site in which communication occurs using audio and visual technologies. Even with the best of technologies, physical gatherings remain an essential part of the work processes. To be sure, there is nothing better than a welcome hug from a long-time colleague or the welcoming hand extended to a new member of the team. As the organization moves forward, efforts will continue to determine how best to optimize human gatherings and the available technology. New assumptions about physical space will focus on value, flexibility, and multipurpose use for both individuals and teams.

Redefining Time

Traditionally, work is accomplished at the workplace during specified hours. With the widespread availability of the Internet, shared files, and social networks, work can occur at any time in any location across the globe. Waiting time for global dialogue is nearly nonexistent. The assumptions specific to the management of schedules and the availability of several individuals simultaneously are being reversed with the technology of real-time communication and data transfer. No longer is the individual waiting for the mail to arrive—the e-mail is waiting for the individual!

Further, traditional shift times and lengths may be even more flexible as virtual care is integrated with physical, on-site care. Research on fatigue for caregivers identified issues of compromised competence near 12½ hours in a 24-hour period or 40 hours in 1 week (Rogers, 2002). Different shift lengths or rest period intervals may be required with increased screen monitoring work.

More Thoughts on Structure, Media, Space, and Time

To be sure, the dismantling of traditional structures and processes has increased the chaos in healthcare organizations. Necessarily, the evolving organizational infrastructure becomes the framework to support multiple realities. The available digital world requires leaders to continually challenge assumptions related to organizational structures, information transfer media, physical workspace, and time for transactions. New realities in these context elements significantly alter interactions from every perspective.

It is important to remember the role of innovation leaders, and the need for evidence to support effective behaviors is relatively new but critical to organizational effectiveness. Creating evidence to support the evolving assumptions about structure, media, space, and time is emerging and yet to be conclusive and instructive—if it ever will be! The choice for transformational modalities or complete elimination of a traditional modality is never an exclusive choice. Rather, the choice is about selecting the best modality for the circumstances. Sometimes, face-to-face communication or a handwritten note is the most appropriate for the situation.

> *"I think one's feelings waste themselves in words; they ought all to be distilled into actions which bring results."*
>
> —FLORENCE NIGHTINGALE

In the next section cultural changes for the trimodal organization are discussed. Necessarily, sustainable changes in the culture require time—a luxury that is less available in the rapidly moving digital world. Now, the innovation leader equipped with multiple tools for communication must advance work to assist individuals to more rapidly adopt cultural changes. Waiting for the laggards to become engaged and enthusiastic about new ideas may not be reasonable for the overall good and sustainability of the organization.

CULTURE AND INNOVATION

According to Kotter and Schlesinger (2008), the ability of organizations to respond to environmental change is of critical concern for the future. The behaviors and norms supportive of this new culture include a vision and infrastructure that continually support and develop the capacity to change, the capacity to evaluate and integrate changes resulting from the digital innovations, increased communication access, media management, and expedited workflow.

Stability is no longer the goal for the healthcare leader; the goals now support continual evaluation of new ideas while ensuring that competent and safe patient care is provided. The emphasis on high-reliability organizations is now more actively tempered with the notion of focus and accountability on the work being done with the understanding that procedures necessarily will change. The emphasis must not be on completing high-reliability checklists and redundancies; the emphasis, or *time out,* needs to focus on defining the team's goal—What is it doing and is it the right thing __ we using the most contemporary approach for the work we are doing?

Now, the challenge for the leader is how to facilitate the development of roles, accountabilities, competence, and expectations in team members for excellence in patient care services and simultaneously ensure flexibility and openness to new processes. The new culture in health care is no longer able to support cultures of rote performance based on standards, practices, and technology developed yesterday and achieve optimal outcomes. The continual evaluation and introduction of new work processes and technology require higher levels of presence and engagement than ever thought possible.

In addition to the expectations for evolving work processes, the patients cared for in a global, virtual world are now increasingly diverse. Caregiver knowledge of multiple cultural traditions, beliefs, and values is foundational. An increasing challenge is for the caregiver to sublimate personal values in deference to the patient's unique values. Providing patient care services from the perspective of one's social obligation as a provider now assumes more significance in the global world. Preferences for treatment modalities, family involvement, life and death rituals, and the role of the caregiver now also vary more widely based on the individual patient. Now more than ever the expectation for patient-centered care is a reality that cannot be ignored. The best decisions for the patient based on his or her beliefs and values must now be supported by structures and processes in the healthcare system as the norm rather than the exception.

To address the environmental changes described and to assist leaders in expanding their competencies as innovation leaders, the following cultural attributes are needed:

- A high regard for and valuing of creativity
- An openness to new ideas
- An expectation to challenge assumptions
- A strong change management process that includes course correction for unsuccessful events
- Positive conflict utilization
- Understanding of the business case for innovation
- The availability of financial resources for innovation work

These cultural attributes are realized in organizational structure and processes and in the behaviors of the leader. A high regard for creativity is realized in an organizational structure that encourages and allows communication freely in the organization. Leader behaviors reflect behaviors that do not require permission from others to collaborate and dialogue with others. There is a spirit of candor and free flow of information without fear of criticism or reprisal. The reality is that some individuals have information at different times, and sharing ideas informally can increase the organization's capacity to solve problems and meet challenges. The goal is to use information to support optimal organizational performance; it is not to gossip or engage in one-upmanship competitions.

Openness necessarily supports and encourages individuals to be creative in a symbiotic way. Behaviors of all individuals reflect communication in an unrestricted manner, interest in new ideas, and willingness to challenge long-held assumptions. The open culture also requires tolerance for the possibility of error and a climate in which errors can be discussed freely and the underlying causes investigated and corrected quickly (Whittingham, 2003). The successful culture is one in which leaders are competent to lead in a trimodal model. Managing the transition between innovation and operations is often overlooked (Figure 2-1). The most critical process for an organization along this continuum is the transition phase. The work to engage individuals, modify the infrastructure for the new work, implement change, and evaluate the results cannot be underestimated. Figure 2-1 includes the continuum of innovations, transition, and operations.

These attributes assume a high level of trust among individuals in the organization. As the culture evolves, greater trust is earned with much effort and consistency of behaviors. The culture is truly brought to life by the leaders of the organization as they role model innovation leadership competencies. To be sure, this is an iterative process of cultural evolution and development of leader expertise. Whereas the following leader competencies focus on those in formal positions in the organization, there is much application for all members of the organization to learn the essence of innovation, personal strengths, and opportunities for growth and as much as possible about the supporting competencies for the organization.

Figure 2-1 Innovation to transition to operations.

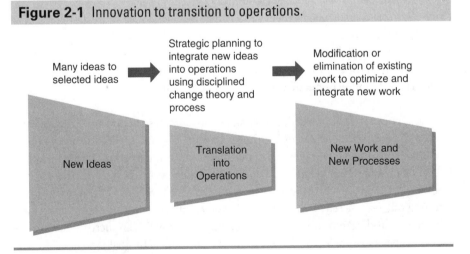

INNOVATION LEADERSHIP

> **Box 2-1** Innovation Leadership
>
> Innovation leadership is not about being an inventor.
>
> Innovation leadership is the work of:
> - Creating the conditions or context for innovation to occur
> - Creating and implementing the roles, decision-making structures, physical space, partnerships, networks, and equipment and technology needed to support innovative thinking and testing
> - Envisioning a better future
> - Having the courage to challenge the status quo
> - Being comfortable with risk taking
> - Having significant ego strength
> - Facilitating and empowering others to be as creative as they can be

As the innovation culture emerges, the role of the innovation leader gains importance in ensuring steady progress for the organization. An innovation culture cannot be sustained without innovation leadership. If innovations are introduced into a traditional culture without adequate transition support and modification of the existing work, the innovations are considered fads and dismissed all too quickly. New ideas are considered burdens rather than opportunities to remain competitive and achieve the highest quality outcomes. Malloch and Porter-O'Grady (2009) describe innovation leadership as *the process of creating the context for innovation to occur; creating and implementing the roles, decision-making structures, physical space, partnerships, networks, and equipment that support innovative thinking and testing.* As previously noted, innovation leaders are now engaged in facilitating the transfer of structure, communication, and space so that the organization can be optimally effective in creating the supportive organizational culture.

Although the traditional leadership skills of planning, organizing, and evaluating remain essential for success, the trimodal culture requires additional competencies. Specifically, leaders must be able to support operations, innovation, and transition management. Competence in the following eight categories is essential for this work (Malloch, 2008). The categories emphasize innovation content, personal innovation competence, and the synthesis of innovation into the traditional leadership roles.

Essence of Innovation

The first competency category focuses on the content of innovation and is described as the *essence of innovation.* Innovation is a frequently used word attached to anything believed new, different, or needing special attention. Numerous descriptions and definitions of innovation (Box 2-2) guide the work of innovation leaders.

What is important to understand is that there are multiple definitions and descriptions of innovation available in both refereed and trade literature. As knowledge in innovation leadership emerges, more descriptions will be presented. The skeptic often dismisses innovation with the belief that nothing new ever really occurs; rather it is only new combinations and iterations of existing products and processes that occur. This approach may indeed be an example of a delaying tactic and does little to address the need for the organization to be contemporary in its work. Becoming entangled in the conceptual precision discussion may serve only to delay meaningful discussion and attention to the future.

Innovation Knowledge

Knowledge and experience in the concepts and processes of innovation is the second competency category. As individuals in organizations generate new ideas, the challenge for

---

Box 2-2 Innovation Descriptions

- The introduction of something new; a new idea, method, or device (Merriam-Webster, 2009).
- Anything that creates new resources, processes, or values or improves a company's existing resources, processes, or values (Christensen, Anthony, & Ross, 2004).
- The power to define the industry; the effort to create purposeful focused change in an enterprise's economic or social potential (Drucker, 1985).
- The first practical, concrete implementation of an idea done in a way that brings broad based, extrinsic recognition to an individual or organization (Plsek, 1997).
- A slow process of accretion, building small insight upon interesting fact upon tried-and-true process (Janet Rae-Dupree, technology writer, Silicon Valley).
- A new patterning of our experiences of being together as new meaning emerges from ordinary, everyday work conversations; a challenging exciting process of participating with others in the evolution of work (Fonseca, 2002).
- Doing new things that customers ultimately appreciate and value—not only developing new generations of products, services, channels, and customer experience, but also conceiving new business processes and models (Cash, Earl, & Morison, 2008).

the leader is to determine what to do with the ideas: consider, develop, adopt, or ignore them. Healthcare leaders are often unsure when and where to begin changes to better accommodate innovations in the digital age. One thing is certain; doing nothing is not a viable option. Doing nothing, holding on to the past, and working to perfect current practices can only put an organization more out of touch with rapidly emerging technology, new work processes, and information. Numerous innovation resources are available to assist the leader in managing innovations. Box 2-3 provides an overview of common innovation-related concepts.

Many organizations create new roles such as a chief innovation officer or master change agent, whereas others work to integrate the work of expectations within each operational role, believing that innovation transcends functional expertise. There are

---

Box 2-3 Innovation-Related Concepts

- Invention: A new process, machine, or improvement that is recognized as the product of some unique intuition or genius.
- Diffusion: Widespread, scattered, or dispersed; a pull concept.
- Dissemination: To spread widely; a push or top-down concept.
- Entrepreneurship: Practice of starting a new organization or revitalizing a mature organization, particularly new businesses in response to identified opportunities.
- Intrapreneurship: The practice of using entrepreneurial skills without taking on the risks or accountability associated with entrepreneurial activities. It is practiced by employees within an established organization using a business model.
- Process improvement: The activity of elevating the performance of a series of actions, especially that of a business process with regard to its goal.
- Reengineering: A process that emphasizes integration of fragmented tasks and data to decrease costs, decrease cycle time, and increase service.
- Research: Activity based on intellectual application in the investigation of matter. The primary aim for applied research is discovering, interpreting, and the development of methods and systems for the advancement of human knowledge.
- Integration: Making the multiple units, functions, and sites of large organizations work together to increase capacity, improve performance, lower cost structure and discover opportunities for improvement that do not appear until one looks across functions (Cash, Earl, & Morison, 2008).
- Evidence: Includes everything that is used to determine or demonstrate the truth of an assertion.

Source: Wikipedia (2009).

advantages and disadvantages for each approach. What still needs to be emphasized is the significant work of transition, the work between innovation and operations. In addition to knowing the language of innovation, the innovation leader needs to understand and experience the processes of innovation.

> *"In a world that is constantly changing, there is no one subject or set of subjects that will serve you for the foreseeable future, let alone for the rest of your life. The most important skill to acquire now is learning how to learn."*
>
> —JOHN NAISBITT

Knowing and experiencing the tools of innovation is a relatively new leadership expectation. As the need to support innovation evolves, a unique body of information is becoming more available to guide the innovation leader. Given that most healthcare leaders are accountable for performance that encompasses operations, innovation, and transition work, the tools of innovation are very helpful in moving between the three modes of work. Brainstorming, scenario planning, and deep dives are examples of innovation tools. Each tool provides specific strategies to facilitate creative thinking that can be quickly translated into prototypes and pilot studies. Initially, some may see innovation as hyped-up brainstorming or open discussions. However, the processes of innovation are highly formalized and designed to provide structure and focus to optimize the processes of innovation.

A brief overview of change management in an innovation culture, the innovation lab, innovation software, and concepts of disruptive innovation, such as thinking inside the box, positive deviance, and design thinking, is provided below.

Change Management

For the innovation leader there are multiple change management strategies rather than a single common approach for change. Instead, the strategy to manage the change is based on the specific resistance the organization is expected to encounter. The resistance or obstacle to innovations varies widely and is unique to each organization. Managing resistance can focus on fear, survival, involvement, or uncertainty. The innovation leader spends significant time in diagnosing both the potential and real resistance. Once the believed source is identified, the team develops strategies to address and minimize the resistance.

*Diffusion of Innovation: "We must become the change we wish
to see in the world."*

—MAHATMA GANDHI

The Innovation Lab

In addition to knowledge and competence in the processes of innovation, a dedicated
physical space is quite useful. The workspace for innovation is unique and focused on
creativity, brainstorming, simulation, prototyping, and testing new ideas. This space,
also known as an innovation lab or workspace for idea generation, dialogue, prototyping, scenario testing, and evaluation of new ideas, provides a dedicated and safe place
for creativity and innovation. It is also a safe place to test new ideas without fear of negative consequences. The characteristics of an innovation lab include small tables for
group work, significant vertical wall space for writing and drawing, electrical outlets
for power cords, and support for audio and visual projection. An innovation toolbox also includes flip charts, markers, software for simulation, mind mapping, and
prototyping tools.

Software Applications

Applications to document, monitor, and prototype innovations are introduced to the
marketplace regularly. Mind mapping tools, one of the more frequently used software
tools, have become increasing effective to document and share complex systems
or projects. This tool is a diagram in which topics are created in a clockwise fashion
representing ideas, groups, problems, and structures and can include video, Internet,
and text attachments. The mind map can also be shared with others for iterative
contributions.

Applications of the mind map range widely. A cancer center is using the mind map
with patients to identify issues to address and plan for care at home. The patient and staff
can then identify the needs they would like to address and focus on the most important
issues. In the university setting, graduate schools are using mind maps to document a
student's ability to collect, order, and synthesize information. At Arizona State University,
College of Nursing and Healthcare Innovation: Master of Healthcare Innovation program, the final capstone project is documented in the mind map and submitted with
a two-page executive summary to meet this requirement. Many opportunities exist in
performance review documentation, policy and procedure manual documents, and
much more.

Concepts Related to Innovation

Diffusion of innovation processes have been described using the S-curve (or the first half of the bell-shaped curve). The stages of adoption of innovations include knowledge, persuasion, decision, implementation, and confirmation. Individuals are identified as innovators, adopters, early majority, late majority, and laggards (Rogers, 2003). Each stage describes the level of readiness of different groups to embrace the new idea and adopt it into their world. Additional work in the diffusion of innovations has been done by Christensen et al. (2004), Fraser (2006), Fonseca (2002), and Greenlaugh, Robert, Bate, and Macfarlin (2007). This new work provides more depth to innovation as well as increased recognition of the complexity of innovation processes.

Design thinking, or thinking like a designer, offers a unique approach in developing new ideas. The designer integrates art, craft, science, business savvy, and an astute understanding of customer needs and the marketplace (Brown, 2008). Design thinking is a discipline that in many ways descended from the work of Thomas Edison and uses design sensibility and knowledge to match people's needs with what is technologically feasible and what a viable business strategy can convert into value for the customer (Brown, 2008; Gelb & Caldicott, 2007).

> *"Faith is taking the first step even when you don't see the staircase."*
>
> —Martin Luther King, Jr.

The innovation leader borrows heavily from the design discipline and develops sensitivity or empathy for others' situations and needs, integrative thinking, and optimism and experiments often and collaborates within and without the discipline of interest. Collaboration with designers not only serves to enhance the physical space for healing; it also contributes to more robust dialogue and expanded thinking among team members.

Thinking inside the box is a strategy not used often enough. Typically, the efforts to encourage creativity focus on motivating others to think *outside the box,* to think radically different. According to Coyne, Clifford, and Dye (2007), a semistructured approach in one's own team can generate great ideas and may be more effective than free-for-all brainstorming and thinking outside the box. The assumption for thinking inside the box is that great ideas can be identified by those closest to the work and by those who are familiar with the existing challenges and feedback from patients. Also, it is believed that when the right questions are asked (i.e., "what is the biggest hassle about buying or using a product or service that people unnecessarily tolerate without knowing?" or "how would we do things differently if we had perfect information about our customers?"), creative new ideas are born to improve products and services—and the ideas are from within the team rather than external experts or research studies.

As the innovation leader becomes competent in both thinking inside and outside the box, the presence of *positive deviants* becomes apparent. Nurse leaders recently recognized the opportunities to identify and encourage individuals whose behaviors seem on the surface to be deviant from the norm and disruptive to the team. In fact, behaviors of positive deviants that stray from the norm are innovative and tend to get better results than coworkers do with the same resources (Jaramillo & Jenkins, 2008). Innovation leaders actively seek out positive deviants and learn from their ideas and experiences. Box 2-4 lists the common behaviors of inside-the-box positive deviants.

Disruptive innovation is an interesting concept in that the potential for behavior change using this approach is significant. However, this behavior change is difficult to truly achieve because of cultural norms, mental models, and established routines. An innovation is said to be disruptive when it cannot be used by customers in mainstream markets. The disruptive innovation defines a new performance trajectory by introducing new dimensions of performance compared with existing innovations. Disruptive innovations either create new markets by bringing new features to nonconsumers or offer more convenience or lower prices to customers at the low end of an existing market (Christenson et al., 2004).

Scenario planning can be used to stress test the assumptions of an innovation. According to Schoemaker (1995), scenario planning provides the team with a disciplined approach that considers multiple conditions in various orders. It is about testing the "what ifs" of new ideas. Specifically, scenario planning is based on a defined scope, identified stakeholders, basic trends in the environment, key uncertainties, and common themes for the situation. In addition, research needs or gaps can be identified during scenario creation. The goal of thinking through scenarios and the other tools of innovation is to get to failure as quickly as possible and to determine what worked and what did not work so the process can begin again.

Box 2-4 Inside-the-Box Positive Deviants: Behaviors for Innovation

- Recognize that leaders cannot possibly have all the answers.
- Ask the best questions.
- Nurture and encourage others to ask questions.
- Recognize the value of the team.
- Look at others with a different lens.
- Be fully engaged.

Finally, one of the most important tools of innovation is a sense of humor. A hearty belly laugh about the realities of the human condition is good for the mind, body, and soul.

Self-Knowledge and Competence

> *"Leadership is an opportunity to serve. It is not a trumpet call to self-importance."*
>
> —J. DONALD WALTERS, AMERICAN AUTHOR

The third competency category is *self-competence.* As a leader required to create the culture and context that supports and facilitates effective operations, innovation, and transition processes, a clear understanding of one's personal strengths and limitations is essential. Knowing one's profile and attributes related to innovation work is the first and most important step in developing competence. Knowledge of decision-making, communication, and conflict resolution styles is foundational for this role. Myers-Briggs (see http://www.myersbriggs.org) and DISC (see http://www.profiles4u.com/what-is-disc-profile.asp) assessments are examples of helpful assessment tools for individuals. Although the innovation leader often overemphasizes self-assessments to learn about styles, strengths, and limitations, the label or category into which the individual falls should never be the primary focal point. Rather, the information about styles is intended to provide insight into an overall set of behaviors and does not reflect all activities. The ability to understand others and collaborate with multiple styles in multidisciplinary teams is the ultimate goal of the innovation leader.

Innovation leaders also examine their information processing and thinking systems styles as a means to excel as transformational leaders. The relationship between emotions and intellectual content is important in understanding not only one's personal style but also the abilities of others. Consideration is also given to understanding rational and experiential information-processing styles (Cerni, Curtis, & Colmar, 2008). Rational processing is analytical, intentional, logical, and slower, whereas experiential information processing is holistic, automatic, associative, and faster. Necessarily, the innovation leader requires both modes of processing to be effective. Areas of strength and areas of development opportunities are important to know.

In addition to understanding one's persona and processes, the innovation leader's attributes include an overwhelming proactive approach, vulnerability, courage, and a small amount of narcissism.

Proactive Versus Reactive State of Mind

The innovation leader tends to be future oriented, actively planning for a better future. The work is about facilitating and empowering others rather than directing and doing; it is about understanding others using multiple strategies and approaches. The leader transcends the tacit knowledge management of knowing what and why to do something to self-transcending of knowledge. The leader moves from reliance on historical knowledge to imagining, intuiting, inspiring, and reflecting the present as the means to the future (Scharmer & Kaufer, 2000).

Vulnerability

The innovation leader is comfortable with uncertainty, thrives on finding solutions to difficult problems, embraces change willingly as the best vehicle for a better future, and believes innovation requires many perspectives and skills from many individuals. For the innovation leader vulnerability is about knowing that one can never know everything there is to know and that this *perpetual incompleteness* is a fundamental trait of all individuals. The essential work is connecting and creating meaningful relationships with others who have different areas of expertise. Box 2-5 lists considerations for self-assessment of one's comfort with innovation processes.

Creativity and Courage: "Life is not about waiting for the storms to pass . . . it is about learning how to dance in the rain."

—UNKNOWN

Courage

Courage for the innovation leader is especially significant. As noted, the individual dares to revolutionize health care from the inside out, from one's personal beliefs and

---

Box 2-5 Self-Assessment: How Confident Are You?

How confident are you to . . .

   . . . work on a team to define and prioritize an innovation goal?
   . . . identify and explore mental models?
   . . . assist a team to examine and understand patterns and trends?
   . . . perform process mapping of a care delivery model?
   . . . lead a brainstorming session?

behaviors. Being daring to eliminate obsolete healthcare dogma and not being afraid of criticism or ridicule are important skills. This courage also guides the innovation leader in facilitating effective and difficult dialogue. When things are not going well, the innovation leader examines and evaluates the situation and facilitates appropriate course correction quickly. This course correction emphasizes learning from the experience without ascribing blame to anyone.

Self-Care

The expert innovation leader's sense of self is so well developed that attention is focused on others and facilitating their development and contributions to innovation work. Recognition is for others, not for personal adulation. The work of the innovation leader is very demanding and unrelenting. Building the case for others to change or at best consider change requires significant focus and energy. Further, much of the work of the innovation leader may be in teams but not with like-minded innovation leaders. This can be somewhat isolating. Thus there is a need for a little bit of leader narcissism—self-care is essential for energy renewal for the innovation leader. Taking time to balance work with one's personal life is essential to sustain high levels of performance and productivity.

Collaboration

The fourth competency category is *collaboration*. Effective collaboration is based on listening, encouraging feedback, openness, and conflict resolution. Effective collaboration is about moving from a group of assembled individuals to a team of highly interactive, participative, goal-oriented individuals. Trimodal work requires these multiple skill sets and perspectives. In today's environment the innovation leader thrives in multidisciplinary teams—the fundamental unit in the organization. The individual is always considered incomplete because one can never know all there is to know. Working alone or in single discipline dialogue is inefficient and ineffective. Transdisciplinary dialogue is the norm to address issues of complexity and innovation.

Innovation leaders have highly developed *listening* skills; they listen without being asked to listen. In addition to being respectful, the goal is to focus on the speaker and acknowledge what is being said. Their goal is to find common ground with others while avoiding the rubber stamps of conversation. Principles of appreciative inquiry guide interactions.

Team members are encouraged to comment on others' ideas; withholding feedback is considered counterproductive to the entire process. The goal is for *sharing feedback* to be a core behavior rather than optional.

Courage and *openness* are hallmarks of successful innovation leaders, particularly in the group process. Teams often include disparate disciplines such as clinicians, engineers, computer specialists, designers, and representatives from several age generations and ethnic cultures. All individuals are encouraged to be role models in the activities of challenging traditional norms and practices and confronting each other when resistance is evident. The innovation leader is patient, tolerant, and interested in diverse discussion in facilitating teamwork. In fact, innovation leaders seek out those known for strong opinions, ability to challenge others, taking risks, and thinking creatively.

Many obstacles are encountered along the innovation continuum. Individuals, equipment, resources, and time can all be the source of conflict among team members. The innovation leader perceives *conflicts as opportunities* to learn more about the issues and to gain insight into values and beliefs of others. The leader avoids efforts to neutralize or minimize the differing opinions until more information is gained. Necessarily, the innovation leader is a master change facilitator and is able to use conflict as an opportunity to gain further insight of pertinent issues.

Synthesis

The fifth competency category is *synthesis.* In an environment characterized by rapid and continuous introduction of new ideas, processes, technology, and equipment, the innovation leader is expected to manage significant amounts of data and quickly consider the level of evidence, value, and potential outcomes. The effective leader is able to synthesize information from providers, patients, payers, and colleagues expeditiously. It is this body of data that the leader synthesizes to create a comprehensive approach or innovation. The wisdom of all team members is considered and combined into a critical mass of expertise.

The continuum of synthesis begins with integrating concepts within the innovation idea to within the operational structure of the organization (see Figure 1-1). Many ideas, considerations, and disciplines come into alignment to create a valuable innovation. Once a concept is prototyped and accepted as a legitimate process or product for the organization, the innovation leader then facilitates the synthesis of the new work into existing operations. Sustainable innovations become operational standards.

Leadership synthesis requires sensitivity to the trajectory of innovation acceptance or diffusion processes as the foundational knowledge for moving from an innovation to operations. New ideas are introduced after careful analysis and then integrated into the overall work of the organization. This work includes the overall translation of innovative ideas into the operational processes once effectiveness is established.

Innovative processes or products can be considered new or different only for a short time before they are moved from pilot or experimental stage to routine operations or deleted. Further, as new processes are shifted to operational standards, consideration is given to elimination of existing work that might be duplicative or outmoded. Eliminating duplicative or unnecessary work is one of the more difficult tasks for the team. Too often, emotional attachment or personal interest in tasks becomes the primary rationale for retaining duplicative or ineffective processes. At some point in time the team needs to work together to collaboratively abandon those processes. Failing to eliminate unnecessary work obstructs or negates the new work as it becomes burdensome and perceived as an add-on. The mind map, as previously discussed, can be an excellent tool to document new processes including goals, advantages, progress, disadvantages, and obstacles.

Formulation

The sixth competency category is *formulation*. To thrive in an integrated environment, skills in the collection of associated information and also the formulation of documents for innovative healthcare proposals are needed. The documents or information put together necessarily includes available evidence and information from action research initiatives. Using an evidence-based approach, the innovation leader and team members also identify the gaps in evidence (Figure 2-2) to determine if the gap is in formal evidence or in patient needs. A gap can be identified on the basis of a long-standing practice that does not have current research support or from a patient request based on patient success with an intervention not previously considered. The contributions made by innovation leaders in identifying the evidence gaps, testing or prototyping processes, and then transitioning to operations are important to evidence building in health care.

Figure 2-2 Gap identification: evidence-based practice and innovation leadership.

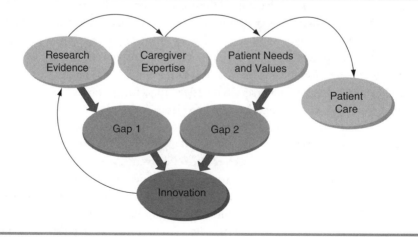

From this evidence-building approach, creation of the business case for the innovation becomes more powerful. A business case or the rationale for expenditure of resources under certain circumstances is essential to support appropriate resource allocations (Burns, 2005). The elements of a strong business case include a description of the new product or service, the intended purpose or goal of the innovation, projection of costs specific to accomplish the innovation, costs excluded from proposal and rationale for exclusion, projected benefits and rationale for valuing of benefits, a timeline for the project from initiation to benefits realization, anticipated profit or loss, nonfinancial benefits expected, anticipated risks and plans to mediate risks, and an overall summary of both short-term and long-term value to the organization and community (see http://www.businesslink.gov.uk/bdotg/action/detail?type=RESOURCES&itemId=1073 792537, retrieved January 5, 2009).

In addition to the traditional elements of the business plan, information specific to the work of innovations must be included, such as issues related to anticipated productivity changes, reductions in cost, market share, patient quality outcomes, new partnerships, and risks for not moving forward, such as losing market share, productivity loss, employee turnover, and profit margin. Further, information that identifies how the innovation could differentiate the organization from competitors, benefit multiple constituencies in the organization, and extend the life of the organization as a value-producing entity are important elements of the business case (Merrifield, Calhoun, & Stevens, 2008).

Necessarily, a business case for an innovation strategy is needed to link the new ideas to the work of the existing organization. Any deviation from the existing mission and vision must be evaluated carefully. Moving forward with an innovation that is not congruent with the mission seriously compromises acceptance and sustainability.

Building the strategic business case for new and untested ideas is challenging because of the unknown outcome of the innovation and the inadequacy of operational tools for innovation. Creating a sustainable budget or projection for an innovation requires knowledge about the past—which may be completely irrelevant—and estimations about the future, which include cost of materials, technology and human resources, and expected revenues. Christensen, Kaufman, and Shih (2008) identified the challenges in creating the business case as the lack of good financial tools to understand the market, build brands, find customers, select employees, organize teams, and develop strategies to advance the work. Specifically, when an organization relies on traditional discounted cash flow and net present value to evaluate investment opportunities, the real returns and benefits are often underestimated. Consideration of fixed and sunk costs using traditional models creates an unfair advantage on challengers and inhibits incumbent firms that attempt to respond. Finally, the emphasis on earnings per share as the primary metric for success diverts resources from investments whose payoff occurs at a much later date. According to Christensen et al. (2008), although these tools are good for operations, they create a systematic bias against innovation. It is very difficult to justify innovation expenses using these analytics. Nevertheless, the case for innovation must be made in such a way that risks are identified and potential enhancements to the mission of the organization are identified.

Managing Knowledge

Managing knowledge is the seventh competency category. Maintaining the focus on work to be done continues to challenge the best leader. As the healthcare community moves from a critical mass of digital immigrants to increasing numbers of digital natives, there are new challenges and opportunities (Prensky, 2001). Box 2-6 lists the characteristics of digital immigrants and digital natives. Digital natives think and process information fundamentally differently from digital immigrants. The analogy between digital natives and immigrants provides a framework from which to under-

---

Box 2-6 Characteristics of Digital Immigrants and Digital Natives

Digital Immigrants
- Are not born in the digital world but are learning to adapt to the digital environment
- Have an "accent," evidenced by turning to the Internet for information second rather than first, or by reading the manual for a program instead of assuming that the program will teach itself to the user
- Are "socialized" differently than digital natives, and are now in the process of learning a new "language." As scientists have said, learning a language later in life uses a different part of the brain.
- Prefer linear, logical processes
- Comfortable in real spaces rather than virtual spaces

Digital Natives
- Have grown up with digital technology and have spent their entire lives surrounded by and using computers, video games, digital music players, video cameras, cell phones, and all the other toys and tools from the digital age
- Are used to receiving information immediately
- Like to parallel process and multitask
- Prefer their graphics before their text as opposed to vice-versa
- Prefer random access (like hypertext)
- Function best when networked
- Thrive on instant gratification and frequent rewards and prefer games to "serious work"

Source: Prensky (2001).

stand these differences and insight as to how to continue to move forward in the health-care world with disparate styles. Translating the work of patient care into the digital native paradigm now requires collaboration and sensitivity not only to natives and immigrants but also to those who have elected not to be digital at all, to remain in the nondigital world as much as possible. For the innovation leader, sensitivity to the disparate perspectives is important because patient care is needed by the older generation, digital immigrants, and digital natives, each group needing specific healthcare knowledge in accessible formats and language.

As new technologies are introduced into the marketplace, the role of the innovation leader as the holder of the vision and mission becomes more important than ever. As an extension of the traditional visioning process, the leader facilitates examination of many new technologies from the perspective of enhancing the organization rather than a perspective focused solely on the new technology. The innovation leader avoids total reliance on technology and at the same time is able to envision a better future.

Managing knowledge can occur in multiple ways from using personal storytelling and interviews to digitally transcribed modalities. Moving to a more digital world is challenging, but it should never take precedence over the fundamental work of patient care. Too often in the recent past, the introduction of clinical documentation systems or medication administration systems has overridden basic patient care practices, and safety has been compromised. Limitations of the new technology should be challenged and modified to support the basic work of patient care rather than changing patient care to practices that delay service or increase the risk for errors.

Coaching

The eighth category is *coaching*. In addition to the traditional coaching for leadership effectiveness in an operational setting, the innovation leader coaches others in the principles of innovation, adult learning, and system change. Most healthcare professionals learn to create a stable and predictable environment as the means to achieve patient outcomes and avoid errors. Changing this paradigm to also support trimodal innovation thinking requires continual dialogue, support, and reinforcement of the value for both stability and innovation. The innovation leader works to empower the *creative genius* in everyone. Creative genius is that part of each individual that has a possibilities-oriented, can-do attitude and way of being that communicates to everyone that anything is possible; it is about being full of excitement, energy, and ideas (McGlade & Pek, 2008). Box 2-7 provides living innovation guidelines.

As a coach, the innovation leader develops a special sensitivity to the errors or the imperfect. Errors are perceived as part of the highway to success; each discovery of what does not work leads to something better. The reality of the human condition and factors that impact behaviors recognize the role of motivation, skill level, experience, and

Box 2-7 Living Innovation Guidelines

1. Be flexible: How do you react to changes in your schedule?
2. Be open: Do you enjoy learning about the activities and accomplishments of others?
3. Embrace failures: How often do you share missteps or failures with others?
4. Be creative: Describe something creative that you did in the last seven days.
5. Abandon your ego: Be sure not to take the credit for teamwork—credit and recognition belong to the team.
6. Explore differences: Work to learn more about individuals who think and act differently than you do.
7. Be resilient: Have you attempted to accomplish something more than five times? (Remember WD-40, the lubricant, so named because the first 39 formulas failed!)
8. Enjoy: How long did it take you to find humor in your last failure?
9. Explore technology: Learn about a device that someone 20 years younger than you is using.
10. Coach: When was the last time you helped someone with an idea or project without giving your advice?

fatigue on work processes. The focus is on creating a culture in which it is not only safe to make errors but in which errors are expected as the normal course of events. Persistent errors that are ignored and permitted to continue are not tolerated.

CONCLUSION

The role of the innovation leader will by nature never be complete. There is always something that needs to be improved, new ideas to be tested, and changing customer demographics that guide the innovation leader in creating an agenda. And, at the same time, safe and effective health care needs to be delivered. It is hoped that the information provided in this chapter will assist leaders in better sorting out this complex work. Also, the guidelines and recommendations to advance both the culture and competencies of leaders are intended to be merely a starting point for this work that is evolving at warp speed. As the acceleration of change continues, it is possible *that less time will be required for traditional operations* and more resources required to manage innovations and transition the selected work into operations. More time will be required to support and role model the transitioning role at the point of service as the means to ensure that patients receive the most appropriate and timely care. Given that most resources are dedicated to operations, the world could be dramatically different in a very short time! Enjoy the journey, share your ideas and dreams—you are your own driver.

REFERENCES

Bennis, W., Goleman, D., & Biederman, W. (2008, Fall). Creating a transparent culture. *Leader to Leader,* 21–27.

Brown, T. (2008). Design thinking. *Harvard Business Review, 86*(6), 84–92.

Burns, L. R. (Ed.). (2005). *The business of healthcare innovation.* New York: Cambridge University Press.

Cash, J. I., Earl, M. J., & Morison, R. (2008). Teaming up to crack innovation and enterprise integration. *Harvard Business Review, 86*(10), 90–99.

Castells, M. (1998). *The information age: Economy, society and culture* (Vol. III). *End of the millennium.* Malden, MA: Blackwell.

Cerni, T., Curtis, G. J., & Colmar, S. H. (2008). Information processing and leadership styles: Constructive thinking and transformational leadership. *Journal of Leadership Studies, 2*(1), 60–73.

Christensen, C. M., Anthony, S. D., & Roth, E. A. (2004). *Seeing what's next: Using the theories of innovation to predict industry change.* Boston: Harvard Business School Press.

Christensen, C. M., Kaufman, S. P., & Shih, W. C. (2008). Innovation killers: How financial tools destroy your capacity to do new things. *Harvard Business Review, 86*(1), 98–105.

Coyne, K. P., Clifford, P. G., & Dye, R. (2007). Breakthrough thinking from inside the box. *Harvard Business Review, 85*(10), 71–78.

Drucker, P. F. (1985, May/June). The discipline of innovation. *Harvard Business Review, 63,* 67–72.

Fonseca, J. (2002). *Complexity and innovation in organizations.* London: Routledge.

Fraser, S. W. (2006). *Undressing the elephant: Why good practice doesn't spread in healthcare.* United Kingdom: Lulu.com.

Gelb, M. J., & Caldicott, S. M. (2007). *Innovate like Edison: The success system of America's greatest inventor.* New York: Dutton.

Greenlaugh, T., Robert, G., Bate, P., & Macfarlin, F. (2007). *Diffusion of innovation in health service organizations: A systematic literature review.* West Sussex, UK: Blackwell.

innovation. (2009). In *Merriam-Webster Online Dictionary.* Retrieved April 9, 2009, from http://www.merriam-webster.com/dictionary/innovation

Jaramillo, B., & Jenkins, C. (2008). Positive deviance: Innovation from the inside out. *Nurse Leader, 6*(2), 30–33.

Kotter, J. P., & Schlesinger, L. A. (2008). Choosing change strategies. *Harvard Business Review, 86*(7), 130–139.

Malloch, K. (2008, November). Empowered for action: Innovation leaders making a difference in health care organizations. *Voice of Nursing Leadership,* 12–13.

Malloch, K., & Porter-O'Grady, T. (2009). *Innovation leader: A practical application for the new world of work.* Sudbury, MA: Jones and Bartlett.

McGlade, J., & Pek, A. (2008, Summer). Spark your creative genius. *Leader to Leader,* 1–15.

Merrifield, R., Calhoun, J., & Stevens, D. (2008). The next revolution in productivity. *Harvard Business Review, 86*(6), 73–80.

Plsek, P. E. (1997). *Creativity, innovation and quality.* Milwaukee, WI: ASQ Quality Press.

Prensky, M. (2001). *Digital natives, digital immigrants.* Retrieved January 5, 2009, from http://www.marcprensky.com/writing/Prensky%20-%20Digital%20Natives,%20Digital%20Immigrants%20-%20Part1.pdf

Rogers, A. E. (2002). Sleep deprivation and the ED night shift. *Journal of Emergency Nursing, 28,* 1–2.

Rogers, E. M. (2003). *Diffusion of innovations* (5th ed.). New York: Free Press.

Scharmer, O., & Kaufer, K. (2000). Universities as the birthplace for the entrepreneuring human being. Retrieved January 5, 2009, from http://www.ottoscharmer.com/docs/articles/2000_Uni21us.pdf

Schoemaker, P. J. H. (1995, Winter). Scenario planning: A tool for strategic thinking. *Sloan Management Review,* 25–40.

Whittingham, R. B. (2003). *The blame machine: Why human error causes accidents.* Boston: Elsevier.

CHAPTER 3

Innovation in Action: A Practical System for Getting Results

Scott Endsley

The state of the U.S. healthcare system cries for change in business practice and in applications of new technologies and for new service models that better meet the needs of the American population. This need for change, as Paul Plsek (1999) has said, "leads directly to the need for ideas for change" (p. 4). Thus innovation is not a backwater domain for a few creative individuals but is rather a central element in the improvement of health systems.

So what is innovation? Innovation is the "first practical, concrete implementation of an idea done in a way that brings broad-based extrinsic recognition to an individual or organization" (Plsek, 1997, p. ii). Innovation is more than creativity; it is a systematic practice for finding testable ideas that can be prototyped and disseminated (Drucker, 2002). Innovation is a discipline that can be learned and mastered.

As you become a master of innovation, there are four mental traps to avoid:

1. Innovations need to be large and have profound impacts. Most successful innovations start small. A few grow into large changes, but most do not start out large. For instance, the urine dipstick was devised as a rapid office-based approach to testing and has now evolved into a wide variety of home and office testing kits.
2. Innovations require the genius of a few talented individuals. Innovation is a team-based discipline that optimally works with the interactions of a diverse group who bring multiple perspectives and talents to the work. In fact, many innovations are the products of what is known as the "Medici effect," which is the creative synergy of multiple disciplines, cultures, and points of view (Johansson, 2006).
3. Innovations are about new ideas. In fact, many innovations are new uses or audiences for existing products or services.
4. Innovations are primarily directed at commercial markets. Innovations are applicable in all settings, including nonprofit, within organizations, or any other endeavor.

Innovation is fundamentally a team sport. Innovations grow from a diversity of perspectives, knowledge, and experiences. It is intersectional, as described by Frans Johansson

(2006) as the Medici effect. The confluence of technical, business, clinical, and social perspectives and skills is the optimum soup for innovations to take shape. As you organize for innovation in your workplace, put a team together that reflects this diversity and skills. Look outside the traditional roles in your organization for other points of views. For instance, the trauma services at Greater Ormond Hospital in London brought in the expertise of race car pit crews to help them redesign the trauma response process.

AN INNOVATION MODEL

This chapter presents a five-step process that is highly iterative, inquiry oriented, practical, and team centric (Figure 3-1). The innovation process has its genesis in defining an existing or new need found in the healthcare environment. A variety of tools and methods is then applied to examine the process as well as the user experience to isolate the potential change points for innovative design. This enhanced understanding of the healthcare challenge generates new ideas to address the challenge from which ideas with the highest potential are harvested and shaped into testable prototypes. Testing of these prototypes answers the question, "will this work?" If the answer is yes, the final step is devising approaches to share this innovation with others, garner support to scale up future applications, and find sustainable business models. The following sections lay out the methods and tools for each of these steps.

Innovation is fundamentally a process of design. Specifically, innovation begins and ends with design for a user based on an understanding of user needs. Technological designers of products in health care start with optimizing feasibility of their product innovation, then work on how to make it useful for people (desirability) and how to make a profit from their product (viability). Business strategists design new business models and services and decide how to effectively integrate technological tools into their offerings. Healthcare designers, on the other hand, use "design thinking," which starts with what people need and desire and then defines the technical and/or service innova-

Figure 3-1 An innovation model.

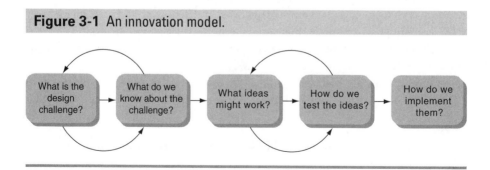

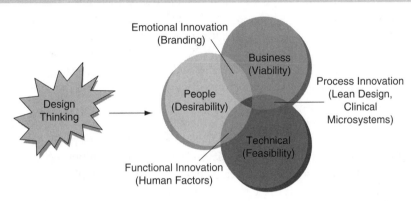

Figure 3-2 Design thinking and innovation.

tions that meet these needs (Brown, 2008). Figure 3-2 presents the relationship between technical innovation, business innovation, and user-centered innovation. Innovation based on design thinking begins with the exploration of what users (people) desire in services and products and then draws as needed technical and business/service elements into the innovation process. The "deep dive," described below, provides an approach to exploring the world of users that informs the design process.

FINDING AN INNOVATION CHALLENGE

Innovation is purpose-driven with the explicit aim of producing value. As you approach your innovation work, a key first step is to define where you want to focus and why it is important to work in this area. This step cannot be emphasized enough and is often neglected in the innovation process. Innovation failure rates are high, with only 4.5% succeeding in the marketplace (Anonymous, 2005). Much of this failure rate can be attributed to poorly framed innovation challenges (Van Gundy, 2008). The forces acting on the direction of innovations include external mandates such as new Medicare requirements; requirements, needs, and preferences of users; definable gaps in care; and the leverage points identified in the epidemiological pattern or clinical logic of a health condition. A four-step method can help you get to where the greatest value might lie in your innovation efforts:

- Step 1: Gather information on mandates, organization requirements and directions, gaps in care, and user needs. There are two nonexclusive approaches to information collection: looking for problems and looking for promise in the system. This step should include interviews with key customers in your health system, including executive management, mid-level managers, front-line staff, and patients. It also includes seeking out literature, information, and reports that are helpful in knowing where the innovation leverage point(s) may lie. Finally, you should consider not only looking backward but also forward in time, using a variety of future-thinking strategies such as scenario planning. The Global Innovation Network (www.gbn.com) has a clear guide on how to conduct a scenario planning session.

- Step 2: Narrow down and prioritize the potential innovation challenges identified in step 1. The nominal group method is a good starting point. Bring your innovation team together and display what has been found in step 1 on a flip chart. Allow the group to label each cluster of themes and topics. Then conduct a silent multivote with each team member using colored dots to indicate which innovation challenge deserves to be pursued. The top one to three innovation challenges are identified through this prioritization strategy.

- Step 3: Write an innovation statement that serves as the focus of the deep dive and idea generation phases. Start with "how might we . . .". A well-crafted innovation statement will have a single objective and will avoid leaping to preconceived solutions or evaluation criteria. The key is to not lock yourself into a premature solution!

- Step 4: Map your innovation strategy based on the identified challenge. Write down the objectives of the innovation challenge for different levels of your organization, including executive management and mid-level management such as head nurses, front-line staff, and patients. Draw lines between objectives if there are linkages that can be made. Figure 3-3 presents a sample innovation strategy map for the challenge of "how might we make it easier for a nurse to administer medications to patients in a safe and timely manner?" The executive-level management objective is to reduce medical errors and the financial/legal consequences of medication errors. This is linked to the nurses' objective of rapid and accurate sorting of medications by patient on the unit, which in turn is linked to the patients' objective of getting their correct medication at the right time. This innovation strategy map is a starting point for where to explore in the deep dive and the type of leverage points that should be observed. Guidance on how to construct an innovation challenge map can be found in Van Gundy's (2008) online monograph.

DOING THE DEEP DIVE

Once you have defined the innovation challenge, the next step is developing a fuller understanding of the challenge. There are four major categories of strategies to use in a deep dive: learn, look, ask, and try. These are described below with suggested tools and

Figure 3-3 Example innovation strategy map.

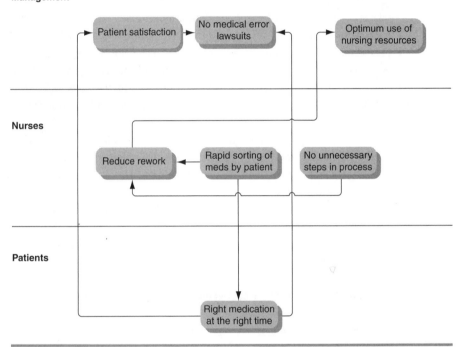

Innovation Challenge Statement

How might we make it easier for a nurse to administer medications to patients in a safe and timely manner?

approaches. The design firm, IDEO, developed a set of deep dive cards called the IDEO Method Cards that portray 51 strategies for learning, looking, asking, and trying (www.ideo.com/work/item/method-cards/). These are very helpful as you initially approach an innovation challenge to plan out a balanced approach to undertaking a deep dive. Select one card from each category for starters.

- *Learn* refers to collecting, synthesizing, and analyzing available information from reports and studies in the published and gray literature as well as reports from your organization, such as annual or quality reports. It also includes information from other related areas such as community served, evidence on procedures and technologies, human resources, and so on.
  - *Tools: PubMed.* The National Library of Medicine (NLM) has an extensive healthcare database of published literature from around the world. Master

innovators visit NLM often through its search engine, called PubMed. An online primer of how to optimize your searching is now available from the NLM (http://www.nlm.nih.gov/pubs/manuals/pm_workbook.pdf).

- *Look* includes a variety of observation methods to capture the experience of users. These include behavioral observation, mapping of patterns, rituals, artifacts, photo or video surveys, and process mapping.

  - *Tools: Photo survey.* Photo montages with annotations allow you to visualize the environments and activities of your users. A photo survey is a scripted photo session of people, processes, and tools that form the core of the user experience in which you are innovating. Create a photo script (where, when, what will be photographed), do the photo shoot, and then display and annotate your photos in a montage with observations, comments, and ideas for innovating.

  - *Tools: Activity mapping (spaghetti diagrams).* Virtually all service and many product innovations require movement. To better understand what is occurring in the existing process or using the existing product, it is highly valuable to track and map the movements of actors within a setting. Draw a physical layout of the environment you are observing; define the usual actors in this environment and assign them a symbol. For a specific process, draw and number lines of specific actor movements, and review with your innovation team to determine where opportunities for streamlining and innovation might occur (and identify in the diagram) (UK National Health Services Institute for Innovation and Improvement, 2008a). Figure 3-4 presents a typical activity map for a hospital unit.

  - *Tools: Behavioral archeology.* Observing and recording activities of people in the environment of interest can reveal patterns of work and the use of tools/artifacts that may serve as the basis for innovation. Find a location in the environment that is out of the way, draw a rough map of the environment (you may use the map from the spaghetti diagram), record the people and activities that occur in this environment, describe the sequence of activities and the implements that are involved, and then share this map and annotated descriptions along with samples of objects with your innovation team to stimulate idea generation.

  - *Tools: Process mapping.* Process maps are visual representations of the steps and activities for a specific process such as a patient visit. They can be simple or complex, depending on the information recorded. For instance, beyond the steps involved, the accuracy and completeness of the activity may also be recorded to estimate the "value" of each step in the overall process. Identify the process to study, define the start and end points, identify all the participants in the process, ask them as a group to define all the steps in the process

Figure 3-4 Spaghetti map of hospital unit.

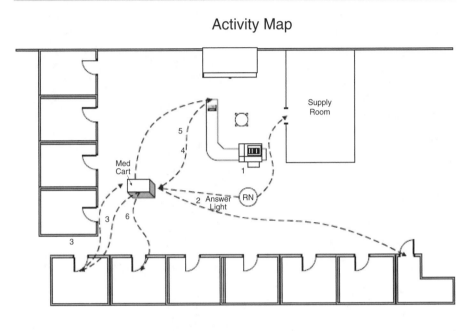

Activity Map

(use sticky notes), ask them to sequence the steps and describe what is occurring at each step (e.g., materials used, information exchanged), and then brainstorm with the group to identify where improvements could be designed into the process. The result is a "future state" map of a new process that can be tested. To learn more about process mapping, the American Society for Quality provides a process mapping guide (www.asq.org/learn-about-quality/process-analysis-tools/overview/flowchart.html). A number of software tools are available that allow construction of a process map. An excellent free tool is available from HealthInsight (www.healthinsight.org/hcp/doqit/workflow.html). Figure 3-5 presents a sample process map for a typical primary care office visit.

- *Ask* encompasses an array of techniques to elicit information from users and others. These can include focus or unfocus groups, activity analysis surveys, knowledge-attitude-practice (KAP) surveys, mind mapping, and body-storming.
  - ■ *Tools: Five whys.* Underlying many opportunities for innovation are unrecognized connections and assumptions. The "five whys" is an easy and rapid technique for diving into the heart of an innovation challenge. With your

Figure 3-5 Process map of office visit.

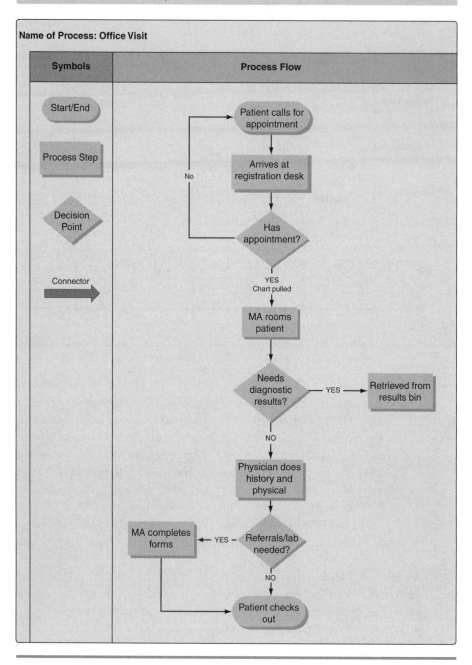

innovation team or with the user group that is helping you construct a process map, state the innovation challenge and ask why this is a challenge. For each subsequent answer or hypothesis, ask why again, record every answer, and repeat for at least five levels. Diagram on a flip chart the sequence of issues and answers and use as a tool for brainstorming ideas for innovation. You often find that the original innovation challenge is not really the core challenge as you dive deeper.

- *Tools: KAP surveys.* KAP surveys are methods to collect a range of data from providers, patients, and others about the innovation challenge. Knowledge refers to what the respondent knows about a disease, a care strategy, a care institution, or provider. KAP surveys are also valuable as a premarketing assessment to determine the viability of a new product or service. Box 3-1 presents a sample KAP survey for chest pain. The American Society for Quality offers a guide on use of surveys for improvement (www.asq.org/data-collection-analysis-tools/overview/survey.html).

- *Tools: Unfocus groups.* Unlike focus groups, which are composed of "typical users," unfocus groups bring together individuals with unique perspectives and passions about the innovation challenge. The goal of an unfocus group is not only to exchange perspectives but also to allow them to interact with a range of materials or service designs and to help you assemble mock-ups. Identify types of individuals who might give a broad and interesting range of perspectives (children are especially good unfocus group participants); organize a group session; ask participants to share their experiences and perspectives with the innovation challenge; solicit ideas for innovation, provide them materials such as drawing paper, and ask them to put together a crude prototype for further discussion or ask them to act out their ideas; and record the feedback, ideas, and perspectives for inclusion in the idea generation phase.

Box 3-1 Sample KAP Survey

Knowledge
  1. Have you heard of the acute coronary syndrome?
  2. What are the symptoms that indicate you should call 911?

Attitude
  3. Do you prefer medications or surgery for blocked blood vessels in your heart?
  4. How likely are you to tell your doctor about your symptoms?

Practice
  5. What is the first thing you do when you get chest pain?
  6. Do you miss taking your medications?

- *Try* is a learning process by doing. Building physical, mathematical, or performance prototypes not only captures your innovative idea for others to see and test but also allows the designer the chance to "build to think" (Brown, 2005). More is described below (see Designing Prototypes), but one key learning tool worth exploring is informance.

  - *Tools: Informance.* Actions speak louder than words. Informance is the acting out of scenarios related to the innovation challenge. They can be performed by the innovation team or by an unfocus group. The benefit is developing a shared understanding of the user experience. Start with a set of actors, define a scenario related to the innovation challenge, ask the actors to act out the experience, and solicit clarifications from the actors as to activities, materials, and experiences encountered. Video record the informance for review during brainstorming.

GENERATING TESTABLE IDEAS

The heart of innovation is the generating and testing of new ideas. This requires the innovator and the innovation team to think differently to move beyond the usual way of thinking or seeing the world. Although there are over 200 published methods for creative idea generation, all come down to three fundamental strategies that include "anything that helps us pay attention in a different way, escape our current mental patterns, and maintain movement in our thoughts" (Plsek, 1999, p. 441). Plsek (1999) identified these three pathways as attention, escape, and movement. Master innovators use both sides of their brains. Left-brain skills enable you to see deeper logical connections and effectively challenge your working assumptions. Right-brain skills enable you to break of out ingrained assumptions and modes of thinking and behaving. A wonderful compendium of techniques for lighting up the right brain has been published by the UK National Health Services Institute for Innovation and Improvement (2008b), called *Thinking Differently,* from which a number of the techniques highlighted in this section are derived. As you explore and develop your skills as a creative idea generator and innovator, it is useful to have some basic rules of thumb in your work. My favorites are Paul Plsek's (1997) eight heuristics for innovative thinking:

1. Make it a habit to purposefully pause and notice things.
2. Focus your creative energies on just a few topics that you care about.
3. Avoid being too narrow in how you define your topic.
4. Try to come up with original and useful ideas by making novel associations among what you already know.
5. When you need creative ideas, remember: attention, escape, and movement.

6. Pause and carefully examine ideas that make you laugh the first time.
7. Recognize that your streams of thought and patterns of judgment are not inherently right or wrong.
8. Make a deliberate effort to harvest, develop, and implement at least a few of the ideas you generate.

"The world we have made as a result of the level of thinking we have done thus far creates problems we cannot solve at the same level of thinking at which we created them."

—ALBERT EINSTEIN

There are two phases of idea generation. The first phase is dedicated to finding an array of ideas through techniques that focus attention, allow us to escape usual thinking, and maintain motion in our imaginations. The second phase involves harvesting these ideas, narrowing down the ideas with the greatest promise, and selecting a small set of ideas to begin prototyping. The first phase is often called *divergence,* as mental patterns expand and evolve, and the second phase *convergence,* as ideas start to get evaluated and sorted (Kelley & Littmann, 2000; Wycoff, 2004). The process of generating innovative ideas is highly iterative with repeated cycles of divergence and convergence before the innovation team is ready to start to build prototypes.

Divergence Tools

The following are a small sample of tools to help you begin expanding your idea horizon. The innovation student is encouraged to consult the work of Edward deBono, especially his seminal book, *Lateral Thinking* (1970). Another valuable resource is the work of Michael Michalko, especially his book, *Thinkertoys* (2006).

- *Tools: Treasure chest.* Some of the best ideas for innovative products and services are derivatives of other ideas. As you move through your world, observe and explore anything that seems innovative—a design, a material, a process. Collect them and store them in a treasure chest, a box or tool cabinet that is able to hold a wide variety of objects. A key aspect of the treasure chest is its ability to separate things of different natures such as photographs, drawings, materials, and objects. Have the treasure chest handy when undertaking unfocus groups or brainstorming to stimulate thinking.

- *Tools: Brainstorming.* Generating ideas as a collective exercise is one of the best ways to generate a lot of ideas. Brainstorming involves assembling your innovation team members, providing them the innovation challenge, and allowing them enough time, tools, and enthusiasm to generate a number of good ideas. A good brainstorming session is able to produce upward of 100 ideas in an hour. Some keys for successful brainstorming identified by IDEO include the following:

  - *Sharpen the focus.* Start with a crisp and simple innovation challenge statement that is high-level enough not to drive the innovation team to a premature solution.

  - *Playful rules.* Rules provide guidance to keep the brainstorming moving forward. These can include "go for quantity," "defer judgment," "encourage wild ideas," and "build on the ideas of others."

  - *Number your ideas.* It allows you to monitor the flow of ideas and to move back and forth between ideas. It also allows easier affinity grouping and prioritization.

  - *Build and jump.* A facilitator encourages taking someone else's ideas and building off of them.

  - *Space remembers.* Capture ideas so everyone can see them. Don't be afraid of covering the walls. Allow participants to wander around the room.

  - *Stretch your mental muscle.* Try a mental warm-up before starting, especially when the group hasn't worked together before. These can be exercises that are word or mind games or pre-work before a brainstorming session such as a Google search. Some great mind games can be found at www.mycoted.com/category:puzzles.

  - *Get physical.* Use a variety of visual techniques to depict and stimulate ideas such as sketches, diagrams, and maps. This is a good time to bring in objects from your treasure chest.

  As you plan and conduct brainstorming sessions to generate innovative ideas, there are some key steps to consider:

  - Assemble a group of participants (5–10) drawn from inside and outside the innovation team. Consider "seeding" the group with a topic expert.

  - Set aside an hour (don't go longer) and arrange a comfortable space.

  - Provide food, toys, and prototyping materials.

  - Facilitator conducts a warm-up exercise (optional).

  - Facilitator presents the innovation challenge.

  - Participants offer ideas written down by the facilitator on flip charts, walls, and so on. Avoid "going around the table" solicitations.

  - Use affinity grouping to cluster ideas into the Big Ideas.

  - Use multivoting to select the best ideas to start prototyping and testing.

  Several tools are available to help you put a productive brainstorming session together. The Institute for Healthcare Improvement has a toolsheet for brain-

storming (www.ihi.org/ihi/topics/improvement/improvementmethods/tools/
brainstorming+affinity+grouping+multivoting.htm). Another helpful resource is
the *Complete Guide to Managing Traditional Brainstorming Events* (www.jpb.com/
creative/brainstorming.pdf).

- *Tools: Body-storming.* Although brainstorming focuses on ideas and sometimes
  prototypes, body-storming focuses on using action to understand and create new
  processes, services, or products. It involves defining a scenario and acting it out
  based on what is understood about the innovation challenge. Based on information from the innovation deep dive, define one or more scenarios that represent
  the innovation challenge. Have your innovation team select actors, and let the
  actors play out the scenario based on what they know. Get feedback and ideas
  from the innovation team on new variations in the scenario and act them out.
  Repeat this cycle until enough ideas are generated. It is helpful to video the scenarios as they are acted out and review them with the innovation team.
- *Tools: Stepping-stones.* This tool is drawn from the UK National Health Services
  Institute for Innovation and Improvement *Thinking Differently* guide (2008b),
  which acts as a catalyst for innovation teams to leap from a seemingly wild idea to
  those that might be buildable. State your innovation challenge, propose an outrageous solution no matter its practicality, list all underlying concepts or assumptions in the idea, and then connect how these concepts or assumptions can be
  applied in the workplace. Box 3-2 provides an example of a stepping-stone exercise.

Box 3-2 Stepping-stone Example

Innovation Challenge: Organization doesn't see the value of innovation in daily
work.

Outrageous Idea: All employees' job descriptions require 20% minimum time
innovating their work.

Underlying Concepts:
- Innovation produces value
- All employees are innovators
- Innovation skills are considered organization competencies
- All work is considered candidate for innovation

Change Ideas:
- Explicitly defining business case for innovation
- Integrating innovation goals into employee performance evaluation
- Employee innovation training program

Convergence Tools

Once you have generated a list of ideas that range from the slightly different to the wildly odd, the master innovator needs to harvest those with the greatest potential for development in the prototyping phase.

- *Tools: Multivoting.* This technique allows each member of the innovation team to express his or her preference for specific ideas. Ask the team to review the ideas and group them based on similarity or affinity. Provide each member with three to five colored dots; each member then sticks the dots next to the idea he or she believes is best. Count the dots and identify the five to seven ideas with the most votes.
- *Tools: Six-hat thinking.* This technique, developed by Edward deBono, provides a way of looking at candidate ideas from different perspectives. Black hats represent risks and cautions, blue hats represent direction and management, yellow hats are benefits, red hats are feelings and intuitions, green hats are creativity and new ideas, and white hats are data and facts. Put on the yellow hat and list the expected benefit of the idea. Next put on the black hat and list the risks of the idea. Then put on the white hat and list what data need to be collected about the idea to know if it would work, and with your red hat on list what gut feelings you have about the idea. Step back and look at the whole picture of benefits, risks, information needs, and gut feelings: Is this an idea you believe worth pursuing? Figure 3-6 presents a six-hat innovation evaluation matrix that is useful as you consider the merits of your top ideas for further prototyping and development.

DESIGNING PROTOTYPES

The ultimate goal of the innovation process is to produce a product or service that improves the lives of the users. Prototypes are mock-ups or models that reflect your idea. They help you think more deeply about the idea and its feasibility, allow you to communicate your idea to others, and to ultimately persuade potential supporters and funders to take the idea to a broader development and dissemination level. It is virtually possible to create a prototype of anything from a procedure to a product. They can be physical, experiential, digital, or mathematical. You never know whether an idea will fly until you make it real and test it in the light of day. Moreover, having something in your hands allows you to see where it could be improved; prototyping is thus iterative and, some say, never ending.

Physical models are the most familiar. We all have built model airplanes or dollhouses. Physical prototypes are quick mock-ups using a wide variety of materials, from Styrofoam, cardboard, wood, clay, or Legos, to name a few (Figure 3-7). Keep in mind that the goal is not a finished product but a rapid yet convincing model that communicates your idea. It is helpful to have on your innovation team someone with craft or con-

Figure 3-6 A six-hat innovation evaluation matrix.

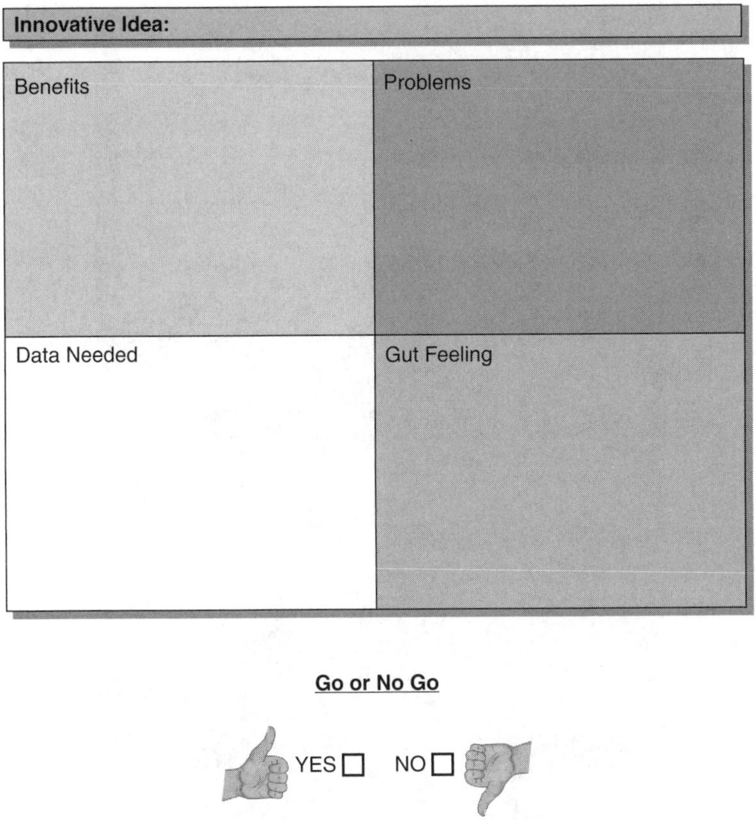

Innovative Idea:	
Benefits	Problems
Data Needed	Gut Feeling

Go or No Go

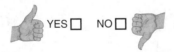 YES ☐   NO ☐

Source: de Bono (2000).

struction skills. Physical models start with a sketch that can take the form of "napkin sketches," stick figures, schematics, flowcharts, or storyboards (Figure 3-8). The guide written by Hanks and Belliston, *Rapid Viz* (1990), is a great place to learn techniques to put a rapid sketch together. Once you have a rough sketch to work from, start building with anything you are comfortable working with. Have fun! Don't strive for perfection but something that reflects your idea. Periodically, step back and look at it: Does it reflect what you are thinking; are there functions/parts/design that could be improved? Some common materials (you can find in any kindergarten class) include

- Common printer paper
- Construction paper

Figure 3-7 Lego robot prototypes.

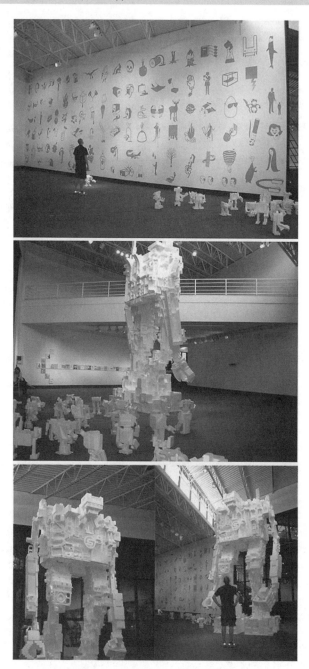

Figure 3-8 Alexander Graham Bell's actual pencil sketch of the telephone concept.

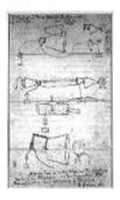

- Bristol board
- Cardboard
- Modeling clay
- Toilet paper rolls
- Paper towel rolls
- Wooden dowels
- Foam-core board
- Beaded Styrofoam
- X-Acto knife
- Hot glue gun
- Urethane foam
- Tic-tacs (for buttons)
- Plywood
- MDF (medium density fiberboard)
- Wire coat hangers
- Plastic wrap
- Fun-foam
- Toothpicks
- Wood glue
- Play-Doh (seriously)

Have fun with this stage. Go a little crazy. This is usually a fun experience, and the fun of it all can lead you to observations that may have been overlooked in the "over-5-year-old" world. Remember, there is *no* wrong way to approach this phase of design.

With the advent of high-speed computing, prototypes can be rapidly constructed within a virtual environment. *Computer-assisted design* applications are software programs that produce two- or three-dimensional representations. Further, these applications can also create virtual environments for these designs, allowing you to walk around. Computer-assisted manufacturing are electronic systems that translate the computer-assisted design into a physical model.

Paper prototyping extends the concept of sketching into near-world applications. The two most common paper prototyping methods are storyboarding and process mapping. Storyboarding, commonly used in the creative arts such as film making, takes action or scene sketches and puts them into a "story." The Institute for Healthcare Improvement developed a tool to help design a storyboard (www.ihi.org/topics/improvementmethods/tools/storyboards.htm). Process mapping as described in the deep dive section lays out the sequence or flow of materials and information through a defined process. This allows not only better understanding of the current practice but also allows the users to redesign the process in testable ways.

Experience prototyping uses idea representations that allow the user to interact and experience the idea. They can be extensions of physical prototypes or can be scenarios of service innovations. They can be set up as a "museum exhibition" to allow the user to walk through the idea. They can also be short video productions that capture the idea. These are particularly effective methods for conveying ideas to someone foreign to the process, such as the chief executive officer or others who decide whether to support further development. Key steps are (1) define the innovation idea, (2) describe the scenario in which the user can experience the physical prototype or the service innovation, (3) set up the scenario with appropriate space and props, (4) provide opportunity for potential users and others to interact, and (5) observe the user interactions and collect their feedback. As an example of use of experience prototyping, Nokia developed a prototype of an image capture and transmittal device for children (now part of their cell phone technology). They provided these working mock-ups to children and let them carry them during their normal day. They subsequently collected information from the children on interest, use and usability, and experience of carrying an image system around with them.

Mathematical models can be used for innovation ideas that may be so small or so large as not to be easily prototyped using physical or experimental methods. For example, a large public health innovation that impacts the spread of disease in large populations may best be modeled in mathematical form. Models may be linear or nonlinear and deterministic or probabilistic. Although it is beyond this chapter to fully detail statistical methods, all mathematical modeling involves the following steps. First, define the variables, those that change and those that stay constant in the analysis. Second, determine the type of mathematical model that is most applicable. Third, compute the model using analysis software. Finally, examine the results of the analysis to determine the variables and the effect level on the outcome of interest. For the interested student there are a large number of statistical textbooks. One useful starting point is Michael McLaughlin's free online monograph "The Very Game . . . A Tutorial on Mathematical Modeling" (www.causascientia.org/math_stat/tutorial.pdf).

Before taking your innovative idea that you've prototyped to your funders and supporters, consider testing it so that you have some pilot data that demonstrate that it works. *Rapid cycle tests* of change are a part of a larger quality improvement set of strategies with which many healthcare organizations are familiar. The keys to these tests are small scale and rapid deployment. In a sense they are a variation of the experience prototype. For instance, select one provider to use the innovation prototype on a small handful of patients for a day or a week. Measure whether the provider and/or patients detect a positive change and how easy or difficult the prototype is to use/do. As you plan and conduct your rapid cycle tests, keep in mind the following tips:

- *Stay a cycle ahead.* When designing a test, imagine at the start what the subsequent test or two might be, given the various possible findings.
- *Scale down the scope of tests.* Dimensions that can be scaled down include the number of patients, doctors, others in the test, and the location and duration of the test.
- *Pick willing volunteers.* Work with those who want to work with you.
- *Avoid the need for consensus, buy-in, or political solutions.* They come later. Choose processes or environments that do not require a long process of approval.
- *Pick easy changes to try.* Look for ideas that seem the most feasible (ideas that green hats like) and might have the greatest impact.
- *Avoid technical slowdowns.* Don't wait for the computer to arrive. Use paper and pencil as needed.
- *Reflect on the results of every change.* Ask what did we expect to happen? What did happen? Were there surprises or unforeseen consequences? What was the best thing about this change? What might we do next? Remember that teams often learn the most from failed tests of change.

To help you organize and learn from conducting a rapid cycle test, Figure 3-9 provides a useful tracking form.

CREATING YOUR PLAN FOR DIFFUSION

Now that you have created a prototype and perhaps have tested it on a small scale, it is time to create a plan for spreading it within your organization or within the marketplace (or both). It is key to understanding the nature of innovation diffusion as well as the role of social networks in this process. With this knowledge and application to your

Figure 3-9 Example of a rapid cycle tool.

Aim: (overall goal you wish to achieve)

Every goal will require multiple smaller tests of change

Describe your first (or next) test of change:	Person responsible:	When to be done:	Where to be done:

Plan:

List the tasks needed to set up this test of change:	Person responsible:	When to be done:	Where to be done:

Predict what will happen when the test is carried out:	Measures to determine if prediction succeeds:

Do: Describe what actually happened when you ran the test.

Study: Describe the measured results and how they compared to the predictions.

Act: Describe what modifications to the plan will be made for the next cycle from what you learned.

innovation, you can create a diffusion plan to guide you in getting your innovation used throughout your organization. When you present your innovation and its prototype to your chief executive officer, board, or other supporters, having an action-oriented diffusion plan demonstrates how thoughtful you are about the future of the innovation.

Dynamics of Innovation Diffusion

The work of Everett Rogers over the last 50 years laid the foundation for how people look at the spread of innovations (Rogers, 1995). He suggested that innovations spread slowly at first, used primarily by the innovators themselves and a small number of "early adopters," then hit a "tipping point" at 15% to 20% use rates where they take off and spread through larger numbers of more cautious adopters, called the early and late majorities. This adoption pattern follows a classic "S" curve and has been demonstrated for a wide variety of innovation histories. Rogers also identified 10 factors that influence how rapidly and widely innovations spread:

1. *Relative advantage.* This is the perceived or real value that the innovation provides to the user in comparison with current practice or products.
2. *Triability.* This is the ability of potential users to try out the innovation without commitment.
3. *Observability.* This is the degree to which potential users see others using the innovation.
4. *Communication channels.* This is the use of specific channels through which opinion leaders and early adopters can transmit their experience, outcomes, and opinions to others in their local social networks and more distant connections.
5. *Homophilous groups.* How homogenous are target user groups based on key characteristics? Innovations spread more rapidly in high homophilous groups.
6. *Pace of innovation/reinvention.* This is the degree to which the innovation evolves through the diffusion process and how easy it is for users to adapt it to their own needs and circumstances.
7. *Norms, roles, social networks.* How connected are user groups in their relationships both within the homophilous group and in distant connections?
8. *Opinion leaders.* This is the presence and influence of individuals who are respected leaders in their homophilous group.
9. *Compatibility.* This is the extent to which the innovation is aligned with the user's current knowledge, skills, attitudes, and beliefs.
10. *Infrastructure support.* This is the presence of existing support infrastructure and process. For example, computed tomographies depend on computers and software.

National Health Services Innovation Diffusion Model

More recently, the UK National Health Services Institute for Innovation and Improvement published a systematic review of innovation diffusion factors and a diffusion model (Greenhalgh, Robert, Bate, Macfarlane, & Kyriakidou, 2005). Similar to Rogers (1995), they suggest that the factors influencing the diffusion process include the nature of the innovation, the dissemination strategies used, the attributes and readiness of the potential user system, the external environment (regulatory, financial), and the linkages between the potential user system and the innovators and supporting infrastructure (Figure 3-10).

Figure 3-10 Factors influencing the diffusion process.

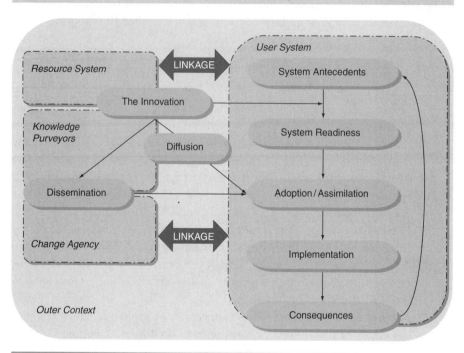

Innovations in Social Networks

There is a considerable body of evidence that suggests that innovation diffusion is strongly influenced by the configuration and functional relationships within social networks (Coleman, Menzel, & Katz, 1957). This occurs through three possible mechanisms (McGrath & Krackhardt, 2003). First, linkages between individuals from different groups might serve to pollinate each cluster with innovations. One benefit, for example, of state medical society meetings is to allow networking of acquaintances from across the state to share their experiences and possibly new ideas. Second, innovations introduced by peripheral members of a densely linked group (e.g., medical directors) might percolate effectively throughout the group. Third, innovations introduced by highly linked individuals diffuse innovations to the many connection networks to which they are tied. This is known as a scale-free network. Google uses this network principle to run its Internet search engine, producing search results in nanoseconds by starting the search with the most connected sites.

As you build your diffusion plan, you must first target a user group that can utilize your innovation. The user group you target determines what types of network diffusion strategies might work. For instance, hospital nursing staff and hospital physician staff are very different in social network configurations. A study from the United Kingdom suggested that nursing staffs, especially head nurses, were very centrally organized, which suggests that innovations might effectively be introduced by head nurses (West, Barron, Dowsett, & Newton, 1999). On the other hand, physician staff were less hierarchically linked to each other but tended to be linked with highly dense clusters with high degrees of connectedness. In this instance the diffusion interventions built on the first and second network configurations will be more effective in physician networks. A classic case of this network method is the opinion leader research on new cesarian section guidelines promoted by the Canadian Society of Obstetrics and Gynecology. The results of this study suggest that opinion leaders/physician champions were the most effective means by which to change practice. Interestingly, the opinion leader does not need to be an early adopter but simply a respected individual who is knowledgeable and believable in his or her innovation promotion.

Creating Your Diffusion Plan

A diffusion plan is a component of the larger business plan that you present to your leadership or potential supporters and funders. The diffusion plan takes into account the key factors influencing the diffusion with special focus on the key characteristics of your innovation and the key characteristics of your target audience. Innovation characteristics include the relative advantage of your innovation over existing products and services; the complexity/ease of use of the innovation; how adaptable it is by potential users; how compatible your innovation is with current work processes, technologies, and interpersonal interactions; and the dependence of your innovation on other existing technologies or work processes. Key characteristics of your target audience to plan for include their demographics (age, sex, position in the healthcare system), the homogeneity/homophile of the group, how they are linked both within the group and to other clusters of people within the organization, healthcare system or medical community, and the characteristics that define how ready they might be to adopt your innovation. The above factors may not be fully known as you develop your plan, so stay flexible in your approaches and learn in the process of trying to disseminate your innovation. Put your strategy into a document that can be shared by your organization's leadership and potential funders.

Creating Your Story

You need to make a compelling case for why your innovation will make a difference. Because diffusion is people dependent, a compelling story is essential. You need to catch and hold the attention of individuals and groups who are your target audience. This can be done through design of a good story that communicates the value and relevance of your innovation and is memorable so that your potential users can retell the story to others. This is known as viral marketing. The best place to craft your story is during your deep dive as you listen and observe the needs, values, preferences, and stories of people who are your target audience. What would you want these networks of people to say about your service or product? How does it make their lives better? Consider the following as you write your innovation story:

- What is the strong, central theme? Can you express it in one line?
- What does the main character(s) share with your target audience?
- In what kind of setting/environment does your story take place?
- What kind of "zing" can you insert (e.g., humor, surprise, outrageousness, the unusual, secrets)?

Communicating Your Innovation

With your innovation prototype, its story, and a diffusion plan in hand, how can you communicate them to leadership and potential funders? Two common strategies previously discussed are storyboards and video presentations. Both are effective vehicles to talk about your innovation and the story that goes with it. For storyboards, make them colorful, highly graphical, and focused on your innovation and its benefits. They should "catch the eye" and communicate at a glance. For video presentations, keep them short (5–8 minutes in length). Write out a script based on your story, rehearse it, and then film it. Try to maintain the "zing" of the story.

- *Tools: Storyboard.* A storyboard is a graphical presentation that enables the innovator to describe the innovation, its uses, and its benefits. When coupled with the actual physical prototype, it can be a compelling way to communicate the development and future of your innovation. There are numerous formats for creating a storyboard. Some key elements to include are
  - Name of the innovation
  - Innovation team (names, photos)
  - Innovation sponsors
  - Statement of the innovation challenge
  - Assessment strategies used and results
  - Description of the innovation
  - Projected future of the innovation

    Great storyboards are brief; highly graphical, mixing images, data, and text together; and focused on how the innovation meets the innovation challenge. They also allow interaction with the innovation if possible through a physical or experience prototype. Draw out the proposed format of the storyboard. Obtain a storyboard (from any office supply store). Assemble the defined elements (images, graphs, text boxes). On a flat surface lay the storyboard down and place elements where you would want them to go. If the team is in agreement, proceed with affixing these elements to the storyboard. Prepare a presentation that highlights the elements on the storyboard. Conduct the presentation to the sponsor, funder, or producer. Figure 3-11 shows a sample storyboard.

Figure 3-11 Example of a storyboard.

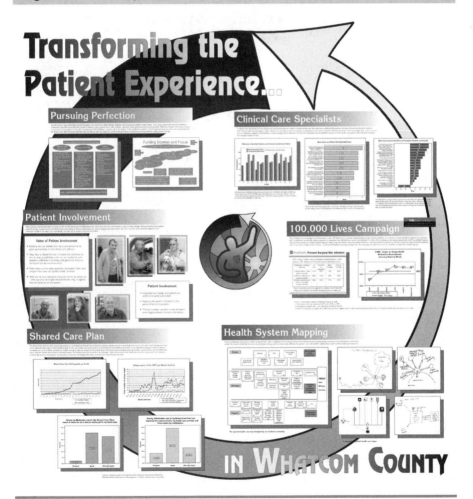

Figure 3-12 Balanced scorecard approach.

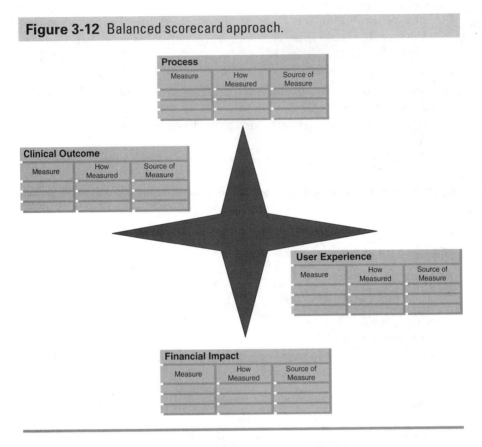

Measuring the Reach and Impact of Your Innovation

As your innovation begins to get disseminated in your organization or in the market-place, measuring the acceptance, use, and impact is important for improving the inno-vation and/or its diffusion plan. Consider using a balanced scorecard approach that includes metrics on use, clinical impact, financial impact, and user satisfaction as a good way to start (Kaplan & Norton, 1996). Figure 3-12 is an example of a balanced score-card approach for measuring the impact of your innovation.

CONCLUSION

Innovation is a systematic, learned process that follows a five-phase process that is highly iterative. The first step defines the real innovation challenge through inter-views, information searches, and data analysis with production of a clear, actionable innovation statement. Based on this innovation statement, the master innovator and innovation team take a deep dive into the challenge using a variety of anthropological methods that help the user learn, look, ask, and try. With a deeper and more comprehensive understanding of the innovation challenge, new ideas are generated through divergent thinking strategies such as brainstorming and then narrowed to a select few for prototyping, using convergent thinking strategies such as multivoting and six-hat prioritization. These select few ideas are ready to be built and tested using physical, experience, digital, or mathematical prototyping methods, then tested on a small scale. Once you have a product or service that has been prototyped, it is time to take it to your leadership for consideration for internal spread and, perhaps, an eventual introduction into the marketplace. Put a diffusion plan together that captures the innovation and a compelling story that addresses the key characteristics of the innovation and its target audience. Plan to measure acceptance and impact during the diffusion process, and modify the innovation and/or its diffusion plan based on results.

REFERENCES

Anonymous. (2005, August). *Business Week, 72.*

Brown, T. (2005, June). Strategy by design. *Fast Company,* 2–5.

Brown, T. (2008, June). Design thinking. *Harvard Business Review,* 85–92.

Coleman, J. S., Menzel, H., & Katz, E. (1957). The diffusion of an innovation among physicians. *Sociometry, 20*(4), 253–270.

de Bono, E. (1970). *Lateral thinking: Creativity step by step.* New York: Harper and Row.

Drucker, P. F. (2002, August). The discipline of innovation. *Harvard Business Review,* 95–102.

Greenhalgh, T., Robert, G., Bate, P., Macfarlane, F., & Kyriakidou, O. (2005). *Diffusion of innovations in health service organizations: A systematic literature review.* Malden, MA: Blackwell.

Hanks, K., & Belliston, L. (1990). *Rapid viz: A new method for rapid visualization of ideas.* Menlo Park, CA: Crisp Publications.

Johansson, F. (2006). *The Medici effect: What elephants and epidemics can teach us about innovation.* Boston: Harvard Business School Press.

Kaplan, R. S., & Norton, D. P. (1996). *The balanced scorecard: Translating strategy into action.* Boston: Harvard Business School Press.

Kelley, T., & Littmann, J. (2000). *The art of innovation.* New York: Doubleday.

McGrath, C., & Krackhardt, D. (2003). Network conditions for organization change. *Journal of Applied Behavioral Sciences, 39*(3), 324–336.

Michalko, M. (2006). *Thinkertoys.* Berkeley, CA: Ten Speed Press.

Plsek, P. E. (1997). *Creativity, innovation and quality.* Milwaukee, WI: ASQ Quality Press.

Plsek, P. E. (1999). Innovative thinking for the improvement of medical systems. *Annals of Internal Medicine, 131,* 438–444.

Rogers, E. M. (1995). *Diffusion of innovations.* New York: Free Press.

UK National Health Services Institute for Innovation and Improvement. (2008a). Guide for constructing a spaghetti diagram. Retrieved June 8, 2008, from www.nodelayachiever.nhs.uk/serviceimprovement/tools/it215_spaghetti_ diagram.htm

UK National Health Services Institute for Innovation and Improvement. (2008b). Thinking differently. Retrieved June 8, 2008, from www.institute.nhs.uk/building_capability/new_model_for_transforming_ the_nhs/thinking_differently_guide.html

Van Gundy, A. B. (2008). The care and framing of strategic innovation challenges. Retrieved April 15, 2008, from www.jpb.com/creative/vangundyframeinnov.pdf

West, E., Barron, D. N., Dowsett, J., & Newton, J. N. (1999). Hierarchies and cliques in the social networks of health care professionals: Implications for the design of dissemination strategies. *Social Science and Medicine, 48,* 633–646.

Wycoff, J. (2004, August). Creativity made simple: Divergence and convergence are critical to successful ideation. Retrieved June 6, 2008, from www.innovationtools.com/Search/searchdetails.asp?ContentID= 152&sitesearch=convergence

CHAPTER 4

Directed Creativity: How to Generate New Ideas for Transforming Health Care

Paul Plsek

Albert Einstein once pointed out, "You cannot solve a problem using the thinking that got you there." Fortunately, although health care has many well-documented problems (Institute of Medicine, 2001), the need for new thinking is also well recognized. For example, an international review of healthcare policies and plans (Bate, Robert, & Bevan, 2004) noted the following:

> Healthcare systems around the world are engaged in striving to make radical and sustainable changes through various programmatic approaches to improvement. . . . The words . . . leave no doubt that what is being envisaged is big, bold, transformational change. . . . Internationally there is a parallel realization and understanding that the design of the existing healthcare system will not deliver what is required for the future. (p. 62)

But, how does one go about deliberately thinking differently?

Fortunately, this is a well-studied problem (Runco, 2007), and there are many practical tools and methods one can use, alone or in groups, to stimulate the production of creative ideas in focused topic areas (Plsek, 1997a). Contrary to popular belief, creativity is not a special gift that only some people possess (Weisberg, 1993). Rather, the ability to think creatively is a capacity we all possess and can actively direct at the issues we face in health care today (Plsek, 1999a). The deliberate production of creative ideas, and the follow-through required to turn those ideas into concrete innovations, is what I call "directed creativity" (Plsek, 1994, 1997b).

Like the reverse gear on an automobile, creativity is not something we need all the time, or even most of the time. There is great value in conservative thinking in the practice of medicine, and constant novelty in organizational processes would be chaotic. However, like an automobile's reverse gear, the ability to apply directed creative thinking is very handy, and may indeed be essential, in some situations.

We begin this chapter by defining the term "creativity" and then use that definition to set the stage for practical methods for stimulating it. We then look closer at how the mind functions, both in normal thinking and in creative thinking. These insights lead directly to three key principles that lie behind methods for directed creative thinking. Understanding these principles helps us to see better how to use the tools of creativity, tools that might otherwise seem odd at first. We explore a variety of tools and show how they might be applied to common issues in health care.

DEFINING CREATIVITY AND IMPLICATIONS FOR THINKING

Although there are dozens of definitions of creativity in the literature, five underlying themes appear frequently and make up what we commonly mean by the term. These are captured in the following definition (Plsek, 1997a):

> Creativity is the connecting and rearranging of knowledge—in the minds of people who will allow themselves to think flexibly—to generate new, often surprising ideas that others judge to be useful. (p. 1)

The recent development of natural-orifice, no-incision surgery—for example, the removal of a gallbladder through the vagina or a brain tumor through the nose (Peng, 2008)—is a good illustration of the definition of creativity. The ability to remove a diseased internal organ without making an incision is a new, useful idea whose practical benefits include reduced risk of infection and shorter recovery time. You probably smiled, expressed surprise, or maybe were even shocked when you first heard it. However, in hindsight we can see that this idea is simply a logical connection of existing knowledge—laparoscopic instruments can be inserted into small openings and the body has several such natural openings. It makes perfect sense now that we hear it, but coming up with the idea required the mental flexibility and courage to step out of the current paradigm of surgery.

Practical Implications From the Definition of Creativity

Understanding what we mean by "creative" is a big step toward directed creativity in that it tells us what to direct our thinking toward. When we wish to be creative, we should try to come up with an original idea by thinking flexibly and making novel associations among what we already know or observe. It may be helpful to explicitly list what we already know or see to aid this mental process, and, indeed, many creative thinking techniques begin with listing. It may also be helpful to be attentive to and curious about new concepts as a matter of course in our daily lives simply for the purpose of making them available in the mind for later creative connection. Purposefully noticing what is going on around us, rather than being on "autopilot," is a useful habit worth cultivating. Again, several creative thinking tools are based on these ideas.

Cynthia Taylor is a nurse manager in a small, rural hospital who has been asked to organize the hospital's annual flu vaccination campaign for the community. Every year for many years the organization has offered low-cost flu shots in one of the lobbies of the hospital, and every year there are numerous complaints about crowded parking facilities and people wandering the hospital's corridors in search of the vaccination station. "How can we get it to flow better this year?" Cynthia wonders as she drives home from work. Conversations with colleagues during the day produced ideas about a designated parking area, better signage, volunteers to direct people, and alternative locations within the facility. "Those are all good suggestions," she thinks, "but I wonder what else we might try?"

She pulls into the drive-through at her local bank to get some cash from the ATM machine and then through the drive-through of a fast-food restaurant to get a grilled chicken salad, fruit cup, and diet drink for dinner. "I'll have the #9 with light Ranch dressing," she says and is soon back on the road. "Hmmmm," she thinks with a smile to herself, "that was pretty good 'flow' for my trip home from work, wasn't it?" She begins mentally listing the various service delivery concepts she has encountered—self-service via a technology interface, drive-throughs that allow you to get what you want without getting out of your car, and being able to quickly refer to a bundles of things that naturally go together.

Having called to mind what we know, the next practical step suggested by the definition is to search for new connections and be attentive to surprises. Allowing for surprise explains why some creativity techniques suggest that we select concepts at random and try our best to combine them into something useful.

The notion of surprise in the definition of creativity has another important practical implication. When you feel yourself laughing or smiling at an idea, pause on that thought and work with it. It is highly likely that it contains the germ of a creative thought. This is in contrast with what usually happens in organizations when someone expresses an off-the-wall idea in a meeting and everyone laughs at it. Rather than pausing to extract the germ of the creative thought, we often simply dismiss it so we can get back to serious business. This works in direct contradiction to what we know from the definition of creativity. Practically speaking, pausing on a laughable thought may be one of the most productive things we can do when we want creativity. Subsequent chapters in this book have more to say about creating an overall organizational culture that favors innovation.

Cynthia wonders if the annual flu vaccination campaign might make the shot available via a drive-through. She imagines a tent in the parking lot with signs directing people to it. The person administering the shot would complete the usual process while the occupants of the cars stick their arms out the window. She immediately smiles at the idea and wonders if it is silly, but after thinking more about she is convinced that it might not be a bad idea after all. At the hospital the next morning, she begins to explain the drive-through idea to the nursing director, who immediately laughs and says, "You're joking, right?" "No, actually, I'm not," Cynthia replies. The look on the director's face turns immediately from a smile to one of concern.

Finally, in noting that creative ideas must be judged to be useful in the end, we find that the definition of creativity suggests that we must work hard to develop the practical value of our ideas. Creativity is not just about flexible thinking and mental free association; our analytical and logical thinking abilities are also needed. The ability to practically shape and develop an idea is just as important as the ability to imagine the idea in the first place. Imagination and analysis are equal partners in creativity. We have more to say about the application of analytical and practical skills in innovation in this and several other chapters in this book.

Cynthia knows she will have an uphill battle convincing her boss and others to go along with the drive-through flu vaccination idea. For example, questions about liability will be raised with all sorts of worst-case scenarios. She will need to research reactions to the flu vaccine and provide for some observation of patients before letting them drive away. She will also need to point out that patients routinely drive their cars away from the hospital only a few minutes after receiving the flu vaccine under the current system, and no one has questioned the legal liabilities associated with this before. She might need to set up the drive-through on a temporary basis for just a day or 2, or maybe test it out with staff volunteers initially while maintaining the standard station in the hospital lobby. It will be hard work and she knows it. But she is convinced intuitively that it is a good idea, and she has never let the obstacles of other people's thinking stand in her way in the past. (Note: We will say more about the role of intuition in leadership of innovation in a subsequent chapter. Also note that at the time of this writing, innovative drive-through flu vaccination services are being created in many states in the United States [Smith, 2008].)

SOME THEORY FOR DIRECTED CREATIVITY: THE MECHANICS OF THE MIND

If creative thinking can be directed so easily, then why is it so rare? To answer this question we need to understand the underlying mental processes that go into the production of both normal thought and creative ideas.

The bottom line is that creative ideas are relatively rare because our minds are not set up to produce them naturally. Rather, our minds are optimized to store and play back patterns of thought and behavior we learned from the past (Friedenberg & Silverman, 2005). However, an issue occurs when the situation demands that we think of something new and different; that is, when we need to think creatively, we too often find that we can think only of what we have thought of before. So, although we all possess the capacity for creative thought, creative thought is not automatic. We must direct our minds to overcome our usual thinking processes.

Role of Perception, Memory, and Judgment in Thinking

Research over the past 50 years has taught us much about both automatic and creative mental processes. Figure 4-1 provides a high-level systems diagram of some key mental processes. (For more details about mental processes and their relationship to creative thinking, see de Bono, 1969, 1992; Friedenberg & Silverman, 2005; Osherson and Smith, 1990; Plsek 1997a.) Our minds gather inputs from the world around us through the subprocesses of perception. We then retrieve patterns from memory (i.e., our past experiences) to make sense of these inputs. Research shows that our perception processes filter out most of what goes on around us and focus our attention toward signals in the environment that fit our existing patterns of how things should be.

Figure 4-1 A high-level model of the mechanics of the mind.

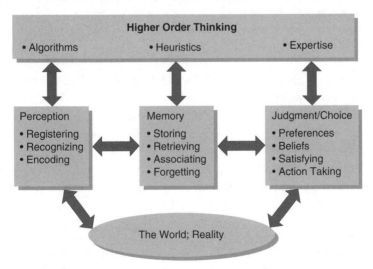

Cynthia had no problem perceiving the drive-throughs at the bank and fast-food restaurant, and she had no problem recalling what to do in order to get the service she needed in those situations. It was just normal, everyday thinking.

Although this perception–memory mechanism is efficient for doing routine tasks, it works against creativity. Our automatic mental processes bias our thinking toward existing ways of doing things and cause us to miss observations that could lead toward a new way.

It is highly likely that Cynthia's colleagues at the hospital have had similar service experiences at the local bank and restaurant. But when their thoughts turned to the problem of designing the annual flu campaign, they naturally thought of the hospital lobby as the venue. Why? Because that is how it had always been done. That was the pattern that corresponded to the situation of the flu campaign, and that was a very different pattern from the one that corresponded to the question of how to get cash from the local bank's ATM.

Directed creativity involves slowing down and redirecting our perception and memory retrieval processes. Though it is not automatic, we can direct our mind to notice things we do not usually notice and to retrieve different mental patterns, or connect to different contexts.

Cynthia's deliberate pause to notice that she was flowing smoothly through her errands on the way home from work, and her deliberate attention to how this could be applied to the context of the flu vaccination campaign, enabled her to go to a different place in her thinking. This was a place that neither she nor colleagues had ever gone to before, despite numerous occasions of receiving drive-through service in the community.

Edward de Bono (1969, 1992) supplies a useful metaphor for the mental mechanics of perception and memory. He suggests that we think of the mind as a rugged landscape with hills, valleys, and streams. The flow of thought in the mind is analogous to the flow of water. The valleys between the hills represent the processes of perception. Just as rainwater is channeled by the valleys into streams at the bottom, so the mental processes of perception channel our thoughts toward existing patterns in memory. de Bono's model is appealing because it corresponds directly to common phrases for mental activity such as "stream of thought" and "mental ruts."

To Cynthia and her colleagues, the mention of the task to "set up the annual flu vaccination campaign" immediately conjures up pictures of the station in the hospital lobby and all the associated problems of parking and lost members of the community. Like rainwater falling in a valley, the hearing of the words channels thinking into the existing mental valley of "the annual flu vaccination campaign" and further thought naturally flows on from that starting point.

In this model memory is a mental rut. When we learn about or see something for the first time, we carve another rut (valley) into our mental landscape. The more frequently we access that memory and repeat the pattern, the deeper the rut (like soil erosion). The deeper the rut, the more automatic is our thinking, creating habits that are hard to break.

So automatic was the idea of setting up the flu vaccination station in the lobby that conversations Cynthia had with colleagues before her drive home about how to do it better simply yielded marginal suggestions for a designated parking area, better signage, volunteers to direct people, and alternative locations within the facility. No one questioned the basic notion that the station would be located somewhere within the hospital and that patients would have to find it by walking through the corridors.

It is important to note that this mental channeling mechanism is not bad. In fact, it gives us many positive and useful human abilities that we take for granted. For example, it enables a clinician to make a preliminary diagnosis based on an initial review of the patient's symptoms. The patient's symptoms fall like raindrops onto the clinician's mental landscape. The clinician has seen the pattern of symptoms before and, therefore, has a well-defined mental valley encoded with the name of the underlying disease. The observation of the symptoms is thereby translated into a stream of thought that identifies the disease. We call this natural mental ability "experience." The mental mechanism is the same whether we are preparing a budget, designing a new healthcare process, or just trying to get out of bed in the morning. We use the past experiences stored in our memory as a guide for how to proceed forward. There is nothing wrong with this.

Although this self-organizing, channeling system is great for doing the repetitive tasks of daily life, it is clearly not optimal when we want creative ideas. Creative thinking requires that we "think outside the box," away from or beyond our current mental valleys, toward new patterns. Creative thinking involves slowing down and redirecting our perception processes instead of letting them flow automatically into the usual mental valleys. It involves connecting to and exploring mental valleys that we do not normally access in the context we find ourselves in at the moment.

Cynthia's mindfulness on her drive home enabled her to connect the mental valleys of banks and fast-food restaurants, where drive-throughs are a common thing, to the mental valley of the annual flu campaign. It was a creative connection that had not been made before. Cynthia allowed her mind to play with the connection, rather than simply remaining in the valley associated with the way the campaign had always been done in the past.

When we need a creative idea, it therefore does little good to tell ourselves and others to just "think harder," simply "suspend judgment" (as in brainstorming), or merely "be playful." Although it is indeed helpful to think hard, suspend judgment, and be playful during creative thinking, these simple suggestions fall short by failing to provide a new *direction* for our thinking. If we remain in our current mental valley, we may find that we are able to come up with only small variations on the mental patterns we already have.

Although perception and memory mechanisms define our thoughts, judgment and choice are the mental processes that stand between our thoughts and actions (refer back to Figure 4-1). Our automatic judgment processes are also channeled toward existing patterns from the past. Research shows that we automatically work to preserve our beliefs, justify our past preferences, and avoid taking risks (Osherson & Smith, 1990; Tversky & Kahneman, 1973, 1981).

So, our judgment processes are also mental patterns, but flavored with emotions. Our mental valleys are comfortable places in our thinking. Suggestions that we move out of these comfort zones tend to trigger emotions of fear and anxiety that lead us to immediately see the new idea as somewhat dangerous. Hence, we can understand the often-observed group behavior that new ideas are greeted with challenging questions and references to the worst-case scenarios that might result from applying them. Creative thinking involves temporarily, but purposefully, suspending these judgments, abandoning the need to justify our past patterns, and risking the expression of new ideas to see where they take us.

The reaction of Cynthia's director ("You're joking right?") and that of well-meaning colleagues who questioned the wisdom of letting patients drive away after receiving the flu vaccine even though for years they had been driving away safely in the current design illustrates these natural, emotional, not-completely-rational reactions.

It is important to note that creative thinking does not suggest that we never apply critical judgment and logical thinking. How could we possibly get to the concrete implementation required to reap the rewards of innovation without critical judgment? Rather, we simply need to hold judgment off a little longer than we are accustomed to when using our automatic mental processes. We can do it. But we must direct our mind to do it.

Three Principles Behind All Tools for Directed Creativity

Books and other resources by Black (1995), de Bono (1992), Higgins (1994), Maher, Plsek, Garrett, & Bevan (2008), McGartland (1994), Michalko (2006), and Plsek (1997a) collectively suggest hundreds of tools that can help us overcome the limitations of these mental processes. A closer look reveals that all these methods are based on three simple principles that help redirect the mechanism of mind: *attention, escape,* and *movement* (Plsek, 1997a).

> *Cynthia Taylor paid uncommon **attention** to how well she was flowing through her routine errands on her way home. She **escaped** the past pattern of how the flu vaccination campaign had been run and how we do things in general in a hospital setting. Rather than allowing her internal judgment to simply dismiss the thought of a drive-through flu vaccination station as a silly idea, she practiced mental **movement** in thinking through how it might work.*

The order of the three is not fixed, but the presence of all three is required somewhere along the way to a creative idea. For example, the idea of the drive-through flu shot could have been just as easily generated by the use of the tool of mental benchmarking (explained below in Mental Benchmarking or Be Someone Else, under Tools for Directed Creativity). Here, we first escape our usual mental valley by selecting other businesses or organizations at random. Banks or fast-food restaurants might have been two industries on which we were asked to focus. The tool then asks us to focus attention on some aspect of the selected business. In the context of wanting creative ideas for our annual flu campaign, we might have focused on how customers flow and receive service in these other settings, and the drive-through concept would have surely come up on our list. The final aspect of mental benchmarking suggests that we take the listed flow and service concepts from other contexts and move in our thinking to imagine how they might be adapted to our setting of the annual flu campaign.

The key point is that we can use deliberate attention, escape, and movement whenever we need to be creative on demand. The principles suggest a potentially infinite number of ways to direct ourselves toward creative thoughts, and this explains why there are so many different tools in the literature. In fact, by using these principles you could invent your own methods for directed creativity to fit the various situations you encounter.

Understanding these three principles also helps us to see the difference between directed creativity and the usual brainstorming session in an organization. Typically, in a brainstorming session the leader reviews the rules of brainstorming—suspend judgment and criticism, freewheel in your thinking, go for quantity, and build on the ideas of others (Osborn, 1953)—with the group and then simply says, "Okay, so what ideas do you have." Judgment is suspended and creative ideas are encouraged, thus creating the conditions for mental movement, *but there is no new direction for thinking.* The theory of directed creativity acknowledges the need to escape the current mental valley and pay attention to alternatives.

Box 4-1 Basic Heuristics for Innovative Thinking

1. Make it a habit to purposefully pause and notice things.
2. Focus your creative energies on just a few topic areas that you genuinely care about and work on these purposefully for several weeks or months.
3. Avoid being too narrow in the way you define your problem or topic area; purposefully try broader definitions and see what insights you gain.
4. Try to come up with original and useful ideas by making novel associations among what you already know or can observe.
5. When you need creative ideas, remember: attention, escape, and movement.
6. Pause and carefully examine ideas that make you laugh the first time you hear them.
7. Recognize that your current streams of thought and patterns of judgment are not inherently right or wrong; they are just what you think now based primarily on patterns from your past.
8. Make a deliberate effort to harvest, develop, and implement at least a few of the ideas you generate.

Source: Reproduced from Plsek, P. E. (1997a). *Creativity, innovation, and quality.* Milwaukee, WI: ASQ Quality Press. © 1997 Paul E. Plsek.

Summary: Heuristics for Directed Creativity

Research indicates that experts in a given area do more effective thinking primarily because they have better heuristics than novices (Gigerenzer & Todd, 1999). Heuristics are general principles that provide productive direction for thought and action, without specifying an exact method or solution. Box 4-1 provides a short list of heuristic advice for innovative thinking based on common themes found in the innovation literature (Plsek, 1997a) and the insights that we gain by understanding the definition of creativity and the mental processes and principles described above.

TOOLS FOR DIRECTED CREATIVITY

In Chapter 3 Endsley presented a five-step model for the innovation process. This model suggests that we need directed creativity tools to prepare our minds for creative thought, to generate new ideas, and to help us further develop the best ideas (Table 4-1).

Tools for preparation support heuristics 1 to 3 in Box 4-1 and primarily use the principles of attention and escape as a prelude to the mental movement that occurs during idea

Table 4-1 Three Types of Directed Creativity Tools Support the Innovation Process

We Need Directed Creativity Tools For:	At These Steps in the Innovation Process Described in Chapter 3:
Preparation	What is the design challenge? What do we know about the challenge?
Idea generation	What might work? (developing alternatives)
Development	What might work? (selecting among alternatives) How to test ideas? How to implement?

generation. In preparation, the goals are to reframe the challenge, examine our current patterns of thinking, identify useful concepts, and create provocative questions that stimulate the imagination. Tools for idea generation generally support heuristics 4 to 7 in Box 4-1 and use a variety of combinations of attention, escape, and movement, with the goal of piling up many ideas without premature judgment. The tools for idea development are linked to heuristic 8. They help us gradually apply judgment, pulling us back a bit from the mental escape that we have been enjoying and focusing attention and movement on what we might need to do to achieve the ultimate goal of turning our ideas into reality.

In this section we look at examples of several tools spanning these three categories. Additional tools and methods can be found in other chapters of this book and in the several books and articles previously referenced. The application of these methods in health care has been documented in the United States (Plsek, 1999b) and the United Kingdom (Maher et al., 2008).

Purpose Hierarchy

It is important in the early phases of the innovation process to avoid prematurely locking-in to a narrowly defined statement of the challenge (Box 4-1, heuristic 3). Nadler and Hibino's (1994) purpose hierarchy is one tool that supports broad thinking about a topic.

To construct a purpose hierarchy, write down an initial statement of the problem, opportunity, or creative challenge and ask, "Why are we interested in this anyway? What's the purpose or point behind it?" Identify several such purpose statements by repeatedly asking these questions. Arrange these in some rational order; for example, from large to small, strategic to operational, crass to noble, whatever seems to fit the situation. Finally, use each of these statements as a starting point to generate creative alternatives for accomplishing that purpose. Also, step back from the list and see what overall insights you get into your original problem or creative challenge.

For example, consider a team that has been given a formal charter by senior management to "Develop innovative process designs to use in our new suburban primary care clinic." We can begin refocusing this topic by asking, "Why do we want to do this?" One answer is "So that we can develop an innovative model of care for replication in our other clinics." We can further refocus by asking again, "But why do we want to do that?" Through repeated questioning and exploring larger and smaller statements of purpose, the team generates the following purpose hierarchy:

- Beat the competition
- Surprise and attract customers
- Get a reputation for being innovative
- Be a showcase for innovation in healthcare delivery
- Be a test site or model for innovation that could be spread to other clinics
- **INITIAL:** innovative process designs for new suburban medical clinic
- Improve a few key processes in our new suburban medical clinic
- Create a sense of excitement among staff that might rub off in better service
- Be creative and innovative

(A purpose hierarchy is best read from the bottom-up, using the items to complete the recursive statement: We want to *item,* so that we can *item,* so that we can *item,* and so on.)

Later, these items can be used, collectively or individually, by various groups to generate alternative ideas based on the statements. For example, we could ask one group to come up with 20 ways that a business might "surprise and attract customers." Another group might be asked to think about ways to "create a sense of excitement among staff that will rub off in better service."

Creative Word Play

Another way to focus attention and some degree of escape from usual thinking in preparation for idea generation is to play directly with the language that we are using to define the challenge initially. One way is to substitute new words to escape our current mental valleys and move in our thinking to search for creative connections in other mental valleys. Pick out key words, jargon, or overly specific words and seek more general words from which we can explore alternatives.

For example, consider a group whose initial statement of challenge reads, "We need creative ideas on the topic of patient access to services." The word "access" is a key word in the statement that is, frankly, jargon. (I mean, really, is that a word you use in everyday conversation outside health care?) A facilitator might ask the group, "What do we mean by 'access'? What are other ways of expressing that?" Claiming to be an alien from Mars who doesn't understand is another way to get at this. This might generate the plainer English phrase "getting the patient and provider together." Now we can ask, "What are various ways of getting patients and providers together?" Ideas about the innovative use of the telephone, e-mail, Web sites, video links, and so on as ways to provide service flow more freely from this challenge statement than from the original one. We could similarly explore other words in the original statement, like "patient," "provider," or "services." The goal is to escape the usual valley of health care thinking and explore the topic in more general terms.

Another approach to word play, and one that opens up more of the possibility of surprise through randomness, involves selecting key words from alternative statements of the challenge and randomly pairing them up to see what thoughts these pairs generate. For example, let's circle key words in each of the statements in the previous purpose hierarchy example regarding the design of a new suburban primary care clinic and randomly select two at a time. Three such pairs might be

suburban–process
beat–showcase
innovate–customer

As with many of the tools of creative thinking, this seems at first a completely nonsensical thing to do. However, when we understand how the mind uses patterns in thinking and that creative ideas occur when we make novel associations among established patterns, we see that such a random pairing of words makes perfect sense for directed creativity. For example, suburban–process might lead the team to think that it would be interesting to follow suburbanites through a typical day, looking for ways to make health services more accessible. This might lead us to consider such innovative ideas as sponsoring stress management education at the half time of soccer games, opening a drop-in women's clinic in a local supermarket, or organizing neighborhood-based health promotion or medication compliance groups.

Mental Benchmarking or Be Someone Else

These closely related tools for idea generation are based on the common observation that people hired from other industries, or friends and family who don't really know too much about health care, often bring with them novel points of view and seemingly innovative ideas about ways to do things when they come into our organizations. We can simulate this effect by imagination.

The basic approach is to first escape the mental valleys of health care by putting oneself into another's mindset, pay attention to what that other person might think, and then finally move to make novel connections back to health care. Generally speaking, the creativity literature uses the term "mental benchmarking" when the alternative mindset is that of a specific business or industry and terms like "be someone else" or "fresh eyes" when the alternative mindset can be anything (e.g., a chef, a 6-year-old child, a horse) (Maher et al., 2008).

Cynthia Taylor in the previous example about the drive-through flu shot clinic was practicing mental benchmarking when she paid attention to the service delivery concepts common in banks and fast-food restaurants and moved in her thinking to apply these to health care. Although she did this by purposefully pausing and noticing during her daily drive home from work (Box 4-1, heuristic 1), the effect could have been just as easily stimulated in a conference room with a team and a facilitator who randomly asks, "How do banks and fast-food restaurants deal with customer flow without having to build larger and larger parking lots?"

As a slightly more elaborate example of a group process, and of the more general tool of "be someone else," imagine a meeting of a dozen physicians, nurses, managers, secretaries, and technologists associated with the challenge to create an innovative suburban primary care clinic. The team leader (or facilitator) spends the first 15 minutes of the session orienting the group and explaining basic mental mechanics: that creative ideas are the combination of mental patterns and that different people have different patterns of thought (heuristics 4 and 7). She then tells the group she is going to read off a list of types of people and occupations. Each person has a pad of paper. When they hear the person or occupation, they are to try to imagine what that person would say or think if asked to help design processes in the new clinic, and then jot these thoughts down on a sheet of paper. Outrageous or laughable thoughts are welcomed (per heuristic 6). After 2 minutes of thinking, each person is to put his or her ideas into the box in the middle of the table. The nurse-manager then reads off another person or occupation and repeats the process for 2 more minutes of silent idea generation. After eight rounds of this (about 15–20 minutes), group members randomly select sheets from the pile and read off the ideas. Participants have the opportunity to contribute new ideas as they think of them. (The team leader has chosen to use this silent brainstorming method because of her past experience with dominating members in such mixed groups. In another setting it might have been easier to just have participants call out ideas for posting on an easel sheet as in a typical brainstorming session.)

Examples of provocations and potential ideas might include the following:

- A 6-year-old child? (fun, active things to occupy my mind; so, how about a medical information computer that patients can access and learn from?)
- A hotel manager? (valet service, rapid check-in for frequent guests; maybe we could apply these concepts in our clinic?)
- A telephone operator? (I have your billing record, name, and address on a computer screen in front of me before I even speak to you; could we do something similar with health and billing information?)

- An Indy 500 racing car pit crew? (instead of a single doctor, a group of doctors and nurses, each with a narrowly defined task to perform, descend on the patient and the entire visit is completed in a matter of seconds).
- A horse? (something to munch on, space to exercise; would patient satisfaction improve if we provided these?)
- A mail-order catalogue manager? (what clinic services can we provide over the phone?)

With 12 participants imagining eight different people and occupations, we will easily have 100+ ideas after only 15–20 minutes. Allowing for duplicates, we should still have at least several dozen ideas from this one session alone.

Notice also that some of the ideas are quite specific (a medical information computer that patients can access), whereas others are rather vague (what clinic services can we provide over the phone?). This is fine. About two-thirds of the way through the time allotted, the group will review all the ideas and identify areas that need more thinking. The vague ideas generated in one round might serve as the central theme for more specific idea generation in another round.

Several books provide tables that list businesses, industries, and others from which one can either randomly or purposefully select points of view to provoke creative thinking (Maher et al., 2008; Plsek, 1997a).

Stepping-stones

Stepping-stones are ideas or wild scenarios that are offbeat but may serve as catalysts or "stepping-stones" for us to make an intuitive leap to a really good idea. Roger Von Oech (1983) suggests that by beginning with an outrageous thought, useful concepts and ideas can subsequently be extracted. By starting with the outrageous (attention), we are able to suspend judgment and think more freely (escape), making connections or associations between seemingly unrelated pieces of information (movement). Edward de Bono (1992) describes this type of tool as a provocation, something that seems utterly impossible, from which we can create new ideas.

Chapter 3 on the innovation process provided one example of a stepping-stone provocation, one that started with an extreme or outrageous approach to the issue at hand. A second type of stepping-stone that is also quite useful in health care starts instead with an extreme or outrageous *scenario* that presents us with the necessity to completely redefine how we approach the issue at hand. Here we are using the same sequence of escape, attention, and movement plus we are picking up on the old adage that "necessity is the mother of invention" and using to our advantage the general observation that healthcare professionals often enjoy rising to the occasion of a crisis.

To construct this second type of stepping-stone provocation, select elements of the system that seem central to the way people currently think about the issue. A good way to identify these is to pay close attention to the things that people tend to say we need more or less of to meet the challenge. For example, typically when we think about meeting the rising demand for emergency services, we think about the need for more doctors, nurses, equipment, and ambulances, or larger emergency departments.

Now create a scenario that exaggerates these elements (by, for example, eliminating them entirely or dramatically reducing them) and challenges people to come up with some approach to the crisis. You can do this by passing a new law or regulation, inventing a mysterious and selective virus, discovering some environmental hazard that forces facilities closure, describing some otherwise unimaginable blunder in thinking . . . anything that creates a crisis of any sort!

Consider these examples, each of which has been used with real teams in health care working on innovative approaches to the provision of emergency services:

- A mysterious virus has wiped out every primary care doctor in the country. Everyone else is completely unaffected. How can we design a direct and speedy flow to hospital emergency departments that channels only those patients who really do need the skills and expertise available in the emergency department while directing the rest to other resources?
- An inspection agency has noted the presence of a mysterious chemical in the hospital's emergency department and has ordered it shut down and sealed off for an indefinite period of time. The nearest other emergency department is 200 miles away. You are in charge of the emergency services network that serves this community: what are you going to do to provide access to emergency care?
- You have reported for your first day on your new, very high-paying job as Director of Patient Flow for a newly constructed hospital, and you now see why they would not let you walk through the facility during the interview. In an incredible oversight, someone has designed this new hospital without allowing any space for the emergency services department! You find an unclaimed space the size of a conference room that you can have, but that is it. How will you handle the inflow of patients who are typically admitted through the emergency department?

Using the last scenario, for example, a hospital team completely reconceptualized the approach to flow through the emergency department to create an 8-minute care path that rapidly assessed incoming patients using a team of professionals and point-of-use testing and then sent the patient immediately to other, appropriate areas of the hospital. The idea was further extended to work more closely with incoming ambulances to triage and perform a workup on patients before they arrive so that when they do they can be immediately taken to more appropriate areas of the hospital (e.g., cardiac patients go immediately to the Cardiac Services area and bypass the emergency department completely).

In constructing the provocation, take time to think through a good list of things in the system that people believe are central to approaching the issue today and take time to carefully craft the challenge to avoid making the new approach too obvious. Create several stepping-stones to make sure that the ideas don't just substitute one taken-for-granted resource for another.

Be prepared for initial incredulity; group members will simply stare back at you blankly and say things like, "That can't possibly happen." Stick with it; insist they deal with it: "No really, it did just happen, now what are you going to do, you can't just sit there, you have to do something." You might want to point out to the group that this reaction is exactly what many people experience in times of crisis, but then they have to get on with it and do something.

Teams tend to have a good bit of fun with this tool. It is meant to be playful and tongue-in-cheek. But this is play with a purpose (Schrage, 2000). The goal is to explore the outrageous suggestion or scenario but to come back to reality with some new ideas on the topic at hand.

Breaking the Rules

This directed creativity tool for imagination involves identifying the underlying assumptions and mental models that maintain the status quo approach to things and then deliberately thinking around them. By definition, an innovation violates the currently accepted assumptions and mental models. In essence, an innovation is such precisely because it "breaks the rules" of the status quo.

For example, consider the mental model that "intensive care" is a specific place in the hospital. It is therefore an innovative idea to consider providing intensive care services through a team of clinicians who can be called into any portion of the hospital to set up intensive care equipment that can then be remotely monitored by a colleague, who might be located just about anywhere there is a high-speed data network connection.

This tool is often used in conjunction with other directed creativity and process improvement tools. The simple, three-step process below both describes the method and shows how it can be supplemented by the use of other tools to stimulate creative thinking for idea generation.

- Step 1: Identify the current assumptions and rules (attention). There are a variety of ways to do this:
  - Simply list them through group discussion.

- Step through a process map (flowchart) and at each step ask, "Why is that step here?" or "What seem to be the underlying mental models behind what is going on here?"
- Tell stories of normal occurrences within the system and ask the questions above.
- Step 2: Creatively challenge the assumptions and "rules" (escape). Again, there are several ways to do this:
  - Propose an alternative assumption or rule.
  - Suggest a stepping-stones provocation. For example, say that the government has passed a law making the current rule illegal ("It is illegal to have a permanent place where intensive care is delivered.") and ask, "What would we do under those circumstances?"
  - Magically make something appear ("The status of every patient in every intensive care unit bed is shown on a big board where everyone can see.") and ask how one would redesign the process if that were true.
  - Be someone else and ask how that person might think about a particular rule. "How might a banker or a store owner think about this rule? How might they state it or modify it? Now, what ideas does that give us for what we might do?"
- Step 3: Walk around in the new world and see what new ideas you can generate (movement). Play out the scenario as to what you would do if the mental models or rules were suddenly altered; capture ideas as the discussion proceeds.

This is a potentially powerful tool for conceptualizing how one might transform a process or whole system. It has been used by the Institute of Medicine (2001) in the United States in the report, *Crossing the Quality Chasm,* and by the National Health Services Institute for Innovation and Improvement in the United Kingdom in efforts to create new thinking about access to secondary care (Rogers, Maher, & Plsek, 2008).

As noted previously, the creativity and innovation literature provides numerous tools for idea generation. The sample above provides insight into the variety of approaches that one can use. The key concepts here are as follows:

- Thinking is naturally channeled into mental valleys that come about through learning over time and that can come to be seen as the only way to do something.
- Creative thinking involves attention, escape, and movement.
- Whereas the traditional rules of brainstorming create the conditions for mental movement, they are not sufficient because they do not specifically address the provision of new attention points and the escape from current patterns of thinking.

- The tools of directed creativity build on what we know about how the mind works and specifically provide attention and escape to add to the mental movement provided by traditional approaches to brainstorming.

Idea Development Checklist

The final directed creativity tool we explore is associated with the third category described in Table 4-1—idea development. Recall from the definition of creativity that creative ideas must ultimately be judged to be useful by others. Unfortunately, rarely do creative ideas emerge in full bloom from a rapid-fire idea-generation session.

In Chapter 3 Endsley described the convergence tools of multivoting and six thinking hats for use in initially harvesting the most promising ideas from among the hundreds that might be generated on a given topic. Still, although we now have fewer, better ideas, the observation above remains true: Rarely do creative ideas emerge in full bloom from a rapid-fire idea-generation session.

Creativity expert Edward de Bono (1992) suggests a series of questions that, in his experience, are often not asked or thoroughly addressed as people press on to test their creative ideas in the innovation process. These questions direct our thinking to consider emotional and people-related issues, the strengths and weaknesses of the idea, systems effects and consequences, and the need for trials and prototypes (Box 4-2).

Box 4-2 Idea Development Checklist

Shaping: How can we modify the idea to address objections that would otherwise cause rejection?

Tailoring: Can we modify the idea to even better fit our needs?

Strengthening: How can we increase the power or value of the idea?

Reinforcing: What can we do about weak points?

Looking toward implementation: What can we do to the idea to enhance the probability of implementation? Who must be involved?

Comparison with current: How does the idea compare with what it is replacing? Should we do further enhancement, expand or scale back the idea?

Potential faults or defects: What could possibly go wrong with this idea? What can we do?

Consequences: What are the immediate and long-term consequences of putting the idea into action?

Testability and prototyping: How can we try the idea on a small scale?

Preevaluation: How can we further modify the idea to meet the needs of those who will evaluate it next?

The questions are meant to be taken as a whole. Start anywhere on the list, consider multiple questions at the same time, and be prepared to reevaluate your work on earlier questions as you go along. When you believe you are done, go through the list one final time to make sure you have not missed anything.

Expect to spend some time in idea development. This work might involve anywhere from 2 to 200 hours of thoughtful work, perhaps spread out over several weeks. Shortcutting development is a common pitfall, leading to half-baked ideas that fail. Of course, overdoing development can be equally problematic. We will have difficulty implementing in the later steps of the innovation process if we load down our ideas with too many clever features.

The product of our work here is a set of more well-thought-out ideas. Although the development questions guide us to critical thinking, we should maintain an overall positive attitude throughout this activity. We want to do everything we can to see that our ideas are accepted by all stakeholders and successfully implemented in the final steps of the innovation process.

CONCLUSION

Directed creativity is an approach to creative thinking that rests solidly on research from the cognitive sciences and decades of experience in a variety of industries. It is an approach that anyone can use; no special gift or genius is required. We described three key principles, eight simple heuristics, and a sample of seven tools and methods.

The ability to think creatively is as strategically important to health care today as the ability to manage finances or deliver good clinical outcomes. Financial management and outcomes management have specific tools that organizations use deliberately. It is now time for healthcare leaders and professionals to become as deliberate about creativity.

REFERENCES

Bate, P., Robert, G., & Bevan, H. (2004). The next phase of healthcare improvement: What can we learn from social movements? *Quality and Safety in Health Care, 13*(1), 62–66.

Black, R. A. (1995). *Broken crayon: Break your crayons and draw outside the lines.* Dubuque, IA: Kendall/Hunt Publishing.

de Bono, E. (1969). *Mechanism of mind.* London: Penguin Books.

de Bono, E. (1992). *Serious creativity.* New York: Harper-Collins.

Friedenberg, J. D., & Silverman, G. (2005). *Cognitive science: An introduction to the study of mind.* San Francisco: Sage.

Gigerenzer, G., & Todd, P. M. (1999). *Simple heuristics that make us smart.* New York: Oxford University Press.

Higgins, J. M. (1994). *101 Creative problem solving techniques.* Winter Park, FL: New Management Publishing.

Institute of Medicine. (2001). *Crossing the quality chasm: A new health care system for the 21st century.* Washington, DC: National Academy Press.

Maher, L. M., Plsek, P. E., Garrett, S., & Bevan, H. (2008). *Thinking differently.* London: NHS Institute for Innovation and Improvement.

McGartland, G. (1994). *Thunderbolt thinking.* Austin, TX: Bernard-Davis.

Michalko, M. (2006). *Thinkpak: A brainstorming card deck* (2nd ed.). Berkeley, CA: Ten Speed Press.

Nadler, G., & Hibino, S. (1994). *Breakthrough thinking* (2nd ed.). Roklin, CA: Prima.

Osborn, A. (1953). *Applied imagination.* New York: Charles Scribner.

Osherson, D. N., & Smith, E. E. (Eds.). (1990). *An invitation to cognitive science: Thinking* (Volume 3). Cambridge, MA: MIT Press.

Peng, T. (2008, April 14). Open wide. No, wider: Are we ready for an era of natural-orifice surgery? *Newsweek,* 19.

Plsek, P. E. (1994). Directed creativity. *Quality Management in Health Care, 2*(3), 62–76.

Plsek, P. E. (1997a). *Creativity, innovation, and quality.* Milwaukee, WI: ASQ Quality Press.

Plsek, P. E. (1997b). Directed creativity and the management of quality in healthcare. In C. Caldwell (Ed.), *Handbook for managing for change in healthcare.* Milwaukee, WI: ASQ Quality Press.

Plsek, P. E. (1999a, March/April). No special gift needed: Generating creative ideas for health care organizations. *Health Forum Journal,* 24–28.

Plsek, P. E. (1999b). Innovative thinking for the improvement of medical systems. *Annals of Internal Medicine, 131*(6), 438–444.

Rogers, H., Maher, L. M., & Plsek, P. E. (2008). New design rules for driving innovation in access to secondary care in the NHS. *British Medical Journal, 337,* a2321.

Runco, M. A. (2007). *Creativity: Theories and themes. Research, development, and practice.* London: Academic Press.

Schrage, M. (2000). *Serious play: How the world's best companies stimulate innovation.* Cambridge, MA: Harvard Business School Press.

Smith, S. (2008, October 29). Fly-by flu shot: No need to get out of the car—vaccination is available at hospital's drive-through. *Boston Globe,* 20.

Tversky, A., & Kahneman, D. (1973). Judgment under uncertainty: Heuristics and biases. *Science, 185,* 1124–1131.

Tversky, A., & Kahneman, D. (1981). The framing of decisions and the psychology of choice. *Science, 211,* 453–458.

von Oech, R. (1983). *A whack on the side of the head.* New York: Warner Books.

Weisberg, R. W. (1993). *Creativity: Beyond the myth of genius.* New York: W. H. Freeman.

CHAPTER 5

Transdisciplinary Design and Innovation in the Classroom

Prasad Boradkar

> *"To cope with escalating complexity in health care we must abandon linear models, accept unpredictability, respect (and utilise) autonomy and creativity, and respond flexibly to emerging patterns and opportunities."*
>
> PLSEK & GREENHALGH, 1993, P. 628

The recent eminence that innovation has enjoyed in business practice has been beneficial to design. Suddenly, design—a discipline that has never truly enjoyed center stage with business (barring a few exceptions)—has gained more visibility and has become the darling of many a corporation seeking to add value to their goods and services. "Innovation is a management discipline; it does not come about through a random or hit-and-miss approach, but it requires design. . . . Design is central to the practice of management. Design is also central to the practice of innovation" (Gaynor, 2002, p. xiii). Though not all executives may embrace these notions of the primacy of design in practices of innovation, there is no doubt about the increased recognition of the value potential of design.

Innovation can be imagined as a form of thinking, a strategy and a mechanism by which a corporation can sustain competitive advantage. Innovative thinking can help an enterprise generate new ways to deliver products and services, manage its own assets, and enhance the efficacy of its processes and strategies. To do so, it needs to structure itself to foster innovative thinking within its ranks. Each discipline plays a specific role in product, service, process, asset, strategy, and structural innovation (Duening, 2007).

What is the role of design in innovation? Although design (especially industrial design) has traditionally been active primarily within the realm of product innovation, there is growing recognition of its value in creatively thinking of new service offerings as well. In addition, it is now accepted that design thinking has the power to influence a corporation's standard processes and strategies to make it much more dynamic and supple in responding to changing needs in the marketplace. Therefore, although the process of doing design (creating things) can directly influence and enhance outcomes of product innovation, design thinking can effectively be applied toward solving a broader range of problems, and therefore can be effective in influencing service innovation, process innovation, asset innovation, and so on. Design's unique contributions to the process of innovation can be summarized in four key characteristics—empathic thinking, transdisciplinary learning, creative problem solving, and the pursuit of tangible outcomes.

EMPATHIC THINKING

Empathic thinking refers to design's emphasis on creating products and services to directly address people's needs. In the past, corporations have too often focused on developing new products that are driven either by styling, new technological capabilities, or market pressures, frequently at the expense of solving the real needs of real people. Styling refers to a tradition in design of creating products that offer a new form factor without added utility. Products designed primarily around a new technology, which may end up having features and functions that nobody wants or cares about, present a different problem. And products designed purely to fill market gaps and fight competition fall short in meeting individual or societal needs. Human-centered design (also referred to as user-centered design) was developed in response to these approaches.

> The user is a central trope for designers and the focus of their professional attention: Identifying and meeting the user's needs and wants is the central mission of designers. Of course, this is never a straightforward process. Consumers have complex, multiple needs, which they are not always able to articulate. Also, designers may create new product ideas that satisfy needs consumers did not know they had. The popularity of Post-it notes is an example. (Wasson, 2000, p. 377)

The rapidly growing field of design research uses such qualitative methods as focus groups, interviews, observations, journaling, and a large number of other ethnographic tools to identify people's articulated and unarticulated needs. Though the tradition of user research has existed in the design discipline for several decades (especially in the work of such visionaries as Robert Propst and Henry Dreyfuss), the explicit use of rapid ethnography is relatively new. Design research has been defined as "a research approach that produces a detailed, in depth observation of people's behavior, beliefs and preferences by observing and interacting with them in a natural environment" (Ireland, 2003, p. 26).

This embrace of user needs is not limited to design. Market researchers use business tools to identify the needs of large segments of target populations. Engineers involved in new product development too have altered the traditional process of designing products from a purely technical focus to one that includes the "voice of the customer."

Widely accepted practices such as total quality management, zero defects, and six sigma take into account customer needs in the process of design.

TRANSDISCIPLINARY LEARNING

"Across all disciplines, at all levels, and throughout the world, health care is becoming more complex" (Plsek & Greenhalgh, 1993, p. 625). To develop comprehensive and appropriate solutions to such complex problems, it is critical to have a team of experts who represent a variety of disciplines and therefore bring the advantage of a diverse set of viewpoints and opinions. One of the primary advantages of interdisciplinarity is its ability to tackle large, complex problems. Interdisciplinarity, multidisciplinarity, and transdisciplinarity are often used interchangeably, but newer definitions of these terms reveal subtle distinctions between them.

Interdisciplinary research (or education) is undertaken when the complexity of a problem necessitates the active engagement of multiple points of view, theories, and methodologies and might require a team approach representing a variety of disciplines. Heavily encouraged in academia today, interdisciplinary approaches are deemed necessary to counter some of the problems of extreme specialization, encourage the generation of creative, nontraditional solutions, and help provide contextual critiques of single disciplines. Interdisciplinarity serves as an umbrella term to include

Figure 5-1 Student teams in the InnovationSpace studio.

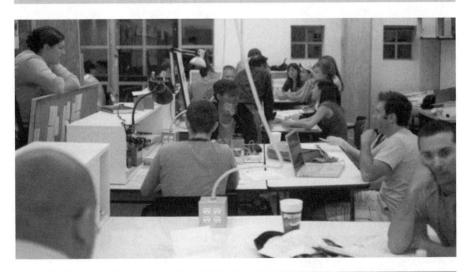

multi- and transdisciplinarity. Generally speaking, in multidisciplinary approaches experts from several disciplines are involved on a research project, but their work may not always intersect. In such situations the problem may be segmented into smaller issues that can then be appropriately handled by single disciplines. On the other hand, transdisciplinarity refers to situations where the knowledge and tools of one discipline influence and redirect the results of another. Much more disruptive and difficult to manage, engagement of this nature typically signals a destruction of disciplinary boundaries with the hope of generating new knowledge that would be impossible to produce by a single discipline.

CREATIVE PROBLEM SOLVING

"Creative and critical thinking are often seen (or stereotyped) as opposites, poles apart and incompatible with one another . . . We hold a different view, believing that creative and critical thinking are two complementary, mutually important ways of thinking. . . . Successful problem solving depends on using both, not just one or the other" (Treffinger, Isaksen, & Stead-Dorval, 2006, p. 3). Design and innovation are both processes of problem solving that involve a series of iterative steps, typically labeled problem definition, research, analysis, idea generation, concept selection, and implementation. Literature in new product development (NPD) presents several variations of this process, but the fundamental sequence of activities is similar (Belliveau, Griffin, & Somermeyer, 2002; Rosenau, 1996). Throughout this process, NPD professionals are required to engage in creative and critical thinking to generate and develop new ideas and then evaluate their potential value. Creative processes involve divergent thinking and the generation of a large number of ideas unfettered by the analysis or evaluation. On the other hand, critical thinking can be referred to as a convergent process in which ideas are assessed on the basis of established criteria. All forms of innovation and problem solving require both forms of thinking—convergent and divergent, critical and creative.

TANGIBLE OUTCOMES

Design involves the translation of verbal instructions into visual materials. In other words, all processes of design generally start with a design brief (generally a written description of a project brief) and lead to the tangible outcomes of sketches, renderings, models, and prototypes. It is important to note that design output is not limited to these visual materials and also includes analyses, budgets, timelines, and product descriptions. The drawings, models, and prototypes serve as means by which to visualize future scenarios in which the new products and services being designed will become accepted components of everyday life.

Exhibit 5-1 Dialog

❧DIALOG

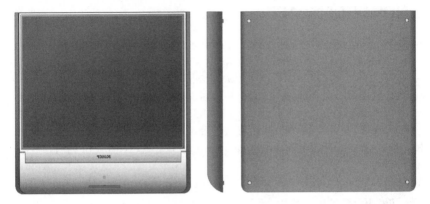

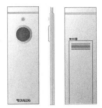

Dialog is a personal diagnostic device for people who require frequent health monitoring. Users, for example, can drop a nanosensor the size of a fingernail into a toilet where it analyzes the content of human waste such as urine. The data are relayed via a wireless connection to a display unit. The device also can be networked with other electronic outputs, including computers and cell phones, to alert remote caretakers, such as the children of aging parents, to potential problems. This project was sponsored by the Center for Nanotechnology in Society at ASU.

Student Team: Thomas Filardo, Industrial Design; Raquel Raney, Visual Communication Design; Jesus Burrola and Jennifer Verdiani, Business; Timothy Shaw, Engineering.

These four characteristics—empathic thinking, transdisciplinary learning, creative problem solving, and the pursuit of tangible outcomes—are design's unique contributions to processes of innovation. These principles are taught to students from design, business, and engineering in InnovationSpace at Arizona State University (ASU).

INNOVATIONSPACE

InnovationSpace is an entrepreneurial joint venture among the College of Design, Ira A. Fulton School of Engineering, and W. P. Carey School of Business at ASU. Now in its fifth year, this transdisciplinary education and research laboratory assembles teams of students from business, engineering, industrial design, and visual communication design to develop products that create market value while serving real societal needs and minimizing impacts on the environment. The program is built on the premise that a traditional, discipline-specific education no longer provides enough expertise or variation in thinking to handle the difficult challenges of 21st century NPD. Faculty in InnovationSpace guide these transdisciplinary teams of students in identifying individual and social needs and thoroughly researching and analyzing the technological, economic, social, and environmental implications of their design solutions. Cross-functional teamwork, a new model of innovation called "integrated innovation," sustainability, and entrepreneurial thinking are the four key ideas that are central to pedagogical structure of InnovationSpace. It is through these four ideas that students learn about and apply practices of innovation.

Cross-Functional Teamwork

Students in InnovationSpace are encouraged to learn from each other. During the fuzzy front end (early stages of NPD) when all students are required to do research to better understand the context of the problem, they take on the role of researchers rather than engineers, designers, or business students. In some cases they do observations and interviews as a team, and at times team members may work individually by focusing on a specific problem that directly relates to their field of expertise and interest.

As the project proceeds and students start gathering information about the market, potential technologies, and social and environmental issues, they dip into their disciplinary toolboxes to analyze the information gathered during research. For example, business students perform SWOT (Strength Weakness Opportunities Threats) analyses of a corporation's market position, whereas engineers might do technology benchmarking. As the information is compiled into one report, all members are required to understand the tools used by others on the team. In such situations there is a significant amount of cross-functional learning. Design students use market mapping to critique products, whereas engineers learn about developing a list of the hierarchy of user needs.

Such cross-functional teamwork is central to the pedagogical approach adopted in InnovationSpace. The presence of faculty members and students from four disciplines creates a diversity that is tremendously beneficial to the class. They bring to class a new set of resources, theoretical approaches, specialized methodologies, and unique tools from these varied disciplines that advance the level of general and specific knowledge of the entire group. This prepares the students to be professionals who are not only trained in their disciplines but who quickly learn that other areas of expertise can in fact improve the quality, depth, and impact of their own work.

Integrated Innovation

Central to the InnovationSpace curriculum is a new model of product development known as integrated innovation. Using this model, students systematically explore and resolve four key questions (Figure 5-2):

1. What is valuable to people?
2. What is possible through engineering?
3. What is desirable to the corporation?
4. What is good for society and the environment?

Figure 5-2 The integrated innovation model.

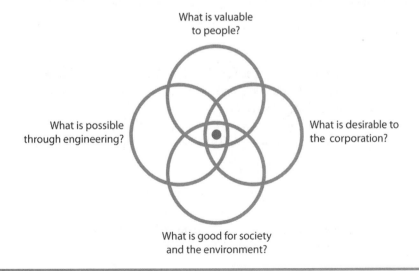

Exhibit 5-2 Cy: Accessible Supply Solutions

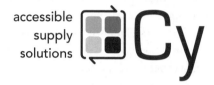

accessible supply solutions Cy

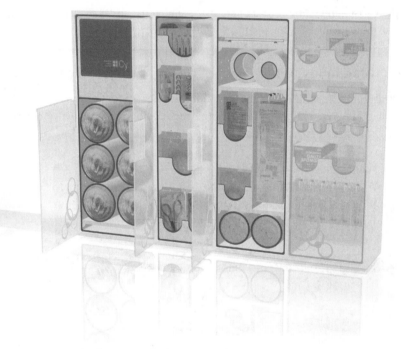

Cy is a two-way supply closet installed on the wall between the patient room and the hallway in hospitals. The closet is accessed for restocking from the hallway but can be opened from inside the patient room. This system not only keeps materials sanitary, but also provides nurses easier access to inventory without having to disturb the patient by entering the room. This project was sponsored by Herman Miller, Inc.

Student Team: Kristina Funck, Industrial Design; Eric Perkins, Visual Communication Design; Megan Lee, Business; Trevor Pirtle, Engineering

The integrated innovation model prompts students to think about sustainability in unexpected ways. For example, by asking the question "What is valuable to people?", the student teams probe real—rather than superfluous—human needs. Any product solution that meets these needs, however, must be examined against the question "What is good for society and the environment?" Even the most environmentally benign products are not sustainable in the long run if, for example, they rely on child labor in their manufacturing or serve only select consumers who can afford them. Students also start to recognize the dynamic tensions that exist between factors that influence innovation and realize that design involves making trade-offs. For example, certain commodity plastics may possess the right material properties and meet manufacturing requirements, but they also may pose higher risks due to human and environmental toxicity. Or, certain executive decisions, such as business process offshoring to poorer nations that have economic advantage for the corporation, may not always translate into positive societal impacts for the workers in those countries.

This model of innovation emphasizes that responsible design involves the delicate task of negotiating the tensions that exist between what is valuable to people, what is desirable to corporations, what is possible through engineering, and what is good for society and the environment. It is also important to recognize that trade-offs extend beyond the scale of design—such as material capabilities versus formal decisions or appropriate ergonomics versus compactness—to larger scale compromises involving such business decisions as outsourced labor cost versus corporate social responsibility, brand strategy versus advertising budget, and so on. This also helps the industrial design students realize quickly that the birth and development of a product involves the expertise of several disciplines and compromises are central to moving products to market.

Integrated innovation guides them in identifying pressing social needs and thoroughly analyzing the technological, economic, social, and environmental implications of their design solutions. This model serves as a framework that guides student research and analysis and helps them collect information about existing and potential users, the market, emerging technologies, and critical social and environmental issues. In addition, as they start generating product ideas, this model also serves as an evaluative tool, helping students gauge the efficacy of their solutions for all stakeholders. This model serves as a very effective teaching tool because it is simple and encourages in-depth exploration of all constituencies that will be positively and negatively impacted by their solutions.

Sustainability

In his book, *Cannibals with Forks,* John Elkington (1997) proposed a definition of sustainable development that asked corporations to consider issues of social equity and environmental responsibility along with those of economic prosperity. This premise, referred to as the triple bottom line, serves as the framework for sustainability that

Figure 5-3 Ecodesign strategy wheel.

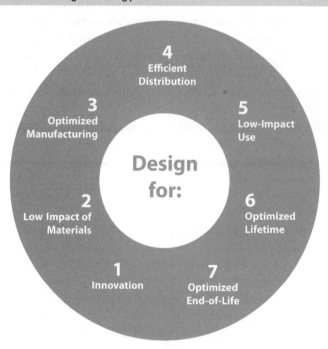

Source: From the Okala Learning Ecological Design Course Guide (White, Belletire, & St. Pierre [2007]).

students use throughout the InnovationSpace program. In each stage of the product-development process, students are introduced to sustainability methodologies that help them meet the triple bottom line. During the concept-development phase, for example, student teams use the ecodesign strategy wheel as a means of improving the environmental and social performance of their product ideas (Figure 5-3). Loosely structured around life-cycle assessment, the ecodesign strategy wheel encourages students to consider low-impact materials, optimized manufacturing, efficient distribution, low-impact use, optimized product lifetime, and optimized end of life.

As the product concepts starts taking form, the engineering and design students make material choices, develop component specifications, and calculate energy usage to minimize the environmental impact of the product. At the same time business students start to establish parameters and guidelines for upstream and downstream supply-chain management that includes everything from the procurement of components and materials to their proper disposal. In the course of this research, students learn, for example, that transporting raw materials and goods by rail and water has a significantly lower ecological impact than transporting raw materials and goods by air. In their business plans students also recommend that corporations align their labor guidelines for vendors with the code of conduct developed by the Fair Labor Association. During this time graphic design students learn about environmentally friendly practices, such as minimizing the weight of packing materials, reducing material variation for ease of recycling, and specifying soy-based inks for printing.

As the design is finalized and a bill of materials is created, the engineering and industrial design students use the Okala Impact Factor Assessment tool developed by ecodesign strategists Philip White, Louise St. Pierre, and Steve Belletire (2007). The Okala process requires them to estimate the total life of the product and its packaging, calculate the weight and size of each component, and compute the total expected energy usage. After some calculations, they are able to quantify the ecological impact of the new product in Okala millipoints. The students also calculate the Okala impact of an existing competitor product by taking it apart and weighing all its components. The goal of the exercise is to compare impacts and ensure that the new design indeed minimizes damage to the environment. At the end, the team summarizes its efforts in the form of a list of reasonable and justifiable social and environmental claims for the product.

In this competitive climate of new product innovation, some argue that devoting resources to sustainability concerns is a pricey diversion that may be good for a company's cache and conscience but an anchor on creativity and the bottom line. The InnovationSpace program at ASU turns this thinking on its head. Using environmental strategies that are integrated into the program's transdisciplinary curriculum, InnovationSpace has demonstrated that sustainability can become a driver that lowers the environmental profiles of products without sacrificing innovation.

Curriculum

The integrated innovation curriculum is delivered over two semesters for a total of 10 student credit hours. The transdisciplinary teams are comprised of students from design, engineering, and business. Each team is also assigned to a project as specified by corporate and research institute sponsors. Student teams are given the parameters of the project and are then free to pursue a design solution utilizing the integrated innovation model as a guide. Integrated innovation guides the teams in identifying viable products, and thoroughly analyzing the technological, economic, social, and environmental contexts and implications of their design solutions. The two-semester curriculum is organized into seven distinct phases. Student teams are expected to complete each phase by a prespecified deadline, further mimicking the pressures and challenges of new product development within the enterprise. The seven phases are organized and defined below.

Exhibit 5-3 InReach

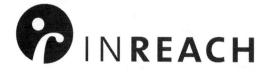

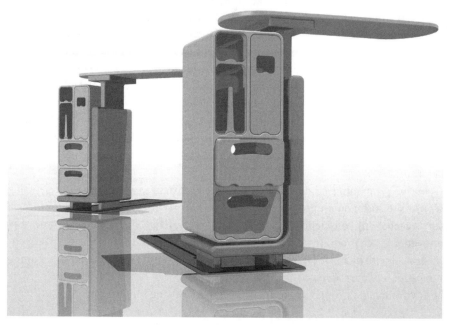

InReach takes a new look at reducing the clutter and improving the utility of bedside furnishings in hospital patient rooms. Combining the functions of both bedside and overbed tables, InReach provides patients with a collapsible horizontal surface for activities such as eating and writing as well as a flexible and customizable unit for storage. Attached to tracks embedded in the floor, InReach can be quickly moved aside at the touch of a finger. This project was sponsored by Herman Miller, Inc.

Student Team: Lindsey Culpepper, Industrial Design; Angela Melzer, Visual Communication Design; Rachel Springer & Bradley Butterfield, Business; James Leos, Engineering

Phase 1: Collecting Information

The fall semester in InnovationSpace starts with the formation of student teams and definition of the problem statement. Students are urged to set aside their disciplinary biases and adopt the roles of researchers intent on discovering the context for which they are to create product solutions. The first phase involves primary and secondary research into discovering needs and opportunities presented by all stakeholders (the user, the technology, the market, society, and the environment). Teams seek answers to the following questions:

- How are the users, purchasers, and influencers affected by the problem?
- What are the needs, attitudes, behaviors, and personalities of the users?
- What are some existing technologies/products in this market space?
- What are some emerging technologies?
- How do these technologies compare with each other and how are they expected to develop in the future?
- What is the nature of the market competition?
- What are the existing products/services in the market?
- What are the hurdles in entering this market?
- What is the company position in relation to this market?
- What are some key social and environmental issues relevant to this context and how are these expected to unfold over time?
- What are the user attitudes toward sustainability?
- Should the corporation be aware of governmental or industry regulations that will influence product development in this area?

Students use primary research techniques of rapid ethnography (interviews, observations, shadowing, etc.) as well as secondary research methods of literature reviews (journal articles, books, etc.) to develop a clear understanding of the context (Figure 5-4). This information is organized in a research binder.

Phase 2: Making Discoveries

The primary goal of the second phase of the InnovationSpace product development process is the production of a research insights report, organized around the four components of integrated innovation (Figure 5-5). Student teams develop actionable insights derived by developing an understanding of (1) users' needs, (2) potentialities presented by existing and emerging technologies, (3) opportunities presented by the market, and (4) key social and environmental issues to be considered. Student teams use a range of analytical tools, including industry competitive analysis, storyboarding, product and technology benchmarking and user needs listing in developing the insights. This helps the student teams develop a knowledge foundation on

Figure 5-4 Phase 1—Conducting research and collecting information.

In phase 1, teams conduct extensive field research. In this case, for the redesign of patient transfer systems, InnovationSpace team Kando did ride-alongs with ambulance drivers and paramedics. Project sponsored by Herman Miller, Inc. and developed by students Eric Fields, Erik Mertz, Kiri Miller, Matt Porembski, Jennifer Rechlin, and Scott Richins.

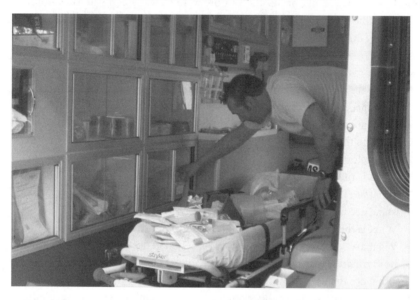

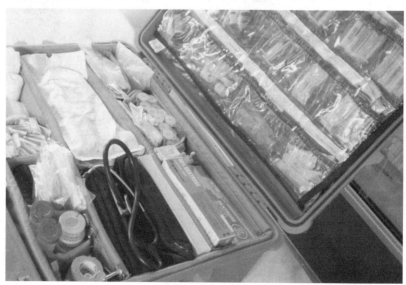

Figure 5-5 Phase 2—Research insights report.

Prepared by Eric Fields, Erik Mertz, Kiri Miller, Matt Porembski, Jennifer Rechlin, and Scott Richins. The report included an overview of user needs, an analysis of the industry and the competition, a list of the technical challenges, and an overview of the social and environmental issues.

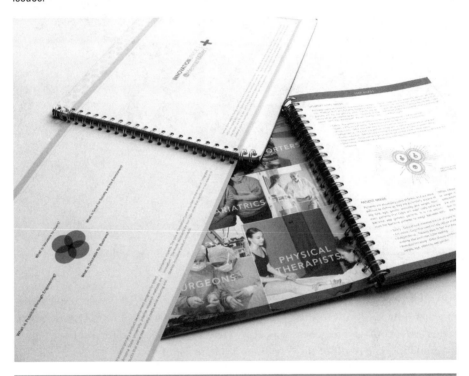

which to draw meaningful conclusions for subsequent analysis and concept exploration. The research insights are further developed into a list of product opportunity gaps (problems in need of product solutions) that can then be converted into products and service offerings.

Phase 3: Creating Opportunities

This phase involves the translation of the insights derived from research and analysis into a range of product ideas. Each team selects the most critical product opportunity gaps and generates ideas through a series of brainstorming exercises (Figure 5-6). The participants in these brainstorming sessions include, in addition to the students, graduate students, faculty members, subject matter experts (nurses, for instance) and

Figure 5-6 Phase 3—Brainstorming sessions and concept ideation.

Gretchen Gscheidle, Research Lead of Herman Miller, Inc. conducting a brainstorming session in InnovationSpace.

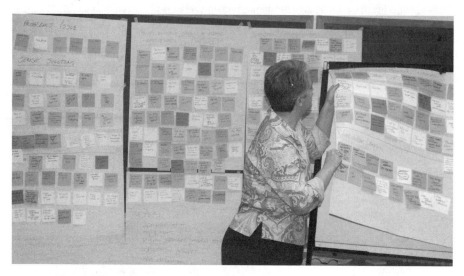

potential users. The project sponsors participate in the sessions and assist the students in generating solutions to the problems. As is the case with all brainstorming, the teams are encouraged to generate as many creative ideas as possible without judging their quality. The result of these sessions is a long list of potential product ideas for selected problems.

The next stage in the process involves narrowing down these lists to a few that have the potential of being valuable to users, desirable to the sponsoring corporation, possible through engineering, and good for society and the environment. At this stage the teams start rapidly visualizing the most promising ideas through sketching (Figure 5-7). By the end of this phase each team has three key ideas selected for further development.

Phase 4: Documentation and Presentation

During this phase students do further engineering, design, brand, and business development around the three selected ideas. By the end of this phase, each team prepares a preliminary innovation proposal, which documents all work completed during the semester. This includes preliminary business plans, initial engineering feasibility assessments, an early product design direction, and a rough brand concept for the three top

Figure 5-7 Phase 3—Concept development: Product idea sketches.

Concept ideation sketches by Eric Fields for patient transfer systems.

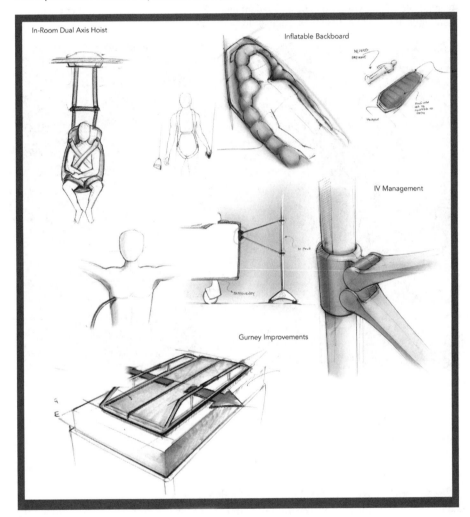

Figure 5-8 Phase 4—Concept development: Product Idea 1 for a patient transfer system.

An inflatable backboard. Design by InnovationSpace team Eric Fields, Erik Mertz, Kiri Miller, Matt Porembski, and Scott Richins. Sponsored by Herman Miller, Inc.

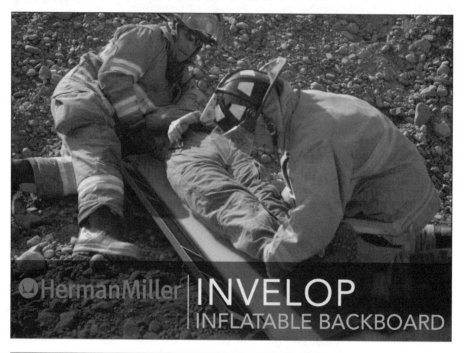

concepts. In addition to the proposal, the teams also design an exhibit and display the three product concepts through rough models, sketch books, and explanatory posters (Figures 5-8, 5-9, 5-10).

Phase 5: Developing Selected Product Concepts

Phase 5 is the first phase of spring semester, and one of the first tasks is the selection of one product for further development. The selection process involves evaluation of the three product ideas by the faculty team, the student team, and the sponsors. The integrated innovation model serves as the evaluative tool to ensure that the selected product idea provides value to all stakeholders. Once a single idea is selected, the students take on individual responsibilities according to their disciplinary expertise. The engineering students start the process of developing technical specifications and planning the construction of the proof-of-concept prototype, whereas the industrial design students start creating a new

Figure 5-9 Phase 4—Concept development: Product Idea 2 for a patient transfer system.

A mobile IV mechanism. Design by InnovationSpace team Eric Fields, Erik Mertz, Kiri Miller, Matt Porembski, and Scott Richins. Sponsored by Herman Miller, Inc.

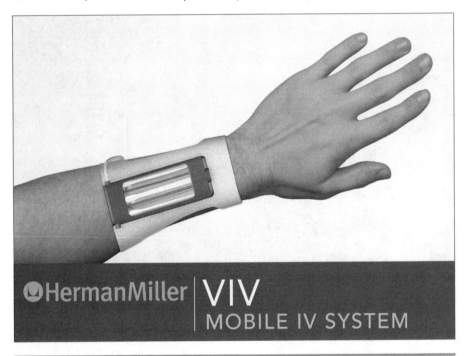

design language (Figure 5-11). The business students start the process of outlining a strategic plan necessary to take the product to market, whereas the graphic design students begin the process of developing a brand strategy (Figure 5-12).

Phase 6: Finalizing Product Concepts

At this stage of the process, students develop the one selected product idea with the goal of making it functional, aesthetically appropriate, well engineered, sustainable, socially responsible, and market-worthy. Most decisions regarding features and functions, aesthetic direction, brand language, and marketing are solidified at this time. Whereas phase 5 is about developing the concept, phase 6 is about finalizing details of that specific concept (Figure 5-13). The engineers and industrial designers collaborate closely to match components with product form, whereas the graphic designers work closely with the business students to align the brand strategy with market strategy.

Figure 5-10 Phase 4—Concept development: Product Idea 3 for a patient transfer system.

A dual-axis patient hoist. Design by InnovationSpace team Eric Fields, Erik Mertz, Kiri Miller, Matt Porembski, and Scott Richins. Sponsored by Herman Miller, Inc.

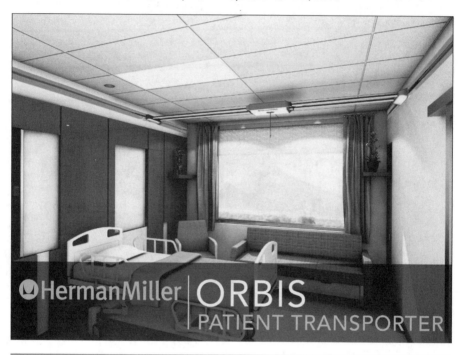

Phase 7: Documentation and Presentation

Once the design is finalized, the industrial designers build an appearance model, whereas the engineers develop the prototype. Graphic design students finalize the brand strategy and create posters and magazine advertising for the product. The business plan is fleshed out completely at this time as well. All materials created by the student team are collated into a final innovation proposal. This phase concludes with a public presentation and exhibit of the products in a trade show format. Corporate sponsors, members of the ASU academic community, and local designers and businesspeople are invited to the latter event.

Several corporate and ASU sponsors provide financial support and ongoing mentorship for the student teams. To date, the roster of corporate sponsors has included such companies as Herman Miller, Inc., Procter & Gamble, and Intel Corporation.

Figure 5-11 Phase 5—Aesthetic concept development for a patient transfer system.

Sketches by Eric Fields.

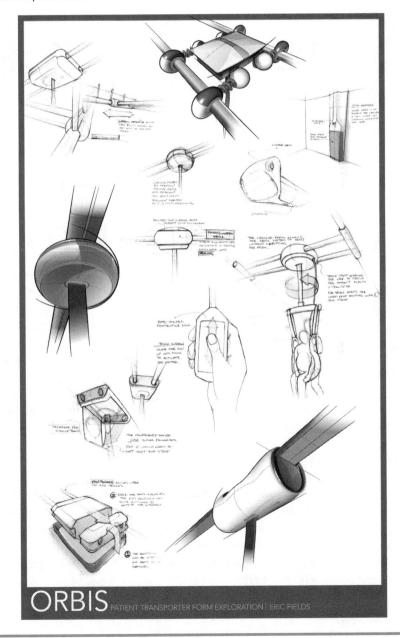

Figure 5-12 Phase 5—Logo designs for Orbis: The Patient Transfer System.

Sketches by Matt Porembski.

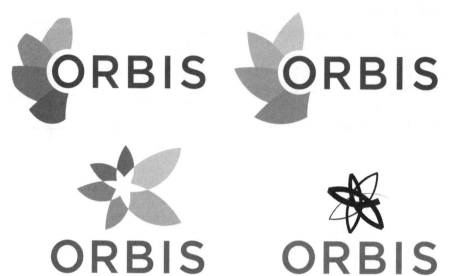

InnovationSpace also partners with researchers and departments at ASU to help imagine potential product solutions for their technologies. ASU sponsors include the Center for Nanotechnology in Society, Flexible Display Center, and Center for Ubiquitous Cognitive Computing. As outlined below, each project with a sponsor is structured around a specific research topic:

- *Arizona Business Accelerator:* Product concepts that improve the daily lives of aging baby boomers
- *Intel Corporation:* Product concepts that increase the comfort and safety of independent living situations for elders
- *Herman Miller, Inc.:* Product concepts that improve acute-care and ambulatory-care environments for patients and healthcare providers
- *Procter & Gamble:* Product concepts that improve the lives of women over age 65 and people who are blind
- *Center for Cognitive Ubiquitous Computing* (ASU): Product concepts that expand access to printed materials for people who are blind

Figure 5-13 Phase 6—Final Design for Orbis: The Patient Transfer System.

Rendering by Eric Fields.

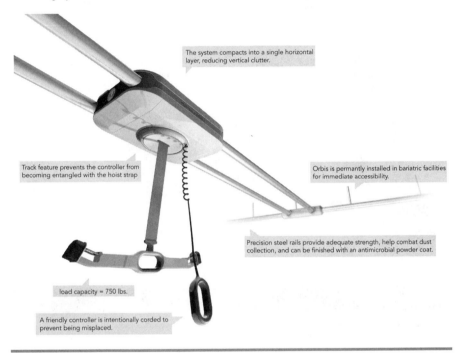

- *Center for Nanotechnology in Society* (ASU): Product concepts that assist individuals with disabilities with everyday tasks
- *Flexible Display Center* (ASU): Product concepts that increase the safety and efficiency of emergency medical responders.

Entrepreneurship

Design entrepreneurship refers to the formation of two types of new ventures—those that provide design services only and those that, in addition to design, manufacture what they design. Over the last 5 years there has been a steady increase in the number of design students creating their own ventures almost immediately after finishing up their bachelor's degrees. The firms they start are typically referred to as design consultancies, and they generally involve two to three partners. In some cases they provide design services as well as find sufficient investment to take their designs into production.

Figure 5-14 Phase 7—Final Design for Orbis.

Design showing all components for Orbis: The Patient Transfer System. Rendering by Eric Fields.

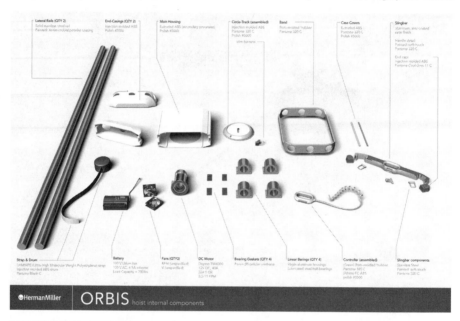

Traditionally, industrial designers and graphic designers have sought employment with in-house design teams of large corporations or with established small- to mid-size design consultancies, but becoming entrepreneurs soon after graduation is a relatively new trend in design.

InnovationSpace offers students some of the basic skills and knowledge necessary to launch their own ventures. While traditional means of education—lectures, assignments, exams, and readings—are important to introduce students to the basic concepts that all entrepreneurs should know, the fundamental concepts of venture creation are emphasized through projects where students are required to apply the knowledge gained through lectures. In InnovationSpace, students have the opportunity to work on NPD projects sponsored by corporations, local entrepreneurs, or research organizations, and as the teams develop new products, they also write business plans, create brand strategies, write marketing plans, and create financial statements for these products. This form of application has high educational value. Also, representatives from the sponsoring institutions provide feedback and guidance

Figure 5-15 Phase 7—Proof-of-concept prototype for Orbis: The Patient Transfer System.

Built by Scott Richins and Eric Fields, with Herman Miller's Doug Bazuin in the harness.

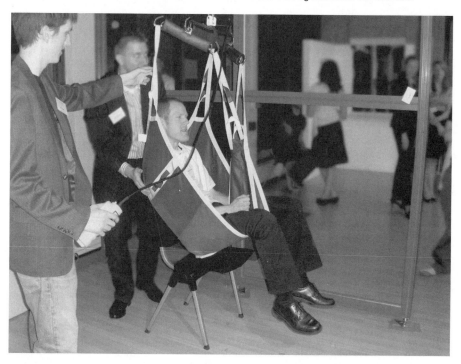

throughout the duration of the project. Although faculty do provide critical feedback, the type of practice-inspired perspective that design entrepreneurs possess can be tremendously beneficial to students interested in starting their own ventures.

CONCLUSION

To devise solutions to the challenges facing our world today (world poverty, child malnutrition, clean drinking water, access to health care, climate change, renewable energy sources, and so on), we need creative and innovative design thinking. Educational programs should prepare young students by providing them with tools they can use in their professional careers to be able to tackle these issues. The primary objective of ASU's

InnovationSpace program is to equip young designers, business professionals, and engineers with the knowledge and skills needed for innovation, so that they can make the world a better place, by design.

Note:

Sections of this chapter have appeared in two other articles: "A Green Dream Team," by Dosun Shin, Prasad Boradkar and Adelheid Fischer, which was published in the *Design Management Review* (Volume 19, Number 4, pp. 49–55), and in "InnovationSpace: A Community of Learners," by Prasad Boradkar, which was published in *Innovation* (Winter 2008, pp. 32–35). The images in this chapter have been used with the permission of Herman Miller, Inc. A special thanks to Eric Fields who provided most of the images for the Orbis Patient Transfer System.

REFERENCES

Belliveau, P., Griffin, A., & Somermeyer, S. (2002). *The PDMA toolbook for new product development.* New York: Wiley.

Boradkar, P. (2008, Winter). InnovationSpace: A community of learners. *Innovation*, 32–35.

Duening, T. (2007). Enterprise process innovation: The ingredients are well known, but what is the recipe? *International Journal of Innovation and Technology Management*, 4(1), 87–101.

Elkington, J. (1997). *Cannibals with forks: Triple bottom line for 21st century business.* Oxford: Capstone.

Gaynor, G. (2002). *Innovation by design: What it takes to keep your company on the cutting edge.* New York: AMACOM Division, American Management Association.

Ireland, C. (2003). Qualitative methods: From boring to brilliant. In B. Laurel (Ed.), *Design research: Methods and perspectives.* Cambridge, MA: MIT Press.

Plsek, P., & Greenhalgh, T. (1993). Complexity science: The challenge of complexity in health care. *British Medical Journal, 323,* 625–628.

Rosenau, M. (1996). *The PDMA handbook of new product development.* New York: Wiley.

Shin, D., Boradkar, P., & Fischer, A. (2008). A green dream team. *Design Management Review, 19*(4), 49–55.

Treffinger, D., Isaksen, S., & Stead-Dorval, B. (2006). *Creative problem solving: An introduction.* Waco, TX: Prufrock Press.

Wasson, C. (2000). Ethnography in the field of design. *Human Organization, 59*(4), 377–388.

White, P., St. Pierre, L., & Belletire, S. (2007). *Okala: Learning ecological design* (2nd ed.). Dulles, VA: Industrial Designers Society of America.

CHAPTER 6

Launch Pad: Creating the Business Case for Innovation

Gerald D. O'Neill, Jr., Sharon C. Ballard,
and Jonathan Levie

The need for innovation to play a major role in the transformation of the U.S. and global healthcare systems has been extensively discussed in society and in this book. Previous chapters discussed the critical role that leadership plays in the innovation process, how one can become an innovator, and the how of innovation, at general and detail levels. A plan for diffusion of an innovation was previously identified as a critical component of the innovation process. It was noted that a diffusion plan was an element of the larger business plan.

At times, an innovation can be developed and spread without development of a new line of business, significant investment, or formal business planning. Often, however, innovation requires significant resources that are beyond the current control or capacity of the innovator. To diffuse the innovation, the innovator must assemble resources that might be controlled by others, such as the management of a large hospital system, outside investors or donors, or other healthcare system stakeholders. To successfully diffuse an innovation may require the creation of a new "venture," whether that venture is a project or an ongoing business, inside an existing organization, or a new start-up. This venture creation process must usually be supported by a business plan, whether formally written or in the collective head of the entrepreneurial team. The business plan encapsulates the business model and plan that will deliver the innovation to the market within a compelling story. The business plan, in the various forms we discuss in this chapter, is often a prerequisite to acquiring the resources needed to successfully diffuse the innovation in the target market.

The primary vehicle for venture creation and innovation is entrepreneurship, the steward of which is the entrepreneur. As a result, there have been repeated calls over the last few decades for increased entrepreneurship and its close cousin, intrapreneurship, in the healthcare system. Experts have issued the call for hospitals, medical practices, doctors, and nurses to become more innovative and entrepreneurial. The consensus seems to be that the state of the U.S. healthcare system needs entrepreneurship, because it is perceived to be the primary vehicle for the creative destruction of innovation. Entrepreneurship, in turn, is often dependent on the creation of compelling new business models, plans, and stories. The purpose of this chapter is to investigate the nature of the entrepreneurship and business planning and storytelling. To begin with the end in mind, entrepreneurs have a tendency to be effective storytellers, and their stories are of opportunity and value creation.

ENTREPRENEURSHIP

What is entrepreneurship? There are many definitions. Much of current academic literature references the work of Venkataraman and his definition: "entrepreneurship as a scholarly field *seeks to understand how opportunities to bring into existence 'future' goods and services are discovered, created, and exploited, by whom, and with what consequences*" (Venkataraman, 1997, p. 120 [italics in original]). In their review Austin, Stevenson, and Wei-Skillern (2006) note that entrepreneurship is researched and taught from three perspectives: the entrepreneur, the "how" of entrepreneurship and the results of entrepreneurship. This book has touched on each of these perspectives in many ways. Through business model, plan, and story development, this chapter takes both the "how" perspective of entrepreneurship, by offering a process model of entrepreneurship and business story development, and the results of entrepreneurship, which are embodied in the value that the innovator-entrepreneur generates for all stakeholders touched by his or her innovation. To these perspectives we add the storytelling perspective of entrepreneurship.

RESULTS PERSPECTIVE OF ENTREPRENEURSHIP: VALUE

Central to most definitions of entrepreneurship are the concepts of opportunity, venture creation, innovation, and value generation. The simplest definition of entrepreneurship might be "entrepreneurs create value." Value creation is the concept that ties venture performance to economic growth and meeting the many of needs of society. Value creation by the firm is a much-researched and discussed concept. In their recent review of the value literature, Lepack, Smith, and Taylor (2007) discuss value in its traditional, monetary sense. They show that value must be understood from the perspectives of value creation, capture, and slippage and from the perspectives of the multiple stakeholders involved.

More recently, the traditional concepts of entrepreneurship and value generation have been extended from this historical, monetary for-profit meaning to include many forms of venture creation, innovation, and value generation. These include the concepts of social entrepreneurship (e.g., Austin et al., 2006), which primarily seeks to create value along the social dimension; eco-entrepreneurship (e.g., Shaper, 2002), which primarily aims to create value along the environmental dimension; and the emerging concept of sustainability entrepreneurship (e.g., Young & Tilley, 2006), which aims to create value simultaneously along the three dimensions of sustainability: economic, social, and environmental.

In their article on social entrepreneurship, Austin et al. (2006) extend a prior model of entrepreneurship created by Sahlman (1996). Sahlman modeled entrepreneurship as a combination of opportunity, people, capital, and deal. Austin et al. extended this framework and adjusted it for social entrepreneurship by placing the opportunity, capital, and people within a context and replacing the concept of deal with the notion of a "social value proposition" at the heart of the venture. This seems a useful model for illustrating that the concept of value generation, in the form of a "value proposition," is at the heart of any entrepreneurial venture.

O'Neill, Hershauer, and Golden (2009) built on the social value proposition of Austin et al. to define the concept of a "holistic value proposition" (HVP), in which the value that is created and captured by each stakeholder in a value network is defined along the three dimensions of sustainability: economic, environmental, and social. By defining the HVP, an entrepreneur develops the answer to the question, "What's in it for me?", for all stakeholders in the network, from the society at large to the individual patient, doctor, or nurse.

In all the above cases, the primary raison d'être of the entrepreneur is value creation. Certainly, transformation through innovation and entrepreneurship of the healthcare system in the manner many envision will result in tremendous new value creation along all three dimensions of the HVP.

"HOW" PERSPECTIVE OF ENTREPRENEURSHIP: VALUE CREATION

A single individual or a team within a large corporation can apply a disciplined, systematic process to entrepreneurship. In fact, Sahlman (1996) and Austin et al. (2006) proposed their models in the context of the "how" of entrepreneurship. They used them to describe how an entrepreneurial venture pursues an opportunity through the application of resources, specifically people and capital. At all levels of economic activity (economy, firm, individual, etc.) are found the concepts of "stocks" and "flows." At the economy level it is "capital stocks" and "income flows." At the venture level it is the balance sheet, which values stocks of capital in the form of assets, liabilities, and equity, and income-cash flow statements, which value flows in the form of revenues, expenses, profits, and cash. Similar paradigms exist for environmental and social forms of stocks and flows. The model of Austin et al. can be seen as a "stocks" model of entrepreneurship that requires the innovation-entrepreneurship process to create value flows.

Execution of the entrepreneurial process is required for the realization of some or the entire HVP of the venture. We suggest a process model of entrepreneurship (Figure 6-1), first created for an introduction to entrepreneurship module at Arizona State University (ASU, 2007). The model can be seen as using capital stocks available to the entrepreneurial team to address the identified opportunity resulting in value creation and capture.

Opportunity Identification

A defining characteristic of the entrepreneur is the ability to identify, analyze, and select opportunities well. Whether resulting from a market imperfection or some other source, the sustainable entrepreneur identifies a new opportunity to create value.

Opportunity-Capability Mapping

As part of the opportunity analysis and selection process, the entrepreneur maps the capabilities of the venture team, whether existing or potential, to the opportunity and makes an informed decision as to whether or not to proceed.

Figure 6-1 Process model of enterpreneurship.

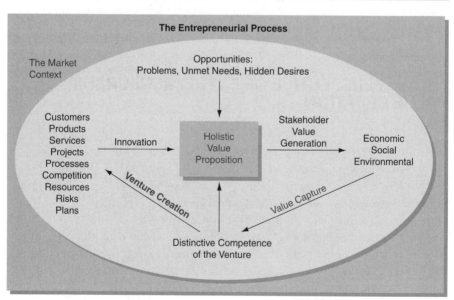

Source: ASU (2007).

Venture Creation and Evolution

Having decided to proceed, the entrepreneur creates the venture, assembling the resources necessary to build the envisioned capability required to address the opportunity. After entry into the marketplace, the entrepreneur evolves the venture on an ongoing basis in response to happenings in the market.

Strategy and Plan Formation

The sustainable entrepreneur forms a strategy to address the opportunity with the venture's capabilities. Much has been written about strategy, which has many definitions and perspectives. For our purpose, strategy defines the target market, customer, products and services, technologies, the HVP, competition, competitive advantage, pricing, promotion, operations, management, alliances, and so on. Plan formation defines specific objectives and milestones overall and by process, the financial and investment plan, and characterizes risks and risk mitigation. The strategy and plan can be well thought out before market entry, or they can emerge as the entrepreneur attempts to innovate and execute. In any case, strategy and plan formation typically become dynamic processes with interaction in the market.

Innovation and Execution

The hallmark of entrepreneurship is innovation, the primary focus of this book. The "something new" can be a product, service, technology, or business model. Entrepreneurs innovate to take advantage of the opportunities created by market imperfections and other sources by introducing new sustainable products, services, technologies, and business models. The successful entrepreneur also executes the strategy, whether explicit or implied, on a daily basis and responds to market changes by identifying new opportunities, assembling new resources, and innovating and executing in the process of ongoing venture evolution.

Holistic Value Proposition

As part of defining the opportunity and the strategy to realize the opportunity, the sustainable entrepreneur defines the value proposition, addressing each of the value creation possibilities for each of the stakeholders in the network. Value creation can exist along the economic, social, and environmental dimension, and the stakeholders can exist at any and all levels of the stakeholder hierarchy and anywhere within the stakeholder network. The value proposition is actualized when the entrepreneur innovates and executes.

Value Creation, Capture, and Slippage

Finally, as a result of innovation and execution, value is realized from the actual delivery of products and services to the end customer through the value network. In our generalized model of value, value can be both "hard" and "soft." The economic value of both can be very easy to very difficult to identify. The entrepreneur captures some portion of the value generated. Even a venture in a nonprofit setting captures value in some form, typically including monetary value, though it may not be from the direct consumer. As they say, "No money, no mission." Stakeholders exchange the various forms of value based on values- and value-informed trade-off decisions. As noted by Lepak et al. (2007), value slippage can occur among stakeholders, reducing the amount of value captured by the stakeholder responsible for the value creation.

Reinvestment and Depletion

Finally, throughout the process capitals are reduced through use, depreciation, obsolescence, and other forms of depletion. The entrepreneur invests some of the captured value back into the stocks of capitals and stakeholders.

Value Network Realization

As a result of execution of the sustainable entrepreneurship flows model, a value network is formed. As previously discussed, this is typically a complex network of stakeholders and flows.

STORYTELLING PERSPECTIVE OF ENTREPRENEURSHIP: BUSINESS MODEL, PLAN, AND STORY

One perspective of entrepreneurship is of the entrepreneur as storyteller (Gartner, 2007). The innovator-entrepreneur uses a variety of discourse, narrative, and story forms to successfully execute many of the steps of the entrepreneurial process, such as gaining resources and selling the offerings of the venture. The entrepreneur tells these stories in written, visual, and, especially, verbal forms. The business plan is one of the most important story forms used by the entrepreneur. The business plan encapsulates the business model and the plan for implementing the venture in the form of a story. The business plan can take several written and verbal manifestations, as discussed below, and is often the primary vehicle used for acquiring resources, such as investment.

COACHING APPROACH TO LAUNCH PAD

In teaching healthcare innovators and entrepreneurs, the authors use a methodology known as Launch Pad. The Launch Pad curriculum and materials were created by Sharon Ballard of Enable Ventures, Inc. and must be licensed from her by a coach or teacher who wishes to use the curriculum. The Launch Pad approach is an innovative, exercise-based approach that helps innovators and entrepreneurs think through and articulate all aspects of the business model, plan, and story required to take their innovation to market.

Launch Pad is based on one of the most important forms of assistance to early-stage entrepreneurs: facilitation or one-to-one coaching coupled with customized assistance for each venture. Coaches are not necessarily professional teachers but often are successful businesspeople with some teaching or public presentation background. Coaches have personal experience in operating a business or at least working in the business world.

What does "coaching" mean in the context of Launch Pad? It is being supportive and encouraging, asking critical and tough questions and showing entrepreneurs how to find the answers to the questions they themselves need to ask. It is a peer-to-peer relationship, clarifying individual and community visions and directions; it is holistic, embracing the whole person and community. Coaching helps people set goals and deadlines. In the specific domain of entrepreneurship, it imparts a gift of skill in viable business creation that entrepreneurs can repeatedly use themselves and pass on to others.

Coaching should not be confused with teaching, which imparts knowledge to the student in cases where the teacher is the expert and can answer questions and evaluate work. Also, coaching should not be confused with forms of advising such as consulting, where experts retain the core skills themselves, or mentoring, where one uses one's personal experience to suggest a specific solution to the mentee's problem. Coaches act as resource facilitators by connecting entrepreneurs to others who can be of value to them. The Launch Pad program draws on the community's assets to address the unique needs that occur with each entrepreneur.

The coaches ask questions and guide business model, plan, and story development efforts by the entrepreneur. They offer specific advice only when asked. Coaches try to avoid creating a dependency with the entrepreneurs. Rather, the coach provides ways of accessing the training, information, and resources the entrepreneur requires for business planning and execution. A good coach holds the entrepreneur accountable to what the entrepreneur says he or she wants to accomplish and checks for consistencies using the facilitation efforts.

The Launch Pad curriculum has been used in a wide variety of innovation, entrepreneurship, and intrapreneurship contexts around the globe, including hi-tech and low-tech, for-profit and not-for-profit, urban and rural, local and global, and across many industries. In terms of the healthcare industry, Launch Pad has been taught in its many forms to a wide variety of innovators and entrepreneurs attempting to bring products, services, and business models to the healthcare industry in an attempt to usher in the disruptive innovation required for a makeover of the industry. The curriculum has, in particular, been used in the groundbreaking Masters of Healthcare Innovation (MHI) program at ASU to teach the principles of entrepreneurship and storytelling to professionals who enter the program with a desire to impact their profession through innovative thinking and action. The remainder of this chapter uses a few examples from the ASU MHI program to illustrate the use of the Launch Pad techniques. The purpose of these examples is not to assert the worthiness of any of the innovation or venture ideas but to illustrate the use of the Launch Pad techniques.

Essence of a Great Business Plan

The fundamental principle of the Launch Pad approach is that a great business story is simply made up of two things: a big opportunity and the answer to the question, "Why are you the person/venture to realize this opportunity?" The big opportunity must elicit a strong gut "I want to be in on this" response in the listener, along one or more of the dimensions of value creation: economic, environmental, or social. The emphasis and mixture of the value proposition depends on the type and focus of the business; for instance, for-profit versus nonprofit, or primarily environmental mission versus social mission versus economic mission (Box 6-1).

Concerning for-profit ventures, the economic motivation is the primary one: Investors are looking for a return on their investment and the entrepreneur must be focused on that. If an opportunity elicits strong reactions in all three dimensions, all the better. The question "Why you?" can also be asked as "What is your ongoing competitive advantage?", which for most early-stage ventures rest on its distinctive competence. Everything else in a business story and plan supports these two fundamental pieces.

The business story is a set of defensible assertions. Almost every statement in a business story is a statement of actual or perceived fact, and these facts must be backed up by research and data. When strung together properly, these defensible assertions should form

---

Box 6-1 Essence of a Great Business Story

- A Big Opportunity
  - A story that creates 'greed,' 'social mission,' and/or 'green response(s)'
- Distinctive Competence
  - Answers the question, 'Why you?'
- Set of Defensible Assertions
- All Other Plan Sections Support These

a story that is compelling, which it will be if it is an interesting opportunity, has a strong answer to the question "Why you?", and is complete, clear, concise, and consistent.

Standard Business Plan Process

The classic approach to a business plan is similar to a phase-by-phase approach to building a work product. First, you begin by doing 6 or more months of research: technology, product, market, and so on. After collecting all your data, you write a 20- to 30-page business plan. While writing the plan, you also develop an integrated set of 3- to 5-year Pro Forma Financials: income statement, balance sheet and cash flow statement, along with an investment scenario and usage of funds.

After completing the plan, you extract an executive summary. Then, you develop a presentation in PowerPoint or a similar medium. Finally, someone challenges you to condense it into a 30-second elevator speech, which can be the hardest task of all.

The funding process then happens in reverse: You meet an investor and give them your elevator pitch, they ask for your executive summary, they invite you in for a presentation, and then (less and less often) they ask to see your business plan and full financials. If they are still interested, they may ask to look at your detailed research, though they are likely to do their own (Figure 6-2).

Compelling Business Story Prototyping Process

Our approach to developing a business model and business plan reverses this process. It uses many of the same principles of innovation explored in previous chapters of this book, with a focus on a prototyping approach to producing the work product: a compelling business story. The business story takes many forms (Figure 6-3).

Figure 6-2 Standard business plan process.

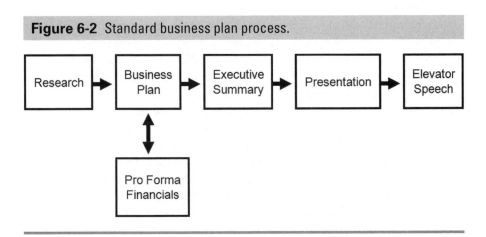

Figure 6-3 Compelling business story prototyping process.

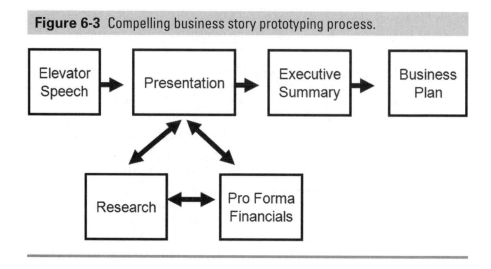

We begin by asking the entrepreneur to express his or her venture's story as a 30-second elevator speech. This forces them from the start to work on the essence of their story: a big opportunity that elicits a response and an answer to the question "why you?". The story might include the value proposition, what you want from the listener (e.g., investment, a partnership, a customer, etc.), or some other highlight.

Then, we begin developing and giving the presentation: right from the start. We do this through a series of exercises that forces the entrepreneur to do the appropriate research to answer typical business plan questions and develop integrated Pro Forma financials. It is critical that the entrepreneur take personal responsibility for this work, including the details of the income statement, balance sheet, and cash flow statement. They must know the numbers behind the story cold.

The prototype presentation is enhanced each week as more is learned about the opportunity and the marketplace and as the plan is developed in more detail. One might ask, "When is the presentation and, thus, the story/plan done?" The simple answer: *Always and never.* It's always done because whenever an entrepreneur presents his or her plan, it is in the state it is in and it is done for that moment. It is never done, because the business plan changes as fast as the world changes around the innovator-entrepreneur.

Because of the way we coach entrepreneurs to develop presentations, they can rapidly produce an executive summary, which basically consists of the verbal messages from the presentation. The entrepreneur can move these messages into a document and, with a bit of editing, have a complete three-page executive summary. Finally, writing the business plan, if required, is a relatively simple process. The entrepreneur turns each of the messages in the executive summary into a paragraph or so that communicates the details and shows the research done. The paragraph is the defense of the assertion embodied in the message. Upon adding the Pro Forma financials developed during the Launch Pad process, the entrepreneur has completed a 20- or 30-page business plan.

This last step may slowly become a relic of the past because we are seeing more investors who don't want to read a 30-page plan—they want to capture the essence of the story, have faith in the team, and do their own due diligence, which they can do from a quality presentation supported by great research and detailed financials. The entire process is iterative. As new things happen, the entrepreneur can use the process and tools to rapidly rethink the business model, story, and plan, resulting in updates to the elevator speech, presentation, research, financials, executive summary, and full business plan.

Launch Pad Curriculum

The Launch Pad curriculum is organized into eight sessions, each with a specific focus. Each session consists of a set of one-page exercises that are deceptive in their simplicity: They are actually quite hard to complete and each typically results in considerable back-up research (Figure 6-4).

Figure 6-4 The launch pad coaching process.

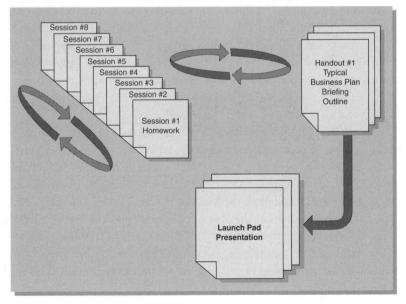

The purpose of the exercises is to develop the answers to questions that an investor expects entrepreneurs to address in a typical business plan presentation. We use one of many outlines that have been given to us over the years by investors. The entrepreneur uses this outline as a general guide to develop his or her specific presentation. Each session results in better answers to the typical questions, which results in a story that is more clear, concise, consistent, and complete and thus more compelling.

The process is organized into an order that has been proven over and over again to be the most effective way of moving an entrepreneur or innovator through his or her thinking about the opportunity and the value they can create and capture by addressing the opportunity with innovative products, services, processes, value network forms, and business models. We begin by asking entrepreneurs to step up from the morass of details that typically deluge them in day-to-day business and to think at the most strategic level about the opportunity, their uniqueness, and how their venture will achieve its overall vision or goal (Figure 6-5).

Next, we have found that the best way to engage most innovators is by thinking about their technology and the products that can come from it. That is why we encourage the entrepreneur to envision what is possible, typically based on many years of expertise working in the healthcare industry. In addition to the many innovation techniques presented elsewhere in this book, we use technology roadmapping and other technology/product focused exercises to begin the planning exercise, with the last steps in the process asking, "What markets should we target?" and "What do we believe our customers will think of our products?"

This leads to a number of marketing and sales exercises focused on understanding the ultimate customer, the value network of firms, organizations and individuals that deliver the product/service bundle to the end customer, the innovator's position within that value network, the marketing and sales process, and early stage product/service delivery and revenue possibilities. The primary emphasis is on talking to real customers and other important market participants and modifying the product/service, business model, and presentation/story based on their feedback.

Then, we move on to understanding the competition in more detail, communicating the competitive differentiator and nailing the HVP. The last two sessions bring it all together by focusing on operations, management, alliances, and financials, although we typically begin discussing financial statements in the first session and weave finance and investment discussions throughout the sessions.

These later sessions support the "big opportunity" and the "Why you?" that is shaped primarily in the first four sessions. They fully articulate the business model that will deliver on the opportunity by using the venture's competitive advantage. Each session consists of a set of one-page exercises, about 60 in all, plus recommended readings that support each session.

Figure 6-5 Launch Pad toolbox and checklist for entrepreneurs.

Session 1 - Introductions, Ground Rules, Strategic Planning
Exercises/Homework

1.1 30-second "Elevator" Message
1.2 Sunflower Exercise
1.3 One-Page Operating Plan Graphic
1.4 One-Page Strategic Business Plan
1.5 Value Proposition Quiz
1.6 Storyboard of 15-minute Presentation
1.7 Opening and Closing Message to Briefing
1.8 Dream List of 20 Briefing Attendees
1.9 One Page Executive Summary for Invitations
1.10 Handouts 1, 2 & 5
1.11 Recommended Readings

Session 2 - Technology, Intellectual Property and Product Plans
Exercises/Homework

2.1 Technology Roadmaps
2.2 Product Feature Roadmap
2.3 Technical Skills Assessment
2.4 Manufacturing Plan, Initial
2.5 Rob's Quality Dog Food Test
2.6 Financial Assumptions for Session #2
2.7 First Cut at all Slides
2.8 Recommended Readings

Session 3 - Marketing and Sales Plans
Exercises/Homework

3.1 Value Chain (food chain) Graphic
3.2 One-page Product Data Sheet
3.3 Purchase Orders or Checks for Deposit
3.4 Price List
3.5 Interview Financial Analyst (Questions in Advance)
3.6 Interview Customer(s) (Questions in Advance; and Customer Reference Letters for Sales Forecasts)
3.7 Sales Process Flow Chart or Timeline
3.8 3-Year Revenue Projections
3.9 Financial Assumptions for Session #3
3.10 Second cut at all Slides
3.11 Recommended Readings

Session 4 - Competition
Exercises/Homework

4.1 Competitive Value Matrices
4.2 Competitive Notebooks
4.3 Competitive Graphic (Summary)
4.4 Value Proposition Refinement
4.5 Financial Assumption for Session #4
4.6 Alliances vs. Competitor Considerations
4.7 "Successful Presentations" by Sharon C. Ballard
4.8 Third Cut at all Slides
4.9 Recommended Readings

Session 5 - Operations, Management, Staffing
Exercises/Homework

5.1 Manufacturing & Operations (final)
5.2 Handout #4 "Start-Up Teams" by Sharon C. Ballard
5.3 "Dream" Board and Advisors
5.4 Organization Charts
5.5 CEO Job Description and Time Sheet
5.6 Wall Street Journal Advertisements for Key Executives
5.7 Recruiting Materials (Executives, Directors, Advisors)
5.8 Financial Assumptions for Session #5
5.9 Fourth Cut at all Slides
5.10 Recommended Readings

Session 6 - Financial Plan
Exercises/Homework

6.1 Revise and Finalize all Financial Assumptions by Plan Section
6.2 Revenues-Ratio Analyses
6.3 One-page Profit/Loss, Cash, Balance Sheets
6.4 Use of Proceeds for all rounds
6.5 Valuation for all Rounds
6.6 Summary Slide
6.7 Executive Summary
6.8 Fifth Cut at all Slides
6.9 Recommended Readings

Session 7 - Dry Run Presentations
Exercises/Homework

7.1 Dress Rehearsal of Presentation
7.2 Dry-Run Feedback
7.3 Executive Summary
7.4 Sixth Cut at all Slides
7.5 Recommended Readings

Session 8 - Final Presentation
Exercises/Homework

8.1 Follow-up Plans
8.2 Lessons Learned
8.3 Skills Assessment
8.4 Recommended Readings

Source: Copyright 2000–2007, EnableVentures, Inc.

Story Development

Beginning with the third or fourth session, the entrepreneur begins doing the presentation at every session. If possible, we put them on film for at least the first dry run, to show them the distance they have to travel, and the last dry run, to show them how well they've traveled that distance. In an iterative way, the entrepreneur prototypes the innovation plan/story by refining and delivering the presentation every week. We begin the first week with a storyboard approach. On one piece of paper the entrepreneur draws 10 to 20 boxes with diagonals between them. The boxes are titled in the order in which the entrepreneur wants to tell the story, guided by our standard business plan briefing layout that, by topic, asks the questions that must be answered in a business plan.

The story begins with an introductory slide that typically follows a form such as Welcome + Thank You + Elevator Speech, which hooks the audience and "tells them what you're going to tell them." The body of the presentation is then a set of major messages or conclusions (which are defensible assertions) that are woven into a compelling story and, thus, "tells them." The Summary and Strategic Issues slides close the story, with the typical format of Major Points in Summary + Thanks Again + Over to You for Discussion, with the hand-off being a focus on the top three to five issues facing the entrepreneur. This is the third and final part: the "tell them what you told them."

By the way, we always emphasize the point that 12 slides in 12 minutes means an average of 1-minute talking time per slide, which is moving pretty fast. So we encourage the entrepreneur to be economical in his or her approach, while being both complete and concise. Like all storyboards, the Launch Pad storyboard is a high-level design and an initial prototype of a story. Each slide in the storyboard takes a specific form. Above the diagonal line of each slide section, the entrepreneur sketches or writes, by hand, how the slide's topic will be represented visually. Below the diagonal line, the entrepreneur writes three to five terse messages or major conclusions he or she wishes the listener to grasp. Only after the storyboard has been refined by hand a few times does the entrepreneur begin to develop the actual slides, transferring the verbal messages to the notes section of the presentation (Figure 6-6).

It is very important to take advantage of both visual and verbal messages. They are very distinct in how they are delivered, the quantity of information in each, the bandwidth on the receiving end, and so on. The opportunity is to be very creative visually and to have the verbal and visual messages amplify one another (Figure 6-7). The alternative is to read off a bunch of text bullets. That makes for the most boring presentation in the world and turns listeners off fast.

Of course, the final slides and story differ from the original storyboard, because each session the entrepreneur is learning more and enhancing the story and, thus, constantly refining the visual and verbal messages. We emphasize that five messages per slide and

Figure 6-6 Storyboard of 12-minute presentation.

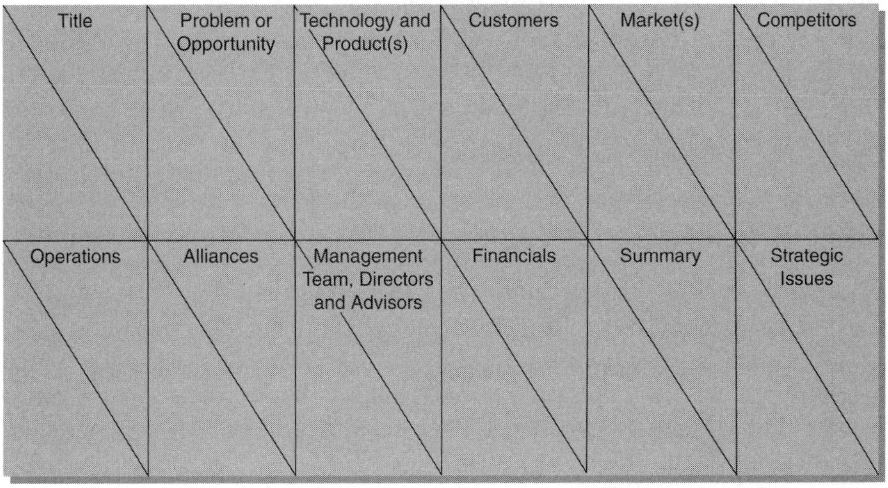

Title	Problem or Opportunity	Technology and Product(s)	Customers	Market(s)	Competitors
Operations	Alliances	Management Team, Directors and Advisors	Financials	Summary	Strategic Issues

12 slides equates to 60 messages, and that's a lot to communicate in 12 minutes. Weaving all this into a compelling story is a challenge. However, once the speaker is in command of the full set of messages, he or she can be spontaneous in his or her delivery by filling out the story with examples, experiences, facts, sources, and other research developed during the process.

Figure 6-7 Ear words and eye words.

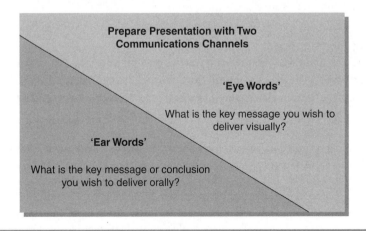

Prepare Presentation with Two
Communications Channels

'Eye Words'
What is the key message you wish to
deliver visually?

'Ear Words'
What is the key message or conclusion
you wish to deliver orally?

If the entrepreneur has done a good job of maintaining the verbal messages in the notes section of the presentation, he or she can copy them into a document very rapidly, thus developing a three-page executive summary. Because all messages are defensible assertions, it is easy to turn each message into a paragraph with research information (the defense) to arrive at a 20- to 30-page business plan. Just add Pro Forma financials developed along the way! Repeat the entire process as one learns more and the market changes.

Strategic Planning

We begin the process by concentrating on high-level strategy and strategic planning exercises. The first session consists of a number of such exercises that ask the innovator to step up from the details of the business and "begin with the end in mind." What will the future look like in 3, 5, or 7 years, if the innovation is successful? How will the innovation impact society? What will be the business result? What is the big objective or goal that the innovation will achieve? What are the major steps required to get from today to that envisioned future?

The first exercise used to begin this strategic thinking is the elevator speech, which we require to be 30 seconds or less. The purpose of the elevator pitch is to gain interest from the listener, from whom an ideal response might be "tell me more." A good elevator speech should include a statement of the problem, solution, and value proposition as an explanation of the big opportunity and one or more assertions that answer the question "Why you?" in such a way that the listener concludes that the innovator, entrepreneur, entrepreneurial team, and/or venture has the potential to be the strongest competitor in the market defined by the opportunity. The elevator speech should also tell listeners what the entrepreneur would like from them and ask for action, such as setting a meeting to further discuss the idea.

Example: Elevator Speech

One student in the ASU MHI program who worked for a large healthcare organization with many hospital sites was the internal innovator leading the charge for a multisite dispatch system that would allocate beds to rural customers across the system from a single control center. Her initial elevator speech was as follows:

> We are in a unique position to meet the varied needs of the rural communities in our state. Currently, our Outreach department provides a one-call concept to improve patient access to care, by providing coordination of physician acceptance, financial/clinical screening, and confirmation of bed availability. We would like to extend this service to our rural customers by providing a central one-call service and supporting information system that

will result in improved response to rural patient needs. Combined with increased market share, this will result in increased revenue and customer reliance on our healthcare system. Could I schedule a meeting to further discuss this with you?

This elevator speech does a decent job of capturing the opportunity and solution. It mentions the value proposition to both the customer and the business. The "Why you?" is based on the proposition that the concept has already been tested in the healthcare system and the project is about extending the project to new customers within the system through the implementation of a new information system. The speech could be improved by dimensioning the opportunity and its impact. For instance, how many customers will be served annually, how much will revenue be increased, and so on?

Product Management Process

Another example of the exercises that comprise the Launch Pad approach to business model, plan, and story development is the sunflower exercise, taken from Rob Ryan's book, *Smartups* (Ryan, 2002). It forces the entrepreneur to articulate the venture's core competency (the center), the general market that the venture addresses (the ground), the major drivers that are calling the venture's core competency into the market (the stem), and the product and service forms in which the core competency will appear (the petals) (Figure 6-8).

An entrepreneur typically identifies *lots* of petals, especially entrepreneurs with horizontal technologies that are capable of doing many things. The last step in the exercise is the most difficult, and it begins to address one of the most difficult challenges faced by many early-stage entrepreneurs: that of focus. We ask the entrepreneur to prioritize the petals in the order he or she imagines they will be rolled out, thus selecting a "beachhead landing" in the marketplace. Of course, this is a complex decision we ask entrepreneurs to make, and this is just a first cut at it. But, we hold their feet to the fire to make a choice and justify it, making the point that they can choose only one item to be first and they must focus on it alone or at maximum a few items that are closely related.

Example: Sunflower Exercise

Another student in the ASU MHI program was interested in starting a consulting company to assist healthcare organizations with understanding and implementing strategies for pursuing sustainability (Box 6-2). She envisioned a number of possible products and services that would engage healthcare companies confronted by serious and difficult environmental challenges.

Figure 6-8 Rob Ryan's sunflower exercise.

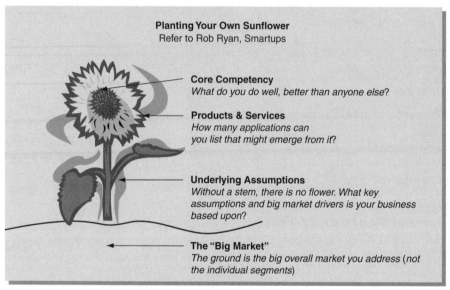

Planting Your Own Sunflower
Refer to Rob Ryan, Smartups

Core Competency
What do you do well, better than anyone else?

Products & Services
*How many applications can
you list that might emerge from it?*

Underlying Assumptions
*Without a stem, there is no flower. What key
assumptions and big market drivers is your business
based upon?*

The "Big Market"
*The ground is the big overall market you address (not
the individual segments)*

Source: Reprinted from *Smartups: Lessons from Rob Ryan's Entrepreneur America Boot Camp for Start-Ups,* by Rob Ryan. Copyright © 2002 by Rob Ryan. Used by permission of the publisher, Cornell University Press. All rights reserved.

Once again, the exercise does a good job of capturing the essence of the company in a one-page exercise. The competency of the organization is captured in a short sentence. A team or organization's distinctive competence can usually be articulated in this manner, with the short statement being emblematic of a set of capabilities that demonstrate that competence. The overall market served by the potential venture is identified in a way that identifies one approach to segmenting the market. The major drivers that call the competency of the venture into the market are crisply articulated. A range of consulting services is envisioned. This exercise stopped short of identifying the order in which the services would be introduced to the marketplace, which is necessary to provide focus for the start-up of the venture.

As an example of how individual exercises fit together to form an overall planning process, consider Session 2, Technology, Intellectual Property, and Product Plans. The sunflower exercise is the first step in technology/product roadmapping, which links markets, products/services, technologies, and research activities over a period of time, typically greater than 5 years (Figure 6-9).

Box 6-2 Sunflower Exercise: Sustainability Consulting Company

Core Competency:
- Analyzing environmental impact of healthcare facilities and processes, and offering plans for decreasing impacts

Products and Services:
- Consulting to individual hospitals or healthcare entities: provide gap analysis and make suggestions
- Software tools to help accomplish that
- Guidebooks to help accomplish that
- Speaking service for motivation and helping institutions to incorporate change
- Networking system for linking entities that are working on these issues

Underlying Assumptions:
- Hospitals need to save money
- Hospitals need public good will
- Hospitals need risk abatement
- Hospitals need staff retention
- Hospitals may have a mission that requests of them good stewardship
- Market and political forces are strong currently to reduce ecological footprint and carbon use

The Big Market:
- All health care entities: hospitals, systems, clinics, governmental agencies

---

The products and services that were numbered in the sunflower exercise go on the roadmap in the order they were prioritized, and the entrepreneur creates a planning diagram that links together the various research and development activities in a time-based critical path manner. This roadmap can serve as the basis for many things: research and development planning and budgeting, technology assessment, access to critical research and technologies, skills assessment, personnel planning, and so on. The roadmap also serves to further the entrepreneur's thinking from technology/product to product/market, thus transitioning to a "market pull" mentality.

The products and services that occur in the first few years are then planned further in a product feature roadmap, in which the major features that generate the value to the customer are planned in annual releases. Finally, the first product for the first market is internally tested by the venture using Rob Ryan's Dog Food Test, which tests the viability and competitiveness of the product along 10 dimensions (2002).

Figure 6-9 An example: Product management process.

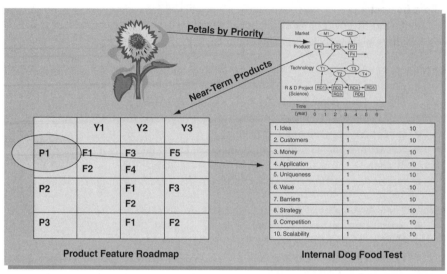

Sources: Sunflower and Internal Dog Food Test: Reprinted from *Smartups: Lessons from Rob Ryan's Entrepreneur America Boot Camp for Start-Ups,* by Rob Ryan. Copyright © 2002 by Rob Ryan. Used by permission of the publisher, Cornell University Press. All rights reserved. Technology roadmap: From Kostoff, R. N., & Schaller, R. R. (2001). Science and technology roadmaps. *IEEE Transactions on Engineering Management, 48*(2), 132–143. © 2001 IEEE.

Marketing and Sales

These exercises then lead into Session 3, Marketing and Sales (Figure 6-10). The product exercises become the basis for a product data sheet and some of the questions to be asked in interviews with customers, analysts, and other value network participants to be identified in Session 3. Value network participants are derived as a result of a value network modeling exercise.

Through the value network modeling exercise, the entrepreneur identifies the key players involved in delivering the "whole product" (Moore, 1999) to the ultimate user in a target market segment. The entrepreneur defines

- Attributes that define the target customer
- Product and service components that comprise the whole product
- Types of organizations and/or individuals involved in the value network
- Specific organizations and individuals of each type
- Financial dynamics of the flow of products and services

Figure 6-10 Value network exercise.

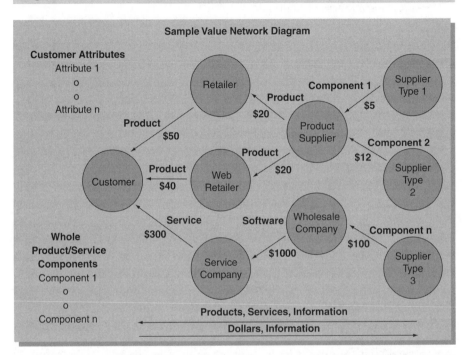

Sample Value Network Diagram

- Information dynamics of the flow of products and service
- Value creation dynamics of the value network

Based on this model, the entrepreneur identifies the most important players in the value network and many of the dynamics that govern its formation, including the dynamics of value creation and capture. Both aspects of the value creation process are important to the value network participants: what value each creates and what value each is able to retain.

Example: Value Network Exercise

Another MHI student envisioned creating a service that would travel to underserved populations as an alternative to clinic-based health care (Figure 6-11). She envisioned a mobile unit that would provide immunizations, health education, and record keeping for such populations.

Her initial value network exercise is comprehensive and captures all steps and players in the process. In fact it is perhaps a bit too detailed. For instance, for her purpose,

Figure 6-11 Value network exercise: Mobile healthcare unit for underserved people.

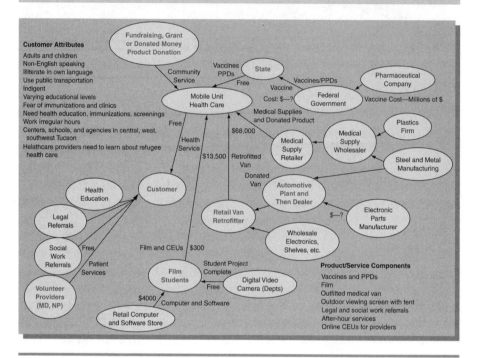

which is to understand the structure of her target market, it is probably of limited usefulness to extend the value network diagram to the providers of steel, metals, plastics, electronic parts, and so on. But the diagram serves to understand and document many of the aspects of the market, including the whole product, the customer served, and the network that the players work in to deliver the whole product to the customer. It also provides initial insight into some of the value dynamics of the network, including some of the cost components of delivering the service to the customer.

Value Proposition

Beginning in the first session and throughout the Launch Pad process, the entrepreneur is asked to reflect on value creation and capture. We repeatedly pose the fundamental question of entrepreneurship: "What value do you create for whom?" Within the HVP framework this can be further stated, "What economic, social and environmental value do you create for each of the players in the stakeholder network that forms around your business?" The Launch Pad value proposition exercises encourage the entrepreneur to think both generally and specifically about value.

The financial value proposition is classically most important to players of the value network (Figure 6-12). The venture's offerings must make financial sense to everyone involved in the network. The Launch Pad financial value proposition asks the entrepreneur to think in terms of the income statement of each participant in the value network, whether the participant is an individual or firm, for-profit or nonprofit. How do the innovator-entrepreneur's offerings increase the bottom line of each type of customer, partner, or supplier involved? By increasing revenues or decreasing expenses or both? Thinking in income statements is the beginning of learning the language of money, which is critically important for the entrepreneur to learn.

Example: Value Proposition Exercise

One student wanted to help her hospital system train new nurses faster while retaining critical "gray matter": the knowledge and capabilities of older nursing talent. She envisioned a specialized nursing unit where new nurses would receive intensive education

Figure 6-12 The financial value proposition.

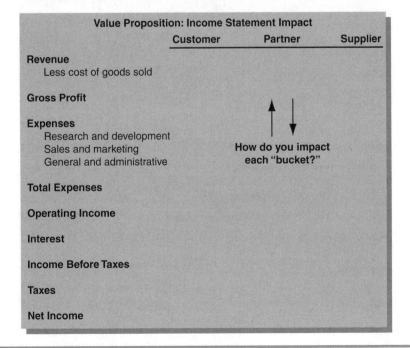

under the guidance of experienced nurses, who might normally leave the business as a result of no longer wanting to deal with the physical rigors of nursing. She envisioned that many of these nurses would remain in their careers longer if they could stay in an educational role. Such a service could have a variety of benefits to those in the value network, including financial. She did an initial project for the two major players in the network: the new training center and the healthcare partners that help create the center and that benefit from the faster, higher volume training of new nurses and retention of older nurses (Figure 6-13).

Thanks to many long years of standardized accounting, the financial value proposition can be understood in well-known terms. That is less true of the social and environmental value propositions, which are becoming increasingly important to society's stakeholders. A number of efforts, such as the Global Reporting Initiative (2009), attempt to stan-

Figure 6-13 Financial value proposition exercise: Old nurse/ new nurse training.

Value Proposition: Income Statement Impact		
	Training Center	**Partners**
Revenue	⇧	⟺
Gross Profit	⇧	⟺
Expenses Research and development	⇧	⇩
Sales and marketing	⟺	⟺
General and administration	⇧	⇩
Total Expenses	⇧	⇩
Net Income Before	⇧	⇧
Taxes and Interest	⟺	⟺
Net Income	⇧	⇧

dardize reporting on the economic, social, and environmental triple bottom line. But, whether standard or not, more and more firms are making efforts to improve their performance to social and environmental measures. In the same manner as the financial value proposition, we ask the entrepreneur to consider how his or her venture impacts the social and environmental "bottom lines" of each value network player. In a similar manner to the financial value proposition, the entrepreneur is asked how its offerings help each player's performance to specific metrics. Each player may have unique goals it is trying to achieve vis-à-vis metrics such as carbon reduction, waste emission, health and safety, community contributions, and so on (Figure 6-14).

Example: Environmental Value Proposition

The student who envisioned a sustainability consulting business for the healthcare industry took a combined view of the environmental and financial value proposition by evaluating how her service would impact the environmental performance of a typical customer. For the purposes of this exercise, she assumed a subscription-based revenue model. Her reasoning, supported by interviews with healthcare providers and her other research, led her to estimate typical energy, waste, and other purchasing benefits that would result from better environmental practices resulting from her consulting services (Table 6-1).

In an extension to the Launch Pad curriculum, O'Neill et al. (2009) also ask the entrepreneur to develop the HVP for their venture. The HVP is an extension of the above

Figure 6-14 The social and environmental value propositions.

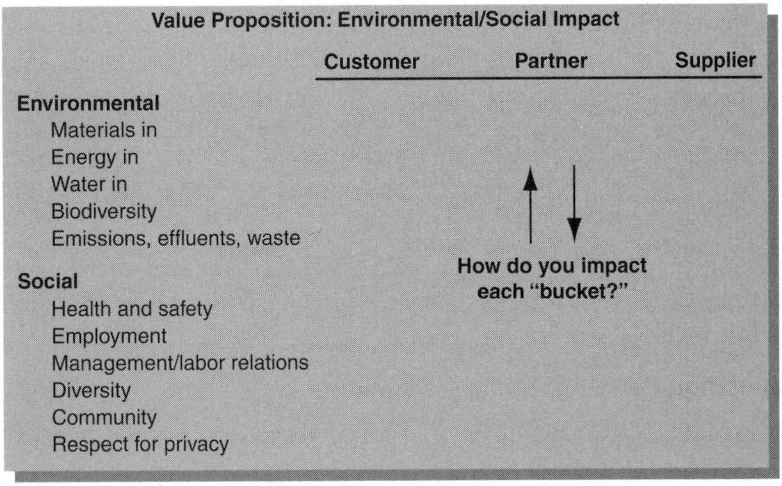

Table 6-1 Value Net Matrix

Per Average Hospital	Cost Before	Cost Now	Savings Per Year	Payback
Energy	$1,200,000	$800,000	$400,000	2 months*
Waste	$400,000	$250,000	$150,000	5 months*
Purchasing	$5,500,000	$5,000,000	$500,000	1.5 months*

*Based on $65,000 subscription rate.

value proposition elements. It requires that the entrepreneur think more broadly in terms of all stakeholders the venture touches, beyond the players that the venture specifically involves in the delivery of products and services. Stakeholders occur at three general levels: the society, the firm, and the individual (Lepak et al., 2007). Some of these are directly involved in the execution of the value network and some are not. Thus the HVP can be represented as a two-dimensional matrix with 12 dimensions of sustainability entrepreneurship opportunity value proposed by the Young and Tilley (2006) model along one dimension and the key stakeholders along the other. In each cell defined by this matrix, statements of value capture can occur that represent what specific value a given stakeholder receives ("captures") in a given dimension of sustainability from participating in the value network of the venture. The HVP provides a comprehensive view of the total value realized by all stakeholders of the entrepreneur's venture (Table 6-2).

With a clear understanding of the structure of the market and an initial understanding of the manner in which the entrepreneur creates value for its stakeholders, the entrepreneur is asked to interact more deeply with customers, partners, suppliers, and other stakeholders. The entrepreneur develops a list of questions he or she would like to ask each type of player in the network. With questions in hand, along with a product data sheet, a prototype or model of the product or service, ideas about pricing and so on, the entrepreneur is encouraged to talk to as many value network players as makes sense for their situation. Based on the feedback received during these marketing-oriented interviews, the entrepreneur modifies aspects of the product, service, business model, or business plan as appropriate. This dance with the market continues until the entrepreneur is convinced that the offerings of the venture are viable in the marketplace.

Competition

Using a distinctive competence to deliver a product/service bundle to a target customer, thus creating a specific value proposition, is the core of venture strategy. Strategy, like entrepreneur, has many definitions. One of our favorites is *the ongoing, never-ending*

Table 6-2 Value Creation Matrix

Value Dimensions	Shades of Economic				Shades of Environmental					Shades of Social		
	Eco-efficiency	Socio-efficiency	Economic Equity	Intergenerational Equity	Eco-effectiveness	Ecological Equity	Environmental Stability	Environmental Sustainability	Socio-effectiveness	Sufficiency	Futurity	Social Responsibility
STAKEHOLDERS												
Society:												
Global												
National												
Regional												
Tribal												
Local												
Community												
Industry												
Value Network:												
Customer												
Partner												
The Sustainable Venture												
Supplier												
Competitors												
Shareholders												
Individuals:												
Employee												
Investor												
Key Public												

Value Creation Statements

search for competitive advantage. A venture's offerings are almost never without competition or, at least, eminent competition. That statement is as true in a not-for-profit setting as it is in a for-profit setting. No matter what the venture, competition must be well understood. Launch Pad exercises that address competition ask the entrepreneur to position the venture's offerings against current and potential future competition in a way that clearly separates it from the competition. The value proposition identified throughout the Launch Pad process is compared with those delivered by the competition in an effort to further differentiate the firm from its competitors.

Example: Competitive Positioning Graphic

A classic way to represent the competitive positioning of an innovation is through the use of a two-dimensional competitive graphic. The purpose of the graphic is to spatially position the innovation or venture in a manner that clearly separates it from the competition. In creating the graphic you can choose whatever dimensions best represent your differentiator. The *x-y* indices can be simple or compound measures. What is important is that you can defend the assertion that is implied by the graphic and choice of measures. One group of MHI students were proposing an "off-the-shelf" innovation methodology and toolkit for healthcare organizations, so employees could learn many of the techniques they were learning in the MHI program, but faster and more cheaply. They positioned their "InnoBox" idea against the competition for healthcare innovation design services in that manner (Figure 6-15).

Figure 6-15 Competitive position: Innovation in a box concept.

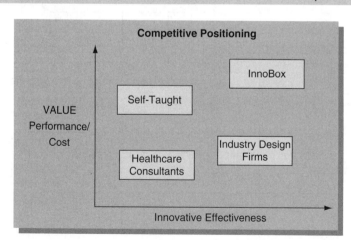

Alliances, Operations, and Management

After defining the fundamentals of the strategy of the venture, the next Launch Pad exercises define the operational model of the firm. Exercises ask the innovator-entrepreneur to think through how he or she will operate the venture on a day-to-day basis. What will the venture do inside the firm? What will be accomplished through alliances? A good way to answer these questions is to return to the value network diagram and to develop a more detailed model of the supply chain by looking at the basic model that starts with inbound logistics and ends with outbound logistics. Which of these steps does the venture do and which will be accomplished through outsourcing, insourcing, or some other supplier or alliance relationship?

Perhaps the most important question concerns what team will be responsible for execution of the plan? To many investors, this is the most important question of all. It has become a cliché that investors will invest in an "A" management team with a "B" innovation before they will invest in a "B" team. The innovator-entrepreneur may or may not have the team in place at the initial stages of the plan. But, he or she must constantly be working toward building the best team possible and must be aware of the holes in the current team at any point in time. The team consists of not only day-to-day management, but also the venture's advisory board and, if a stand-alone venture, the board of directors. Partners are also critical members of the team.

Financials

Money is the language of business. It is incumbent on the innovator-entrepreneur to speak the language. The last module of the Launch Pad curricula teaches the basics of entrepreneurial finance and provides a set of exercises to help the entrepreneur answer basic financial questions: What financial future will the venture create, in terms of revenue, expenses, income, assets, liabilities, equity, and cash flow? The Launch Pad philosophy centers around the income statement, also known as the profit & loss statement. It is one of three statements that make up the basic language of entrepreneurial finance.

The financial aspect of the story tells how the venture is going to survive and prosper by generating positive cash flow. It also tells how much investment is required to make the future happen. Once again, this is critical whether or not the venture is a for-profit or not-for-profit venture. If it is a for-profit venture, investors expect a rate of return commensurate with the expectation set by the entrepreneur and the level of risk inherent in the venture. If it is a not-for-profit venture, investors/donors expect the venture to create a "social return on investment" commensurate with the investment/donation.

The entrepreneur must learn how to speak in terms of the income, balance sheet, and cash flow statements. He or she must develop forward-looking statements, called pro forma statements, for the first 3 to 5 years of the venture. Box 6-3 shows the basic format of these statements.

Box 6-3 Three Financial Statements

Income Statement	Balance Sheet	Cash Flow Statement
Revenue	**Assets**	Net income from operations (+/−)
Cost of goods sold	Cash and equivalents	Depreciation (+)
Gross Profit	Accounts receivable	Amortization (−)
	Inventory	Accounts receivable (−)
Expenses	Other short-term assets	Inventory (−)
Marketing	Property and equipment	Other short-term assets (−)
and sales	Less accumulated	Accounts payable (−)
R&D	depreciation	Other short-term liabilities (+)
G&A	Total property and	Net income adjusted to cash
Total expenses	equipment	
	Other long-term assets	Investing
Net income	Total assets	Plant and equipment (−)
before I & T		Other long-term assets (−)
	Liabilities	
Interest	Accounts payable	Financing
	Other short-term	Long-term liabilities (+)
Taxes	liabilities	Paid-in capital (+)
	Long-term liabilities	
Net income	Total liabilities	Net cash from period
		Beginning cash
	Equity	Ending cash
	Paid-in capital	
	Retained earnings	
	Total equity	
	Total liabilities 1 equity	

The income statement shows the flow of revenue, expense, and income through the venture over a period of time, which can be any period from a day to a year. The income statement shows whether the business creates value in the marketplace, reflected in revenue, which is the customer's willingness to pay, and whether it captures some of that value, reflected in net income.

The balance sheet shows the financial status of the business at a point of time, reflected in assets, which are the things the venture owns, and its liabilities and equity, which is how the firm owns those assets. The income statement, in combination with "balance sheet transactions" such as purchasing equipment, selling stock, or taking out a loan, effectively transitions the beginning balance sheet to the ending balance sheet.

The cash flow statement shows how cash flowed through the business over the same period of time reflected in the income statement. Cash flows in income statement and balance sheet categories as sources (+) and uses (−) of cash. Positive net income results in positive cash growth. Growth in assets uses cash. Growth in liabilities and equity sources cash. The pluses and minuses in Box 6-3 show how the various categories of the income and balance sheet statements typically source or use cash in a growing venture.

When an integrated set of pro forma financials is built for the venture, the entrepreneur will have the answer to the question "How much investment is required to make the envisioned future happen?" The entrepreneur will also be able to answer the companion question, known as usage of funds: "How will the entrepreneur use the investment to make the envisioned future happen?" That is, what income statement and balance sheet categories will be spent? Finally, the entrepreneur can calculate various return on investment measures based on the required investment and profitability. Quantitative social return on investment measures can also be calculated.

The Rest of the Story

Finally, the entrepreneur must discuss details of his or her plan, especially research and development plans and marketing and sales plans. These plans are often discussed in terms of the process that will be used and/or major milestones that will be accomplished.

To show that the entrepreneur is as much a risk-manager as a risk-taker, he or she can list the major known risks in the business and how he or she is going to mitigate those risks by knowing when they emerge and how he or she will deal with them, if and when this happens. When telling his or her story in presentation form, the innovator-entrepreneur summarizes the opportunity and why the venture will deliver on it and asks for a next action step, such as due diligence or investment.

CONCLUSION

The effective entrepreneur is often an effective teller of future stories. With completion of the Launch Pad sessions, the entrepreneur has, at least initially, defined all critical aspects of the new venture: its strategy, offerings, markets, customers, partners, suppliers, competition, operations, management, financial future and investment requirements, along with critical milestones and risk mitigation strategies. If the entrepreneur has done a good job of cataloging these components as effective messages, then she or he can organize them into a variety of story forms to communicate the venture and its offerings to customers, partners, employees, investors, and other stakeholders.

It is then up to the start-up entrepreneur to execute the story, that is, to bring the envisioned future into being. He or she might do so through repeated telling of the venture story and, then, modification of that story, and the venture it represents, as a result of repeated interaction with the marketplace. Throughout the process the entrepreneurial team should never lose sight of the fact that its story must be one of value creation for all of the stakeholders that the venture touches.

REFERENCES

Arizona State University. (2007). Introduction to entrepreneurship. *ASU 101,* Entrepreneurship Module of Introductory course to university life at Arizona State University.

Austin, J., Stevenson, H., & Wei-Skillern, J. (2006). Social and commercial entrepreneurship: Same, different, or both? *Entrepreneurship Theory and Practice, 30*(1), 1–22.

Gartner, W. B. (2007). Entrepreneurial narrative and a science of the imagination. *Journal of Business Venturing, 22,* 613–627.

Global Reporting Initiative. (2009). Retrieved January 26, 2009, from http://www.globalreporting.org/

Kostoff, R. N., & Schaller, R. R. (2001). Science and technology roadmaps. *IEEE Transactions on Engineering Management, 48*(2), 132–143.

Lepak, D., Smith, K., & Taylor, M. S. (2007). Value creation and value capture: A multilevel perspective. *Academy of Management Review, 32*(1), 180–194.

Moore, G. (1999). *Crossing the chasm: Marketing and selling high tech products to mainstream customers.* New York: HarperBusiness Essentials.

O'Neill, G. D., Hershauer, J. C., & Golden, J. S. (2009). The cultural context of sustainability entrepreneurship. *Greener Management International, 55,* 33–46.

Ryan, R. (2002). *Smartups: Lessons from Rob Ryan's entrepreneur America boot camp for start-ups.* Ithaca, NY: Cornell University Press.

Sahlman, W. A. (1996). Some thoughts on business plans. In W. A. Sahlman, H. Stevenson, M. J. Roberts, and A. V. Bhide (Eds.), *The entrepreneurial venture* (pp. 138–176). Boston, MA: Harvard Business School Press.

Shaper, M. (2002). The essence of ecopreneurship. *Greener Management International, 38,* 26–30.

Venkataraman, S. (1997). The distinctive domain of entrepreneurship research: An editor's perspective. In J. Katz & R. Brockhaus (Eds.), *Advances in entrepreneurship research and growth* (Vol. 3, 119–138). Greenwich, CT: JAI Press.

Young, W., & Tilley, F. (2006). Can business move beyond efficiency? The shift toward effectiveness and equity in the corporate sustainability debate. *Business Strategy and the Environment, 15,* 402–415.

CHAPTER 7

Transforming Healthcare Quality Through Innovations in Evidence-Based Practice

Bernadette Mazurek Melnyk, Ellen Fineout-Overholt, Susan B. Stillwell, and Kathleen Williamson

Ongoing innovation, typically defined as the introduction of something new or radical that leads to positive change (Mckeown, 2008), is necessary for transforming the healthcare system and continually improving the quality of care being delivered. Innovations should be empirically supported (i.e., have an evidence base to support them), however, for healthcare administrators, policymakers, and clinicians to place confidence in them. The chances for innovations to be successful and sustained in health care are much greater in an environment with a culture that supports positive deviance (i.e., a different and creative way of thinking that challenges current paradigms and leads to positive change) (Jaramillo et al., 2008), innovation, and evidence-based practice (EBP).

Findings from studies have long supported that EBP leads to a higher quality of care, improved patient outcomes, decreased geographic variation in the delivery of care, reduced healthcare costs, and greater job satisfaction (Heater, Becker, & Olson, 1988; McGinty & Anderson, 2008; Shortell, Rundall, & Hsu, 2007; Williams, 2004). As a result, federal agencies, the Institute of Medicine (IOM), insurers, and leaders in health care advocate for and/or mandate the use of EBP by health professionals (Roundtable on Evidence-Based Medicine, 2008). However, despite its positive outcomes and the current mandates, only a small percentage of clinicians consistently use an evidence-based approach to care (McGinty & Anderson, 2008; Williams, 2004). To reach the IOM's goal that by 2020, 90% of clinical decisions are evidence based (McClellan, McGinnis, Nabel, & Olsen, 2007), there must be rapid transformations in healthcare systems to create environments with cultures that promote and sustain innovative integration of the EBP paradigm.

The main purposes of this chapter are to describe the EBP paradigm and how it can transform healthcare thinking and discuss the role of innovation within the paradigm. Key strategies for building and sustaining innovative EBP cultures within healthcare organizations are also highlighted.

EBP PARADIGM AND THE ROLE OF INNOVATION WITHIN THE PARADIGM

EBP has become a desirable characteristic for healthcare delivery organizations and educational institutions. Agencies have mandated its implementation for accreditation, certification, and recognition (Reigle et al., 2008). However, the challenge lies in the fact that the words "EBP" are present in documents or policies, but the basic paradigm that drives the thinking in organizations has not changed. If the EBP paradigm has not been diffused throughout the entire organization, processes and initiatives are typically approached in the same traditional way, often obtaining less than optimal outcomes. However, there are some clinicians and educators who have fully adopted the EBP paradigm in their care and educational curriculums who are achieving better outcomes for their patients and students. Adoption of the EBP paradigm is truly the seed and foundation for transforming health care to ultimately deliver the highest quality of care and best patient outcomes.

To adopt the EBP paradigm, it must first be understood. To understand the EBP paradigm, clinicians must first know the scope of what is understood as evidence. Evidence is "something that furnishes proof" (Merriam-Webster, 2009). In the EBP paradigm external evidence is that which is generated from well-designed research studies, whereas internal evidence is that generated from practice (e.g., quality improvement, outcomes management, and EBP implementation projects). In 2000, Sackett, Straus, Richardson, Rosenberg, and Haynes defined EBP as the conscientious use of current best evidence in making decisions about patient care. Since then, the definition of EBP has been broadened in scope and is now referred to as a life-long problem-solving approach to clinical practice that integrates (a) a systematic search for, critical appraisal of, and synthesis of the most relevant and best research (i.e., external evidence) to answer a burning clinical question; (b) one's own clinical expertise, which includes internal evidence generated from practice, data from a thorough patient assessment, and the evaluation and subsequent wise use of available resources necessary to achieve desired patient outcomes; and (c) patient values and preferences (Melnyk & Fineout-Overholt, in press) (Figure 7-1). Unlike research that generates new knowledge and external evidence for practice, EBP translates evidence from research into clinical practice to improve the quality of care and patient outcomes.

In the EBP paradigm there is no magic bullet for determining the exact percentage that should be allocated to each of the three EBP components or how they will be blended when making an innovative clinical decision. The weight of each EBP component will vary based on the characteristics of each clinician–patient clinical encounter. The clinician is the key to the integration of research, clinical expertise, and patient preferences to make the best clinical decisions. When patients are not informed, clinicians must provide the evidence to the patient in a manner that can be appreciated. The patient can then discuss how he or she would like to proceed with treatment. For example, evidence from research might support the efficacy of one antibiotic over another in treating pneumo-

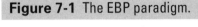

Figure 7-1 The EBP paradigm.

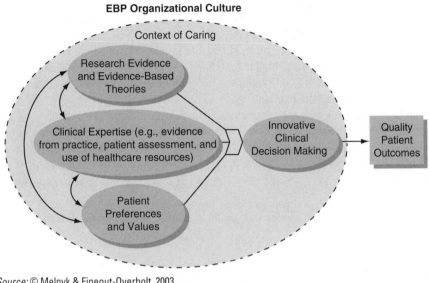

Source: © Melnyk & Fineout-Overholt, 2003.

nia in older adults. However, if the patient is likely to experience adverse side effects from the preferred antibiotic and will likely refuse to take it and there is another antibiotic with similar efficacy, the clinician has a responsibility to discuss these options with the patient. The patient can then decide which medication is the best for him or her. In this case patient preference outweighs the evidence from research and perhaps from clinical expertise. In this case example the healthcare provider and the patient choose an alternative antibiotic with similar efficacy and tolerable potential adverse effects that achieve the outcome of resolving the pneumonia.

The EBP paradigm is the underpinning of the process used to integrate evidence into practice to improve outcomes of care, the EBP process. This process begins with fostering a spirit of inquiry. Innovation in health care must start and is fostered by an environment where inquiry is not only welcome but an expectation. The steps of the EBP process move from asking a searchable, clinical question to disseminating the results of implementing the evidence in practice (Box 7-1). Each step is critical to achieving the best outcomes for the patient for whom the clinician is caring.

Step 0: Cultivating a Spirit of Inquiry

Healthcare provider dissatisfaction with the status quo can be an impetus for innovation (Mumford & Moertl, 2003). Questioning the status quo in the organization provides a

---

Box 7-1 Seven Steps of the EBP Process

Step 0: Cultivate a spirit of inquiry.
Step 1: Ask the burning clinical question in the format that yields the most relevant and best evidence (i.e., PICOT format).
Step 2: Search for and collect the most relevant and best evidence to answer the clinical question (e.g., searching for systematic reviews, including meta-analyses).
Step 3: Critically appraise and synthesize the evidence that has been collected for its validity, reliability, and applicability.
Step 4: Integrate the evidence with one's clinical expertise and the patient's preferences and values to implement a clinical decision.
Step 5: Evaluate outcomes of the practice decision or change based on evidence.
Step 6: Disseminate the outcomes of the evidence-based practice decision or change.

Source: From Melnyk & Fineout-Overholt, in press.

---

climate for clinical curiosity and a spirit of inquiry. Building a spirit of inquiry (i.e., a never-ending questioning attitude within individuals about the best practices to improve patient care and outcomes) is a necessary foundation and first step for both innovation and EBP. Without an inquisitive mind and a constant questioning spirit, innovations in the delivery of health care will not occur. Every day in health care presents opportunities for questioning current practices (e.g., in staff nurses who work in acute care hospitals, how do 8-hour vs. 12-hour shifts affect job performance and medication errors? In children hospitalized on an in-patient psychiatric unit, how does unlimited visiting by parents vs. restricted daily visitation affect the number of prn medications? In stroke patients, how does a new device that supports arm motion lead to improved functioning in the affected arm?). These types of questions lead to innovations and set the groundwork for EBP.

Step 1: Asking the Burning Clinical Question in PICOT Format

An organization that embraces a spirit of inquiry unleashes the EBP paradigm within which to transform healthcare thinking that results in positive changes and improved delivery of care. One needs to move beyond asking questions to gain knowledge only for the sake of gaining knowledge. Gaining knowledge for knowledge's sake does not lead the organization to make positive changes in its healthcare delivery system. Knowledge can be more powerful when it stimulates questions for innovative clinical decision making that leads to improved patient outcomes. These are the burning clinical questions that can lead to sustaining initiatives that transform patient, provider, and systems outcomes. Monitoring of thought processes can provide a context for the types of questions being asked. Healthcare providers can stymie their spirit of inquiry by asking only background type questions. Background questions concern general knowledge and answer such questions as "how" or "why" (Straus, Richardson, Glasziou, & Haynes, 2005). For example, how does exercise affect heart rate or why does raising the head of a patient's bed ease respirations? The answers to background questions are generally found in textbooks. Answers to background questions are important and are essential to foster innovative thinking and formulate foreground questions, which are questions that focus on clinical issues that can be answered from scientific evidence and keep the provider up-to-date in providing quality care (Fineout-Overholt, Nollan, Stephenson, & Sollenberger, 2005).

A foreground question drives the search for specific knowledge that healthcare providers need to make clinical decisions (Fineout-Overholt, Nollan, et al., 2005; Straus et al., 2005) that change the status quo and transform the quality of health care. Clinicians need up-to-date evidence to provide the best care, and they need the information quickly. For example, a patient tells you that he saw an ad for joining a group to help him stop smoking and asks you if group therapy is effective or whether hypnosis is better. Embracing the EBP paradigm leads you to resolve the uncertainty of the best therapy by formulating a foreground question and searching for the evidence that supports the blending of the evidence, patient preferences, and clinical expertise for innovative clinical decision making and a positive outcome. The innovative clinical decision making starts with asking the burning clinical question in the PICOT format.

The following PICOT format elements should be considered for all clinical questions:

- "P" refers to *population* of interest and can include individuals, families, and organizations, for example, teenagers with depression, families of critically ill patients, or Magnet facilities.
- "I" refers to the *intervention* or issue of *interest* (e.g., a treatment such as a medication) or a diagnostic test (e.g., fall prevention program or new glucometer) as well as a condition, such as a chronic condition or new diagnosis (e.g., diabetes or newly diagnosed breast cancer).
- "C" refers to *comparison* intervention (e.g., the treatment or diagnostic test being compared with the intervention) or issue of interest (e.g., acupuncture compared to heat application). "C" may also refer to the usual standard of care.
- "O" refers to the *outcome* of interest (e.g., pain, patient satisfaction or nurse retention rate).
- "T" refers to *time,* such as the length of time it would take for the intervention or issue of interest to impact the outcome. Time may or may not be appropriate for every question.

In the patient–healthcare provider scenario above, the formulated PICOT question might read, "In patients who smoke, how does group therapy compared with hypnosis affect smoking cessation?" This question focuses on specific knowledge that is searchable and answerable to inform clinical decision making with this patient compared with a background question that might read, "What therapies are available to help patients stop smoking?" Different therapies may be gleaned from reading textbooks, which may be outdated and take time to read. However, up-to-date scientific evidence to answer this specific clinical question, group therapy compared with hypnosis, can be found only in reliable sources, such as electronic databases. To be efficient, healthcare providers need to formulate the clinical question to a searchable answerable question that will lead them to a successful search. To construct a focused PICOT question, the healthcare provider can use a systematic and consistent approach with the use of a template (Table 7-1).

Strategies to promote innovative thinking and changing the status quo include having healthcare providers submit burning clinical questions, wear buttons with question marks to provide a constant reminder to question rituals and other practices, develop communities of practice or journal clubs with individuals of like minds who have a passion for improving quality care, and incorporate slack time for healthcare providers to explore and try ideas (Shirey, 2007). Once the healthcare provider has developed a well-constructed PICOT question, searching for the evidence to make an innovative change in practice is the next step in EBP.

Step 2: Searching for and Collecting the Most Relevant and Best Evidence to Answer the Clinical Question

How to find evidence to answer the question about changing the status quo or supporting an innovative culture involves an understanding of the healthcare organization's information architecture and systems that support the healthcare provider at the point of care (Porter-O'Grady & Malloch, 2008). With the rapid change in technology, healthcare providers can access current evidence from a variety of sources. An innovative model to organize evidence-based information services was proposed by Haynes (2007). This model, referred to as the 5S Model, identifies five categories of evidence, all beginning with "S", that are available for use by the clinician. The model levels the services to be accessed and recommends using "Systems" (e.g., computer decision support systems [CDSS]) first, because the CDSS can fully integrate the patient's characteristics with the current best evidence. Thus the clinician does not need to go any further. If a CDSS is not available, clinicians are suggested to use "Summaries." Summaries integrate all the evidence for managing specific health problems, not just one component of the health problem, using evidence from synopses, syntheses, and original studies. Examples of summaries offering evidence information include clinical

Table 7-1 Examples of Types of PICOT Questions

Question Type	Description	Template Example
Therapy or intervention	What treatment or intervention causes the outcome	In family members of critically ill patients (P), how does unrestricted visitation (I) compared to restricted visitation (C) affect family satisfaction (O) within the patient's ICU length of stay (T)?
Prognosis	What predictors are associated with an outcome	In patients with heart failure (P), how does home dobutamine infusion (I) compared to not agreeing to home dobutamine infusion (C) influence the patient's quality of life (O)?
Diagnosis	What test accurately diagnoses the outcome	In adults with wheezing (P) are peak flow and spirometry (I) compared to peak flow alone (C) more accurate in diagnosing asthma (O)?
Etiology	What condition is associated with an outcome	Are women age 70 and older (P) who have osteoporosis (I) compared to those without osteoporosis (C) at increased risk for fractures (O)? (T = not applicable)
Meaning	How an experience affects an outcome	How do nurses in acute care facilities (P) with shared governance (I) perceive their control over patient care delivery (O)? (T = not applicable)

Source: Adapted from Fineout-Overholt & Stillwell (in press).

evidence and DynaMed. "Synopses" provide brief information on a study or systematic review usually found in evidence-based journals. Examples include the American College of Physicians' Journal Club and Essential Evidence Plus. "Syntheses" include systematic reviews or meta-analyses that can be found in PubMed, CINAHL, and the Cochrane Library. "Studies" encompass original research that addresses single healthcare management issues, for example, a randomized control trial that can be found in PubMed or CINAHL databases. Table 7-2 provides other resources for evidence.

Table 7-2 Resources for Evidence

Resource	Description	Example
Systematic reviews	A summary of the literature that uses explicit methods to perform a thorough literature search and critical appraisal of individual studies and that uses appropriate statistical techniques to combine these valid studies. (http://www.medicine.ox.ac.uk/bandolier/booth/diagnos/glossary.html)	Cochrane Reviews (www.cochrane.org/reviews/index.htm) Joanna Briggs Institute (www.joannabriggs.edu.au/about/home.php) Campbell Collaboration (www.campbellcollaboration.org)
Clinical practice guidelines	A systematically developed statement designed to assist clinician and patient decisions about appropriate health care for specific clinical circumstances (http://www.medicine.ox.ac.uk/bandolier/booth/diagnos/glossary.html)	National Heart Lung and Blood Institute (www.nhlbi.nih.gov/guidelines/index.htm) National Guideline Clearinghouse (www.guideline.gov) Agency for Healthcare Research and Quality (www.ahrq.gov/clinic/cpgsix.htm)
Preappraised (prefiltered) evidence	Expert(s) have reviewed and/or appraised the data in the field of study (Guyatt & Rennie, 2002)	ACP Journal Club (www.acpjc.org) American Family Physician (www.aafp.org/afp) Bandolier (www.jr2.ox.ac.uk/bandolier) Evidence-Based Nursing (http://ebn.bmj.com) Worldviews on Evidence-Based Nursing (http://www.wiley.com/bw/journal.asp?ref=1545-102X&site=1) International Journal of Evidence-Based Healthcare (http://www.wiley.com/bw/journal.asp?ref=1744-1595&site=1)
Peer-reviewed (refereed) journals	A process in which papers undergo review by experts; intended to ensure high quality of the subject worthy of publication (Brown, 2009)	Check individual journal; Ulrich's Periodicals Directory provides refereed information (www.ulrichsweb.com)

If evidence services are not available, the EBP paradigm requires innovative searching strategies for relevant information. Databases may include Web-based sites, such as PubMed (www.pubmed.gov) and National Guideline Clearinghouse (www.guideline.gov), or electronic databases, such as MEDLINE (literature of interest to many disciplines), CINAHL (literature specific to nursing), or PsychINFO (literature specific to mental health and psychology). To find the answer to the PICOT question, more than one database can be quickly searched. The keywords in the PICOT question should be used to guide the search process and become the search terms in the database. Thus formulating a well-developed PICOT question drives a precise and effective search. The search is to answer a narrow and specific burning clinical question with relevant evidence to determine if the practice change is safe and produces the best outcome. For example, in the PICOT question, "In *family members of critically ill patients* (P), how does *unrestricted visitation* (I) compared to *restricted visitation* (C) affect *patient physiological stability* (O) during *the patient's ICU length of stay* (T)?", key terms are italicized. To effectively search the database, each term would be searched individually using the database-controlled vocabulary when available (e.g., MeSH terms in MEDLINE or Subject Headings in CINAHL). The controlled vocabulary is an indexing system that provides more power for your search. For example, "unrestricted visitation" was indexed, among others, to "office visits," "home visits," and "visitors to patients." Selecting "visitors to patients" resulted in 1,252 articles. Using the text word "unrestricted visitation" yielded three articles. Depending on the database, not all keywords are indexed or have an appropriate indexing term. Thus using the text word or a synonym is necessary.

Using text words for topics that are new and where little available information in journals is likely would be an appropriate approach to search databases (Fineout-Overholt, Nollan et al., 2005). When each keyword from the PICOT question has been individually searched, the searches should be combined using Boolean connectors to narrow the search to the specific question. Previously, searching the term "visitors to patients" resulted in 1,252 articles—a number unrealistic to review for the busy healthcare provider. Combining the searches may result in a more manageable number of articles that are specific to answer the PICOT question. Therefore the Boolean connector "and" should be used with all relevant searches. One other technique to rapidly search for relevant and manageable evidence is using "limits" (e.g., limit your search to "humans" and the "English" language). Figure 7-2 shows an example of search results searching keywords individually, combining searches, and limiting the search to English.

Note that words in parenthesis are keywords using controlled vocabulary, words in quotation marks are text words, and combined searches are indicated by the search numbers (S9, S6, or S6,S3,S2) connected with the Boolean connector "and." Search S9 yielded 8,414 articles, whereas S6 yielded 4,946 articles. Combining these two individual searches yielded 22 articles, a manageable list of articles to move to the next step of critical appraisal.

Figure 7-2 Sample Search Results

Add to Search	Search ID#	Search Terms	Search Options	Actions
☐	S11	S9 and S6	Limiters – Language: English Search modes – Boolean/Phrase	View Results (22) Revise Search View Details
☐	S10	S9 and S6	Search modes – Boolean/Phrase	View Results (23) Revise Search View Details
☐	S9	"visit"	Search modes – Boolean/Phrase	View Results (8414) Revise Search View Details
☐	S8	S6 and S3 and S2	Search modes – Boolean/Phrase	View Results (2) Revise Search View Details
☐	S7	S6 and S5 and S4	Search modes – Boolean/Phrase	View Results (3) Revise Search View Details
☐	S6	(MH "Critically Ill Patients")	Search modes – Boolean/Phrase	View Results (3946) Revise Search View Details
☐	S5	"family satisfaction"	Search modes – Boolean/Phrase	View Results (204) Revise Search View Details
☐	S4	(MH "Visitors to Patients")	Search modes – Boolean/Phrase	View Results (1252) Revise Search View Details

Step 3: Critical Appraisal and Synthesis of Evidence

Step 3 in the EBP process is appraising research evidence to see if it is well done (i.e., valid), clinicians can expect similar outcomes (i.e., reliable), and it is applicable to the patients for whom the clinician cares. However, the initial appraisal (i.e., evaluation and synthesis of the evidence) for clinicians includes how they think and talk about external evidence (i.e., research). This critical appraisal and synthesis of external evidence is an essential aspect of living the EBP paradigm (Fineout-Overholt, 2008). A quick evaluation of where emphasis is placed in regard to research can assist clinicians in understanding the value they place on research and its use to change practice and improve outcomes. Either clinicians emphasize the conduct of research methods (i.e., the practice of research) or they emphasize how research can be used in practice (i.e., the worth of a study to improving practice outcomes) (Fineout-Overholt, 2008). This type of careful inspection can assist clinicians in determining whether or not research is considered as useful to daily clinical decision making within their clinical environment.

Clinicians may request knowledge/information from sources other than themselves. However, if they do not seek the best available knowledge (i.e., external and internal evidence), their decision making will be off-base with less than quality outcomes. Pravikoff,

Tanner, and Pierce (2005) found that approximately 67% of clinicians used their colleagues as their most likely source of information, not findings from research. This is unfortunate because all information applied to clinical decision making must be valid and reliable. It is challenging at best to hold colleagues' opinions up to scrutiny for their worth to innovative clinical decision making without objective data to support that their opinions are valid and reliable. However, a barrier to seeking out research findings is the ease of their use by clinicians. An innovative approach to incorporating research findings into decision making is required or clinicians simply do not have the time to engage in this sometimes less than user-friendly source of valid and reliable information.

The traditional approach to evaluating whether or not research was usable in practice was to critique it. Critique is defined as the act of criticizing or a critical discussion (*Merriam-Webster,* 2009). The focus of this endeavor often has been to find the errors or flaws. In contrast, critical appraisal is focused on appraising the worth of the research to practice. Diamonds are appraised for their gem quality (i.e., worth). Those that are considered higher in gem value are appraised as having higher worth. Errors in the diamond (i.e., clarity) are considered in the appraisal process, as well as its ability catch the light (i.e., cut), its size (i.e., carat), and its color. All these aspects of the diamond are synthesized into a gestalt recommendation of its worth. Appraisal of research is quite similar. The EBP paradigm requires that clinicians carefully consider the aspects of each study with a focus on how they influence the utility (i.e., applicability) of the research to clinical decision making.

Clinicians practicing based on the EBP paradigm value internal and external evidence for clinical decision making. However, Pravikoff and colleagues (2005) found that the number one personal barrier to practicing based on evidence was a lack of value for research. Such disparity in values provides opportunity for innovation. The EBP paradigm, with its focus on quality patient outcomes that are confidently anticipated, enables clinicians to reevaluate their priorities, values, and investment of time and energy in patient care. Critical appraisal is an investment for a clinician. The appraisal process begins with rapid critical appraisal (RCA) of the final cohort of studies from the search.

Each study, review, or guideline from the search has to be evaluated using standardized criteria to determine if it is valid, reliable, and applicable to the patient for whom the clinician is caring. Checklists have been created to expedite the RCA process (see Box 7-2 for an example of an RCA checklist) (Melnyk & Fineout-Overholt, 2005). The product of the RCA is a narrowed cohort of "keeper" studies that will, at best, answer the clinical question or, at worst, inform the issue (Fineout-Overholt, 2008). Although the RCA process is innovative itself, if there are no studies to apply the process to, further opportunity for innovation occurs. Clinicians without valid, reliable, and applicable external evidence to guide practice cannot rely on tradition to underpin their work. They must determine what practice-generated outcomes exist (i.e., internal evidence) that demonstrate quality outcomes are being achieved.

Box 7-2 Rapid Critical Appraisal Checklist for a Randomized Clinical Trial (RCT)

1. Are the study findings valid?

A. Were the subjects randomly assigned to the experimental and control groups?   Yes   No   Unknown

B. Were the follow-up assessments conducted long enough to fully study the effects of the intervention; Were the outcomes measured with valid and reliable instruments?   Yes   No   Unknown

C. Did at least 80% of the subjects complete the study?   Yes   No   Unknown

D. Was random assignment concealed from the individuals who were first enrolling subjects into the study?   Yes   No   Unknown

E. Were the subjects analyzed in the group to which they were randomly assigned?   Yes   No   Unknown

F. Was the control group appropriate?   Yes   No   Unknown

G. Were the subjects and providers kept blind to study group?   Yes   No   Unknown

H. Were the instruments used to measure the outcomes valid and reliable?   Yes   No   Unknown

I. Were the subjects in each of the groups similar on demographic and baseline clinical variables?   Yes   No   Unknown

2. What are the results of the study and are they important?

A. How large is the intervention or treatment effect (NNT, NNH, Effect size, level of significance)?   _____

B. How precise is the intervention or treatment (Confidence Interval)?   _____

3. Will the results help me in caring for my patients?

A. Are the results applicable to my patients?   Yes   No   Unknown

B. Were all clinically important outcomes measured?   Yes   No   Unknown

C. What are the risks and benefits of the treatment?   _____

D. Is the treatment feasible in my clinical setting?   Yes   No   Unknown

E. What are my patients/family's values and expectations for the outcome that is trying to be prevented and the treatment itself?   _____

Source: Melnyk & Fineout-Overholt, ARCC, Inc.

The level of evidence (i.e., the study design, including whether it is a systematic review, randomized controlled trial, or case-control study) can assist clinicians in determining the study's worth to practice. There are different study designs that best provide evidence to answer specific types of clinical questions. For example, the best design to provide a confident recommendation for what should be the care provided to answer an intervention clinical question is the study design of a systematic review of randomized controlled trials. This is called level I evidence for that type of question (Box 7-3). If the clinical question were asking about the meaning of an experience (e.g., new diagnosis, hospitalization, new baby), the best study to provide an answer would be a synthesis (i.e., systematic review) of qualitative design studies. This would be level I (i.e., the best evidence) for that type of question (Fineout-Overholt & Stillwell, in press). The bottom line for clinicians is the confidence they have in the study findings. To determine whether or not there is enough confidence in the study findings to act on them requires understanding of the level of the evidence and the quality of the evidence (i.e., how well the study is conducted or its validity).

Assessing the validity of a study requires clinicians to understand what constitutes well-conducted research. Flawed methodology of a study can invalidate the findings, rendering them unusable for practice. It must be emphasized that flawed methodology does not mean negative findings. A very well-done study can find that an intervention does not work as the researcher expected it to, and this information is valuable to clinical practice. Often, clinicians and educators focus on studies with positive findings; however, this approach provides only knowledge about what does work, neglecting those studies that inform clinicians about what does not work. Both kinds of studies are valuable to innovative clinical decision making.

Once validity has been established, clinicians focus on the findings of the study. If findings are reliable (i.e., if clinicians do what the researchers did, they will get similar results), then the findings should be put into practice. When study findings are valid and

---

Box 7-3 Levels of Evidence for Intervention Clinical Questions

Level I: Evidence from a systematic review or meta-analysis of all relevant randomized controlled trials
Level II: Evidence obtained from well-designed randomized controlled trials
Level III: Evidence obtained from well-designed controlled trials without randomization
Level IV: Evidence from well-designed case-control and cohort studies
Level V: Evidence from systematic reviews of descriptive and qualitative studies
Level VI: Evidence from single descriptive or qualitative studies
Level VII: Evidence from the opinion of authorities and/or reports of expert committees

Source: From Melnyk & Fineout-Overholt, 2005.

Table 7-3 Example of an Evaluation Table

Citation/ Purpose	Conceptual Framework	Design/ Method	Sample/Setting	Major Variables Studied and Their Definitions	Measurement	Data Analysis	Findings	Level & Quality of Evidence (Strength & Confidence to Act)
EXAMPLE Author Year Title Brief purpose	Theoretical basis for study (e.g., Maslow, Roy's Adaptation Model, Self-regulation Theory)	e.g., Cohort Study (CS), Randomized Controlled Trial (RCT)	Number (N=) of subjects Characteristics (e.g., age—list only pertinent characteristics), Attrition rate (e.g., %)	Independent variables (e.g., IV1 =; IV2 =) Dependent variables (DV)	IV1 = scales used with validity/ reliability information IV2 = scales used with validity and reliability information	What statistics were used to answer the question (e.g., ANOVA)	Statistical findings (e.g., results for your question)	■ Level of evidence ■ Strengths and limitations ■ Benefit compared to risk or harm if implemented ■ Feasibility of use in your practice

Source: Stillwell, S. (2006). *Integrating EBP into the curriculum.* Unpublished manuscript, Arizona State University.

reliable, clinicians can have confidence in getting similar results with their patients. At this point clinicians evaluate the applicability of the findings to their patients (Box 7-3). All these aspects of research studies can be assessed within the RCA checklist.

Once the RCA process has been completed, the keeper studies are entered into the evaluation process for the purpose of synthesizing the evidence to answer the clinical question. An evaluation table has been used effectively for this endeavor (Table 7-3). Aspects of the studies are placed in the table, and as the process moves forward synthesis occurs and commonalities as well as disparities across studies begin to be apparent. Another table can be created that contains pertinent synthesis information (Table 7-4). This table brings the reader along toward the conclusion from the synthesis, which is the clinical recommendation for action on the synthesized evidence.

In addition, an innovative approach to evaluation of the external evidence is concept mapping, also referred to as mind mapping. This meta-cognitive method of appraisal offers clinicians the opportunity to "interrelate isolated concepts [PICOT elements] through visual representations of what they understand [synthesized evidence]" (Conceicao & Taylor, 2007, p. 268). Through this visual representation the relationships among the study aspects (e.g., findings, designs, limitations) and the PICOT question elements take shape and the clinical recommendation (i.e., gestalt of the evidence) becomes apparent (Figure 7-3). The final product of critical appraisal of evidence is whether or not the evidence is sufficient to lead clinicians in confident practice change and subsequent outcome. Whatever the outcome (Figure 7-4) of the appraisal (i.e., adequate well-done evidence or not sufficient or poor-quality evidence), clinicians have the opportunity to innovatively address the improvement of patient outcomes.

When the gestalt is known about the available evidence, whether found in single studies, syntheses, synopses, or summaries, clinicians need to make innovative decisions about how to implement the evidence in the care of their patients.

Step 4: Integrating the Evidence With Clinical Expertise and Patient Preferences and Values to Implement a Clinical Decision

Clinicians often report a lack of time to conduct their practices based on the full EBP process (Funk, Champagne, Wiese, & Tornquist, 1991; Gerrish & Clayton, 2004; Parahoo, 2000). However, it is often unrecognized that clinicians operate daily from the EBP paradigm. Although they may not have the time to search, appraise, and synthesize the literature for every clinical decision, it is reasonable that they incorporate the best empirical knowledge they have with their expertise and their patients' preferences before making a decision about the care of their patients.

Engaging the full seven steps of the EBP process requires forethought about impact and resources. It is important for clinicians to engage this process and for systems to innovatively consider how to cultivate an environment that supports such engagement for those endeavors that bring about confident, sustainable change. However, for daily

Table 7-4 Example of a Synthesis Table

Variables	Studies	Shaneyfelt et al. (2006)	Werb et al. (2004)	Coomarasamy & Khan (2004)	Shorten et al. (2001)	Jacobs et al. (2003)	Barnett et al. (2000)
	Level of Evidence	I	I	I	VI	VI	VI
Dependent variable	Knowledge	X	X	X	X		X
	Skills	X	X	X		X	X
	Attitudes	X	X	X	X		
	Behaviors	X		X			
	Patient outcomes						
	Demonstrated improvement	NA	X	X	X	X	No stats
Independent variables	Problem-based learning or evidence-based learning		X				
	Curriculum-integrated model			X	X	X	X

Sources: Barnett, S. H., Kaiser, S., Morgan, L. K., Sullivant, J., Siu, A., Rose, D., et al. (2000). An integrated program for evidence-based medicine in medical school. Mount Sinai Journal of Medicine, 67(2), 163–168; Coomarasamy, A., & Khan, K. S. (2004). Learning in practice: What is the evidence that postgraduate teaching in evidence based medicine changes anything? A systematic review. British Medical Journal, 329, 1–5; Holloway, R., Nesbit, K., Bordley, D., & Noyes, K. (2004). Teaching and evaluating first and second year medical students' practice of evidence-based medicine. Medical Education, 38, 868–878; Jacobs, S. K., Rosenfeld, P., & Haber, J. (2003). Information literacy as the foundation for evidence-based practice in graduate nursing education: A curriculum-integrated approach. Journal of Professional Nursing, 19(5), 320–328; Shaneyfelt, T., Baum, K. D., Bell, D., Feldstein, D., Houston, T. K., Kaatz, S., et al. (2006). Instruments for evaluating education in evidence-based practice: A systematic review. Journal of the American Medical Association, 296(9), 1116–1127; Shorten, A., Wallace, M. C., & Crookes, P. A. (2001). Developing information literacy: A key to evidence-based nursing. International Council of Nurses International Nursing Review, 48, 86–92; Werb, S. B., & Matear, D. W. (2004). Implementing evidence-based practice in undergraduate teaching clinics: A systematic review and recommendations. Journal of Dental Education, 68(9), 995–1003.

Figure 7-3 PICOT question and evidence.

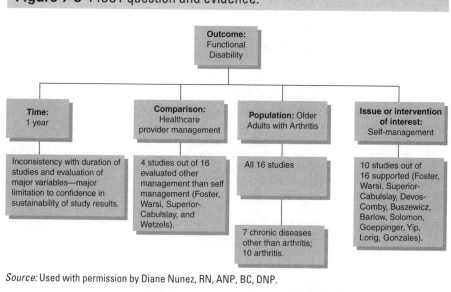

Source: Used with permission by Diane Nunez, RN, ANP, BC, DNP.

decision making, the EBP paradigm is the underpinning for clinical decision making that ensures the small in nature but large in impact decisions (e.g., prioritizing mouth care for the newly intubated patient or advocating for parent participation in a single event of a hospitalized child's care) get made, especially when patient preferences and clinician experience challenge the status quo of care and drive the decision making over and above the science. Barriers to EBP offer an opportunity for innovative care.

Clinical decision making within the EBP paradigm requires the innovative union of evidence with clinical experience and patient preferences. Integration of experiential knowledge within the EBP paradigm is essential for quality outcomes to be achieved. In addition, the integration of empirical knowledge (i.e., blending internal and external evidence) into the EBP paradigm is imperative. This approach can be used in current change methodologies but is not sometimes evident in their descriptions. For example, the plan-do-study-act (PDSA) method may or may not bring in external evidence. Ideally, the data brought into the decision making are a blend of valid research and internal evidence from quality initiatives. However, some use this methodology in a manner that ignores scientific knowledge or, at best, assumes clinicians bring this knowledge to decision making. The findings of Pravikoff and colleagues (2005) refute that assumption. A major force in the healthcare improvement movement is the Institute for Healthcare Improvement (IHI). Don Berwick, one of the nation's leading authorities on healthcare quality and improvement issues, and his colleagues have done an outstanding job of heightening providers' awareness of the need for outcome

Figure 7-4 Innovative clinical decision making within the EBP process.

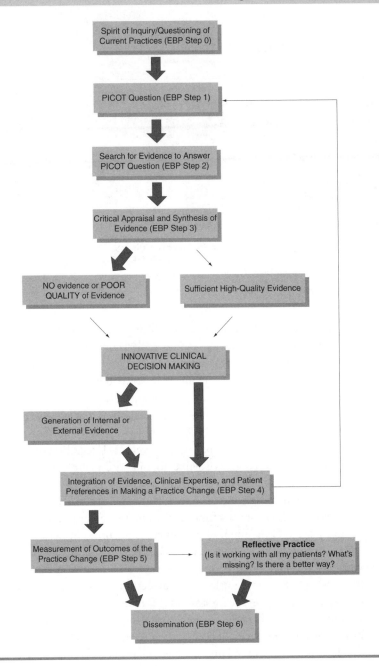

evaluation and the link between action and outcome. However, on the IHI Web site (http://www.ihi.org/IHI/Topics/Improvement/ImprovementMethods/Changes/), the process of rapid cycle change using PDSA is described as follows:

> A change concept is a general notion or approach to change that has been found to be useful in developing specific ideas for changes that lead to improvement. Creatively combining these change concepts with knowledge about specific subjects can help generate ideas for tests of change. After generating ideas, run Plan-Do-Study-Act (PDSA) cycles to test a change or group of changes on a small scale to see if they result in improvement. If they do, expand the tests and gradually incorporate larger and larger samples until you are confident that the changes should be adopted more widely.

For this type of rapid cycle change to be most effective at sustaining quality outcomes, external evidence must be combined with the internal evidence from practice before decisions are made about what should be done. Although change is imperative, we cannot engage in tests of change for which we are not reasonably confident about the outcome. The only valid and reliable source of that confidence is a blend of both scientific and practice-based evidence. The costs are too high to conduct tests of change based solely on ideas generated from experience or best practice in other institutions. Clinical decision making based on small tests of change may incur error that is not acceptable or even unsafe for patients. However, evidence-based rapid cycle change (e.g., using the PDSA method) can bring out quick application of the best we know and demonstrate desirable outcomes in an innovative way that can be sustained.

Some caveats are in order for clinicians who are daily changing practice and making highly influential clinical decisions. First, the notion of harm must be forefront. Clinicians cannot know the margin of harm associated with ideas that are not evidence based. Feasibility of initiatives also is important to sustainability and requires both external and internal evidence to demonstrate what will work in a particular environment. As clinicians evaluate how they make decisions (e.g., based on evidence, status quo [we've always done it this way], experience alone), there is opportunity for innovative decision making.

Step 5: Evaluating the Outcomes of the EBP Change

The fifth step in the EBP process is evaluating the outcomes of the practice decision or change based on evidence (Melnyk & Fineout-Overholt, 2005). According to Fineout-Overholt, Melnyk, and Schultz (2005), "clinicians must carefully consider appropriate outcomes to best reflect the success of evidence implementation" (p. 335). According to Donabedian (2003), outcomes are desirable or undesirable changes in individuals and populations that can be attributed to health care. Outcomes might include changes in health status, knowledge acquired, behavior of patients and family members that may influence future health and care, and satisfaction of patients and family members with the care received and its outcome (Donabedian, 2003). EBP has an effect on patients' clinical, physiological, physical, psychological, and social outcomes as well as on the healthcare system's cost, access, and quality (Donabedian, 2003). Outcomes should be measurable to be evaluated so change and impact on care can be documented.

To understand the impact of an evidence-based implementation project, outcomes need to be collected, analyzed, interpreted, and used to improve practice (Fineout-Overholt & Johnston, 2006). To produce quality patient, provider, and system changes in clinical practice, innovative clinical decision making using valid and reliable outcome data is essential.

Step five of the EBP process helps the clinician to determine if the EBP implementation project was successful, effective, equitable, timely, and needs to be modified or discarded (Gawlinski, 2007). Outcomes flow from the PICO question. For example, in the following PICO question, "In adult ICU patients (P), how does unrestricted visitation (I) versus restricted visitation (C) affect family satisfaction (O)?" Outcomes selected should (a) be relevant to the EBP project objective, (b) reflect what the clinician is aiming to accomplish, (c) be achievable, and (d) be measurable (i.e., the data on the outcome must be available) (Block, 2006; Gawlinski, 2007). Evaluating the impact of an EBP implementation project is important to determine whether the outcomes observed in studies are similar when applied to actual clinical practice (Gawlinski, 2007).

It is important to know how to enter data into a database and analyze data using simple statistics (Fineout-Overholt & Johnston, 2007). The collection of baseline data for the project is needed to understand the background and significance of the problem. During the postimplementation phase of the EBP project, baseline data are used to compare with data collected after implementation to measure impact on the outcome(s).

Healthcare organizations have their own systems that collect, maintain, and analyze data. They collect data in a variety of categories, including length of stay, failure to rescue, number of infant deliveries, complication rates, infection rates, fall rates, vital signs, and pain management, to name just a few. Understanding the structure of the organization (e.g., who holds the data? who generates the data? where are data located and how are data used?) is important to investigate before starting an EBP implementation project. It is important to determine the appropriate outcomes that can be measured to evaluate the impact of an EBP implementation project. Another strategy of locating outcomes is through prior research on the issue and what is expected to change with the evidence-based implementation project (Gawlinski, 2007). Evaluation of outcomes from an EBP implementation project involves following up to determine whether actions or decisions were useful and achieved the desired outcomes (Polit & Beck, 2008). Once the outcomes are identified, it is important to determine how to measure them. Too⌐ ⌐ tion, cost of tool(s) and time, how and who will be involved in collection of the data, anᴅ ensuring inter-rater reliability are important to figure out before implementation (Gawlinski, 2007). According to Gawlinski (2007), it is best to use instruments from the original research that are short, concise, user-friendly, and easy to complete rather than developing new ones. Determining the method and timing of evaluation, such as pre-test–post-test, and for how long the implementation will take for sustainability also are needed before implementation (Gawlinksi, 2007; Melnyk & Fineout-Overholt, 2005).

Data collection should be driven by the outcomes in the EBP implementation project. It is important to ask the right question and be clear about the request for data. Sources of internal evidence, which is locally obtained facts or information, can be located in many areas in an organization (Stetler & Caramanica, 2007) and can include the following:

- Quality management data (incident reports, sentinel events, patient satisfaction and regulatory/accreditation requirements)
- Finances (billing and diagnosis-related groups)
- Human resources (employee and payroll systems)
- Clinical systems (laboratory and point-of-care outcomes)
- Health information management data
- Administration (dashboards, bed flow)
- Electronic medical records (patient records)
- Data collected from outside sources (Agency for Health Research and Quality, National Database of Nursing Quality Indicators, Centers for Medicare and Medicaid Services [CMS], discharge databases, etc.)

Data can stimulate discussions about evidence-based projects, identify groups at risk, and make findings easy to interpret. "Measuring outcomes and linking them to nursing actions is critical in developing an evidence-based practice and in launching high-quality improvement efforts" (Polit & Beck, 2008, p. 323).

In the EBP paradigm, data-driven decision making is making use of data from published research, unpublished research, outcomes management initiatives, quality initiatives, or implementation projects to drive healthcare decisions (Fineout-Overholt and Johnston, 2007). Innovation in the use of collecting, maintaining, analyzing, and interpreting data in health care lies at the heart of redesigning and improving healthcare delivery (Block, 2006). Outcomes are often tied to reimbursement and regulatory issues by organizations such as The Joint Commission, CMS, IHI, and the American Nurse Credentialing Center Magnet Recognition Program (Fineout-Overholt & Johnston, 2007). When a healthcare system provides care that is safe, effective, patient-centered, timely, efficient, and equitable, it is far more successful in meeting patients' needs and improving healthcare outcomes (Block, 2006; IOM, 2001). Patients should receive care that is based on the best evidence, effective, efficient, and delivered in a seamless, coordinated effort (Block, 2006; IOM, 2001). Healthcare systems have a duty to provide evidence-based innovative clinical decision making to produce quality patient outcomes.

Evaluating available resources is an important step in the EBP paradigm. Having the right up-to-date resources can influence point-of-care decision making. Interdisciplinary healthcare professionals and administration should be involved when planning and implementing evidenced-based projects. Necessary training and resources, such as EBP education, technology infrastructure, data mining, and statistical analysis support for successful EBP implementation, should be provided. According to Simpson (2006), nurses cannot shy away from technology and need to contribute and be part of the process to establish their contribution to patient outcomes. The use of electronic health records and computerized physician order entry and dashboards are information-rich resources that provide clinicians with searchable databases to locate outcomes in order to (a) assess whether a problem exists, (b) obtain baseline data before implementing an EBP project, and (c) allow access to important data to evaluate a project's outcomes. To determine if the project is successful and has produced the impact on patient care, outcomes must be measured.

Step 6: Disseminating the Outcomes of the EBP Decision or Change

Step 6 in the EBP process is disseminating outcomes from the implementation change project. So often, healthcare institutions and clinicians do not learn about the success of EBP changes because the findings are not disseminated. Even within the same organization, outcomes generated from executing a successful EBP implementation project on one unit are not shared with other units. As a result of these silos, change and positive outcomes are often isolated, when in reality they could produce more widespread benefits. Healthcare professionals need to be aware of the most recent evidence that can inform best practices (Cheek, Gillham, & Ballantyne, 2005; Oermann et al., 2008).

Oermann and colleagues (2008) state that "When studies reveal new findings and validate nursing interventions and best practices, that information needs to be communicated to nurses who can consider its use in practice" (p. 150). Researchers need to communicate their findings in clinical journals so that clinicians can understand it and for their work to impact clinical practice (Cheek et al., 2005; Melnyk & Cole, 2005; Oermann, Galvin, Floyd, & Roop, 2006; Oermann et al., 2008). Researchers who publish their work can provide information on how findings can be used in clinical practice, collaborate with practitioners by having them review reports for clinical relevance, and present findings at conferences for practitioners (Oermann et al., 2006). Publishing and presenting in clinical journals and conferences promotes the growth of EBP (Oermann et al., 2008), although it is important to note that dissemination of knowledge/

reports from studies and EBP implementation projects alone are usually in changing practice, because clinicians must have sufficient knowledge and skills in EBP to translate published findings into clinical practice.

The EBP paradigm requires out-of-the-box thinking when disseminating the results of an evidence-based change project. Traditional ways of dissemination include developing a manuscript for publication in a clinical journal and presenting a poster/podium presentation at a conference. To influence practice change, communicating the outcomes of an EBP project in other innovative ways is a necessity. Innovative strategies for sharing results of an EBP implementation project with clinicians within a healthcare organization might include using the Intranet to post the results of a project, newsletter articles, journal clubs, staff meetings, EBP rounds, council meetings, and posters in the workplace. Outcomes from the project also can be used to write new guidelines, procedures, and/or policies and workplace competencies (Gawlinski, 2007).

CREATING A CULTURE TO IMPLEMENT AND SUSTAIN EBP INNOVATIONS IN HEALTHCARE SETTINGS

To create an environment and culture that fosters the implementation and sustainability of EBP innovations to transform health care, innovation and EBP must be established as central themes in the vision and purpose of an organization (Melnyk & Davidson, in press). The vision and mission should be displayed prominently throughout the organization as a constant reminder of the high priorities of the institution. When all new clinicians are oriented to an organization, the vision and mission should be highlighted so that the priorities of the institution are clear and individuals understand exactly how they can contribute to them. Performance evaluations and clinical ladder systems also should include expectations for transforming health care through innovative evidence-based decision making and care.

Organizational leaders sometimes forget how critical a common vision, created by a strong leadership team with input from clinicians, is for fostering an environment where innovative evidence-based decision making permeates throughout the institution. In addition, role modeling of innovative best practices by administrators and managers communicates to clinicians that the leadership team is willing to walk the walk themselves and not demand a type of care they are not willing to deliver.

Once the vision is set for creating a culture in which innovative EBP decision making is the norm, the development of a strategic plan that outlines action strategies with timelines and potential barriers with mechanisms to overcome them is necessary (Melnyk & Fineout-Overholt, 2005). Clinicians should be involved in the strategic planning process so they feel ownership of the plan, which typically results in a deeper investment in it and in the institution.

Building a cohesive team who will lead the implementation effort also is key to the success of the project. Informal leaders throughout the organization who do not hold titles but who have strong influence with their peers can be extremely helpful to the success of the strategic plan. These individuals are often champions and can help to overcome barriers, especially negative attitudes by staff, when encountered.

Sustainability is becoming a frequently used buzz word in many arenas (Melnyk, 2007). For sustaining a culture of innovation and EBP, there needs to be mechanisms in place to continue and accelerate the implementation of EBP once it is initiated in a system. It is common for health professionals to become excited about learning EBP knowledge and skills. Unfortunately, that excitement often diminishes as time goes on and clinicians are faced with heavy caseloads and stressful working conditions, which is the reason that many of them say they are unable to provide evidence-based care. In lieu of the stressors in today's healthcare environments, point of care clinicians need a key mechanism to assist them with implementing and sustaining innovative evidence-base care. This key mechanism may very well be an EBP mentor or an advanced practice nurse with in-depth knowledge and skills in EBP as well as in organizational and individual behavioral change strategies, which was first proposed in Melnyk and Fineout-Overholt's

Figure 7-5 Melnyk and Fineout-Overholt's ARCC model.

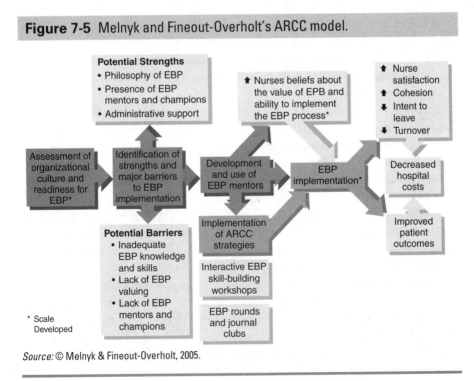

Source: © Melnyk & Fineout-Overholt, 2005.

advancing research and clinical practice through close collaboration (ARCC) model (Figure 7-5) (Melnyk & Fineout-Overholt, 2002). The ARCC model was first conceptualized in 1999 by Melnyk as part of a strategic planning effort to advance system-wide implementation and sustainability of EBP in an academic medical center and progressive healthcare community (Melnyk & Fineout-Overholt, 2002). The very first step in the ARCC model is an organizational assessment of the culture and readiness for EBP so that EBP facilitators and barriers can be identified with a plan to overcome them. EBP mentors are then developed and placed within the healthcare system to work directly with point-of-care staff to foster their knowledge and skills in innovative evidence-based care. Prior research findings have indicated that EBP mentors are key in strengthening clinicians' beliefs about EBP and their ability to implement it (Melnyk & Fineout-Overholt, 2002). Other studies also found that when EBP beliefs are strong, there is greater implementation of EBP (Melnyk et al., 2004). In addition, findings from a randomized, controlled pilot study indicated that nurses who received mentoring from an ARCC EBP mentor, in comparison with those who received mentoring in physical assessment skills, had stronger EBP beliefs/confidence, greater implementation of EBP, and stronger group cohesion (R. F. Levin, Pace University, Lienhard School of Nursing, New York, NY, personal communication, 2006), which is known to be a predictor of nurse satisfaction and turnover rates.

The ARCC model defines key components of the EBP mentor role that include the following:

- Assessing the state of readiness of an organization to sustain an EBP culture, including strengths and limitations
- Stimulating, facilitating, and educating clinical staff toward a culture of EBP, including overcoming barriers to best practice
- Role modeling EBP
- Working with staff to generate internal evidence to guide best practice through outcomes management and facilitating staff involvement in research to generate external evidence
- Using evidence to foster best practice
- Collaborating with interdisciplinary professionals to advance and sustain EBP (Melnyk, 2007).

EBP mentors also have outstanding strategic planning, implementation, and outcomes evaluation skills so they can monitor the impact of their role and overcome barriers in moving to a culture of best practice.

Other strategies for fostering and sustaining an innovative EBP culture include conducting (1) innovation workouts (i.e., sessions where groups of clinicians and leaders convene to brainstorm innovations in evidence-based care); (2) EBP rounds, where the clinical significance of a problem is introduced, followed by presentation of the PICOT question, the search for evidence, critical appraisal of the evidence, and recommendations for a clinical practice change based on the evidence; and (3) journal clubs where clinicians learn the skills of EBP and work together on evidence-based solutions to healthcare problems. Placing PICOT boxes on clinical units can be a constant reminder to staff to continually question their practices. In addition, the formation of EBP councils within healthcare organizations to assess current practices and generate innovative evidence-based solutions to improve practice and patient outcomes can foster a culture of best innovative practices. Providing the resources and tools that clinicians need to implement innovative best practices also is essential, including computers at point of care for searching and release time to work on innovative EBP implementation projects. Finally, recognizing and rewarding individuals on a regular basis who have successfully launched innovations in EBP through annual events or monthly newsletters are key to fostering an innovative EBP culture.

CONCLUSION

Healthcare reform in today's society requires leaders and clinicians who are committed to innovating clinical care through the EBP process. Through EBP innovations, healthcare quality can be improved to provide the best patient outcomes. A culture that supports clinicians to innovate improvements in patient care through EBP is essential to implementing and sustaining this gold standard paradigm.

REFERENCES

Block, D. (2006). *Healthcare outcomes management: Strategies for planning and evaluation.* Sudbury, MA: Jones and Bartlett.

Brown, S. J. (2009). *Evidence-based nursing: The research-practice connection.* Sudbury, MA: Jones and Bartlett.

Cheek, J., Gillham, D., & Ballantyne, A. (2005). Using education to promote research dissemination in nursing. *International Journal of Nursing Education Scholarship, 2*(1), Article 31.

Conceicao, S. C. O., & Taylor, L. D. (2007). Using a constructivist approach with online concept maps: Relationship between theory and nursing education. *Nursing Education Perspectives, 28*(5), 268–275.

Donabedian, A. (2003). *An introduction of quality assurance in health care.* New York: Oxford University Press.

Fineout-Overholt, E. (2008). Synthesizing the evidence: How far can your confidence meter take you? *AACN Advanced Critical Care, 19*(3), 335–339.

Fineout-Overholt, E., & Johnston, L. (2006). Teaching EBP: Implementation of evidence: Moving from the evidence to action. *Worldviews on Evidence-Based Nursing, 3*(4), 194–200.

Fineout-Overholt, E., & Johnston, L. (2007). Evaluation: An essential step to the EBP process. *Worldviews on Evidence-Based Nursing, 4*(1), 54–59.

Fineout-Overholt, E., Melnyk, B. M., & Schultz, A. (2005). Transforming health care from the inside out: Advancing evidence-based practice in the 21st century. *Journal of Professional Nursing, 21*(6), 335–344.

Fineout-Overholt, E., Nollan, R., Stephenson, P., & Sollenberger, J. (2005). Finding relevant evidence. In B. M. Melnyk & E. Fineout-Overholt (Eds.), *Evidence-based practice in nursing and healthcare* (1st ed., pp. 39–68). Philadelphia: Lippincott, Williams & Wilkins.

Fineout-Overholt, E., & Stillwell, S. B. (in press). Asking compelling clinical questions. In B. M. Melnyk & E. Fineout-Overholt (Eds.), *Evidence-based practice in nursing and healthcare* (2nd ed.). Philadelphia: Lippincott, Williams & Wilkins.

Funk, S. G., Champagne, M. T., Wiese, R. A., & Tornquist, E. M. (1991). Barriers to using research findings in practice: The clinician's perspective. *Applied Nursing Research, 4,* 90–95.

Gawlinski, A. (2007). Evidence-based practice changes: Measuring the outcome. *AACN Advanced Critical Care, 18*(3), 320–322.

Gerrish, K., & Clayton, J. (2004). Promoting evidence-based practice: an organizational approach. *Journal of Nursing Management, 12,* 114–123.

Guyatt, G., & Rennie, D. (2002). *Users' guides to the medical literature: A manual for evidence-based clinical practice.* Chicago, IL: American Medical Association.

Haynes, B. (2007). Of studies, syntheses, synopses, summaries, and systems: The "5S" evolution of information services for evidence-based healthcare decisions. *Evidence-Based Nursing, 10,* 6–7.

Heater, B., Becker, A., & Olson, R. (1988). Nursing interventions and patient outcomes: A meta-analysis of studies. *Nursing Research, 37,* 303–307.

Institute of Medicine [IOM]. (2001). *Crossing the quality chasm: A new health system for the 21st century.* Washington, DC: National Academy Press.

Jaramillo, B., Jenkins, C., Kermes, F., Wilson, L., Mazzocco, J., & Longo, T. (2008). Positive deviance: Innovation from the inside out. *Nurse Leader, 6*(2), 30–34.

McClellan, M. B., McGinnis, J. M., Nabel, E. G., & Olsen, L. M. (2007). *Evidence-based medicine and the changing nature of healthcare.* Washington, DC: National Academy Press.

McGinty, J., & Anderson, G. (2008). Predictors of physician compliance with American Heart Association guidelines for acute myocardial infarction. *Critical Care Nursing Quarterly, 31*(2), 161–172.

Mckeown, M. (2008). *The truth about innovation.* Upper Saddle River, New Jersey: Pearson Prentice Hall.

Melnyk, B. M. (2007). The evidence-based practice mentor: A promising strategy for implementing and sustaining EBP in healthcare systems. *Worldviews on Evidence-Based Nursing, 4*(3), 123–125.

Melnyk, B. M., & Cole, R. (2005), Generating evidence through quantitative research. In B. M. Melnyk & E. Fineout-Overholt (Eds.), *Evidence-based practice in nursing & healthcare: A guide to best practice* (1st ed., pp. 239–281). Philadelphia: Lippincott, Williams & Wilkins.

Melnyk, B. M., & Davidson, S. (in press). Creating a culture of innovation in nursing education through shared vision, leadership, interdisciplinary partnerships and positive deviance. *Nursing Administration Quarterly.*

Melnyk, B. M., & Fineout-Overholt, E. (2002). Putting research into practice. Rochester ARCC. *Reflections on Nursing Leadership, 28*(2), 22–25.

Melnyk, B. M., & Fineout-Overholt, E. (2005). *Evidence-based practice in nursing & healthcare* (1st ed.). Philadelphia: Lippincott, Williams & Wilkins.

Melnyk, B. M., & Fineout-Overholt, E. (in press). *Evidence-based practice in nursing & healthcare* (2nd ed.). Philadelphia: Lippincott, Williams & Wilkins.

Melnyk, B. M., Fineout-Overholt, E., Feinstein, N. F., Li, H., Small, L., Wilcox, L., & Kraus, R. (2004). Nurses' perceived knowledge, beliefs, skills, and needs regarding evidence-based practice: Implications for accelerating the paradigm shift. *Worldviews on Evidence-Based Nursing, 1*(3), 185–193.

Merriam-Webster Dictionary. (2009). *Critique.* Retrieved June 4, 2009, from http://www.merriam-webster.com/dictionary/critique

Merriam-Webster Dictionary. (2009). *Evidence.* Retrieved July 24, 2009, from http://www.merriam-webster.com/dictionary/evidence[1]

Mumford, M. D., & Moertl, P. (2003). Cases of social innovation: Lessons from two innovations in the 20th Century. *Creativity Research Journal, 13,* 261–266.

Oermann, M. H., Galvin, E. A., Floyd, J. A., & Roop, J. C. (2006). Presenting research to clinicians: Strategies for writing about research findings. *Nurse Researcher, 13*(4), 66–74.

Oermann, M. H., Nordstrom, C. K., Wilmes, N. A., Denison, D., Webb, S. A., Featherson, D. E., Bednarz, H., Striz, P., Blair, D. A., & Kowalewski, K. (2008). Dissemination of research in clinical nursing journals. *Journal of Clinical Nursing, 17,* 149–156.

Parahoo, K. (2000). Barriers to, and facilitators of, research utilization among nurses in Northern Ireland. *Journal of Advanced Nursing, 31,* 89–98.

Polit, D. F., & Beck, C. T. (2008). *Nursing research: Generating and assessing evidence for nursing practice.* Philadelphia: Lippincott, Williams & Wilkins.

Porter-O'Grady, T., & Malloch, K. (2008). Beyond myth and magic: The future of evidence-based leadership. *Nursing Administration Quarterly, 32,* 176–187.

Pravikoff, D., Tanner, A., & Pierce, S. (2005). Readiness of US nurses for evidence-based practice. *American Journal of Nursing, 105,* 40–51.

Reigle, B. S., Stevens, K. R., Belcher, J. V., Huth, M. M., McGuire, E., Mals, D., & Volz, T. (2008). Evidence-based practice and the road to Magnet status. *Journal of Nursing Administration, 38*(2), 53–102.

Roundtable on Evidence-Based Medicine. (2008). Retrieved July 15, 2008, from http://www.iom.edu/CMS/28312/RT-EBM.aspx

Sackett, D. L., Straus, S., Richardson, S., Rosenberg, W., & Haynes, R. B. (2000). *Evidence-based medicine: How to practice and teach EBM* (2nd ed.). London: Churchill Livingstone.

Shirey, M. R. (2007). Leadership and organizational strategies to increase innovative thinking. *Clinical Nurse Specialist, 21,* 191–194.

Shortell, S. M., Rundall, T. G., & Hsu, J. (2007). Improving patient care by linking evidence-based medicine and evidence-based management. *Journal of the American Medical Association, 298*(6), 673–676.

Simpson, R. (2006). Automation: The vanguard of EBN. *Nursing Management, 37*(6), 13–14.

Stetler, C. B., & Caramanica, L. (2007). Evaluation of an evidence-based practice initiative: Outcomes. Strength and limitations of a retrospective, conceptually-based approach. *Worldviews on Evidence-Based Nursing, 4*(4), 187–199.

Straus, S. E., Richardson, W. S., Glasziou, P., & Haynes, R. B. (2005). *Evidence-based medicine: How to practice and teach EBM.* Philadelphia: Elsevier.

Williams, D. O. (2004). Treatment delayed is treatment denied. *Circulation, 109,* 1806–1808.

CHAPTER 8

Combining Diffusion of Innovation, Complex, Adaptive Healthcare Organizations, and Whole Systems Shared Governance: 21st Century Alchemy

Gregory Crow and Gregory A. DeBourgh

"The real act of discovery consists not in finding new lands, but in seeing with new eyes."

PROUST

It is time for a renaissance in health care in general and in healthcare organizations (HCOs) specifically. During the last Renaissance scientists of the time attempted to transmute, or change, elements of lesser value—such as lead—into elements of greater value—such as gold. They also used alchemy in an attempt to discover an elixir of life. We all know how both scientific endeavors ended—no gold and no elixir.

However, the concept of changing, or transmuting, elements of lesser value into elements of greater value has contemporary application. In the healthcare renaissance we are writing about, we propose that any HCO can transmute, or change, its healthcare practices that are of good value into health care practices of great value and in the process discover an elixir that can sustain any HCO. Moreover, to accomplish this much will need to change, and the rationale for the changes will need to be well explained to all stakeholders.

The alchemy used to design and operate HCOs in the 20th century is not sufficient enough to meet the ever-increasing complexities of health care in the 21st century. According to Porter and Teisberg (2006), HCOs of the past were mainly focused on issues related to the control, prevention, and treatment of infectious diseases and the occasional episode of acute illness. Today's HCOs must contend with those issues as well, with the added burden of managing the complexities of chronic illness with comorbidities in patients who are living longer and therefore require extremely complex care services that are difficult to coordinate. We believe that many HCOs did not redesign their systems of care to accommodate this new reality. The complexities associated with the management of chronic illness, coupled with the ever-increasing complexities of the American healthcare system, demand new organizational arrangements and care processes. HCOs need to be much more nimble and flexible to survive in this new reality. An additional burden is the fact that HCOs will no longer be able to pass on the cost of their preventable mistakes to payers. The 20th century HCOs used the old alchemy of

- Top-down command-and-control management structures
- Fixed, rigid, and overly bureaucratic structures and care processes
- Centralized decision making
- Quality defined by the provider and the HCO
- Care processes based mostly on passed-down wisdom and very little evidence and designed around the needs of the department or provider
- Passing on costs of mistakes to federal and state governments as well as insurance companies
- Physician as the sole arbiter of all things clinical

The value of 20th century HCOs was internally defined and communicated to its community.

The 21st century is demanding a new alchemy that will change, or transmute, the way HCOs are designed, operated, and evaluated. The alchemy of this renaissance includes the concepts and practices of

- Decentralized power, authority, and decision making
- Empowered point-of-service staff and practitioners
- Care value as defined by the patient as well as the provider, the payer, and the HCO
- Evidenced-based care
- Nimble and flexible bureaucracies, responsive to the needs of the point-of-service personnel and allowing innovation to arise from anywhere in the system
- Continuum-based care designed around the needs of the patient
- Managers who lead more with influence than power
- Leaders who can tolerate ambiguity and chaos
- Costs associated with mistakes no longer be passed on to federal and state governments or insurance companies
- Physician as care team member

A 21st century HCO's value to its community is now defined not only by the HCO, but by its community, the healthcare environment in which it operates, and those paying the bills. As a consequence, it must now operate on a completely different set of assumptions.

FROM HERE TO THERE

This is a chapter about complexity, complex adaptive systems, diffusion of innovation (DOI), whole systems shared governance (WSSG), and leadership in the complex world of the American healthcare system. We believe that writing about complex adaptive systems and processes is best explored in a constant comparison and iterative narrative style. Therefore the old ways and new ways of leading are discussed side-by-side so the reader can compare both simultaneously. This chapter is built on the following positions:

- The future is not merely an extension of the past.
- Changes in health care are accelerating and will continue to do so.
- In the last century the American healthcare system shifted from an "open complicated system" to a "complex adaptive system," and many healthcare leaders did not notice.
- Only complex adaptive organizations can adequately meet the challenges of complex adaptive environments.
- Changing organizational structure and empowering staff, managers, and practitioners through WSSG without providing them with knowledge, skills, and abilities to lead will likely make an organization's problems much worse.
- DOI is an excellent vehicle for spreading management and leadership capabilities to those participating in WSSG.

Now more than ever, HCOs are struggling to meet the complex and ever-changing healthcare needs of the patients, families, and communities they serve. HCOs that have the adaptive ability to successfully deal with internal and external environmental chaos and ambiguity are not only more likely to survive and thrive in the present environment but, more importantly, they are likely to thrive into the future. When HCOs were merely complicated organizations operating in the complicated healthcare world of pre–diagnostic-related groups or more recent healthcare reforms, they could rely solely on the vertical hierarchy to manage their resources. They were able to pass on the costs associated with their mistakes to state and federal governments or to insurance companies. Those halcyon days are over. Today's complex healthcare world requires a far more sophisticated and decentralized alchemy of management and leadership techniques that involve staff, practitioners, and managers working in unison to meet the complex healthcare needs of all they serve. The leaders of these HCOs clearly understand that the future is not the past.

This last statement might sound trite; however, many managers, practitioners, and staff assume that the future is merely an extension of the past. Nothing could be further from reality. Burton and Moran (1995, p. 7) state that "future focused organizations are constantly focused on a journey of discovery, and the future is where their fortune and continued existence lies." Leaders of successful HCOs have learned some important survival lessons from the past; things that others ignored, even when their environment was screaming at them to change. These leaders tirelessly work to ensure that their organization is working in harmony with its environment, thereby creating goodness of fit. Successful leaders see goodness of fit as a blend between discovery and purpose that requires a constant blending of capital and knowledge (Burton & Moran, 1995). Successful leaders create goodness of fit by accurately reading and decoding complex, and oftentimes ambiguous, environmental feedback. Accurately decoding feedback allows novel organizational arrangements to emerge that make the HCO a better fit with its environment. Goodness of fit between an organization and its environment is the currency of the 21st century, and the only way to obtain this currency is to adapt. Effective leaders "are not willing to sacrifice tomorrow on the altar of yesterday. They do not avoid activities that build a successful tomorrow to keep yesterday alive a little longer" (Burton & Moran, 1995, p. 12).

Not only is the complexity of patient care increasing, but the rate of change that practitioners and organizations are faced with is accelerating. Because change is a constant companion, practitioners, staff, managers, HCOs, and the administrators who lead them must do a better job of providing structures and processes that facilitate goodness of fit between their organization and the environment in which they operate. Often, the important clues to the way forward are very subtle in nature, in fact, so subtle they can be completely overlooked. Moreover, as Barker (1992), Leonard (1998), and Naisbitt (1984) indicate, if the clues do not fit our mental model, we will outright reject them or dismiss them as unimportant. This lack of understanding about the way forward puts HCOs, one of a community's most valuable resources, at great risk. Barker (1992) tells us that in turbulent times when change is rapid and unrelenting, we often do not have time to react. Rather than react, we have to get much better at anticipating the future. Barker goes on to say that a "significant competitive advantage lies with those who anticipate well in turbulent times" (p. 204).

A leader's ability to anticipate the future partially depends on his or her ability to know where to concentrate his or her attention, and the attention of the entire organization, while in the midst of a tsunami of information. The leader's ability to concentrate his or her attention on the bits of information that have the greatest relevance to the organization's survivability is enhanced by the leader's willingness to explore the many potential futures of the organization. Leaders who can accurately "see and understand" what is happening inside their organization and simultaneously "see and understand" what is happening in the external environment provide the organization an opportunity to foresee, or anticipate, the future (Barker, 1992; Burton & Moran, 1995; Leonard, 1998).

Gardenfors (2006, p. 34) states that "humans are endowed with brains that have the capacity to fill in incomplete patterns in our environment, and this ability helps us to identify behaviors that will make us more successful in the future." This advantage is enhanced if the HCO has fewer and fewer incomplete patterns to fill in. This can be accomplished if staff, practitioners, and managers are empowered and willing to step out of their comfort zone and experience what the future is demanding of them. Decentralized organizations have the added advantage of having many more people helping to fill in incomplete patterns. Leaders who empower staff and encourage them to step out and experience the changing world place their organizations in a good position to take advantage of the future, rather than be a victim of the future.

Many administrators continue to act on assumptions that are out-of-date (Hammer & Champy, 1993). The problem remains that our present states of thinking, and therefore our decision-making processes, have not caught up with the realities we currently face (Barker, 1992; Naisbitt, 1984). HCOs must be willing to examine and change, where necessary, every structure and process in an effort to facilitate goodness of fit.

In addition to changing organizational structures and processes for better environmental goodness of fit, practitioners must also be willing to change their practice for a better goodness of fit between them and their organization. Changing structures and continuing care processes that are often filled with wisdom passed down from the ages, and often lacking contemporary evidence, does little to help either the organization or the patients it serves. We must embed practice changes with the best available evidence to make real and sustained change. The fact remains that many of the changes made in HCOs today turn out to be only marginally effective in dealing with the complexities of the American healthcare system. The costs associated with real change are high; however, we believe it is less expensive than the cost of not changing. Donna Shalala, former U.S. Secretary of Health and Human Services, notes that "health care is inherently less expensive than poor health" (as cited in McClellan, McGinnis, Nabel, & Olsen, 2008, p. 156).

Staff, managers, practitioners, and the organizations in which they work must be willing to adapt and evolve together. However, if not facilitated properly the process of identifying what changes are required to adapt and evolve can result in massive internal confusion and chaos, leading to a lack of cooperation between practitioners, management, and staff. This lack of internal cooperation is perhaps one of the major reasons HCOs are struggling to meet the demands of their environment. When an organization is internally disorganized and misaligned, it is more likely to be out of alignment with its environment, making goodness of fit between the organization and its environment difficult, if not impossible.

What more and more practitioners, staff, and administrators are beginning to understand is that the old mechanistic, hierarchical, and rigid healthcare delivery systems of the past are simply not flexible and nimble enough to meet the challenges of 21st century health care. To be nimble and flexible staff, practitioners, and leaders must have access to internal and external information that flows freely in all directions. The free flow of information is essential so that "the right person(s) can make the right decision(s), in the right place, at the right time and for the right purpose" (Porter-O'Grady & Malloch, 2007, p. 176). Timely decision making at the point-of-service by well-informed and competent staff, managers, and practitioners is essential to organizational success.

Rigid hierarchies slow down information flow in both calm and turbulent times, and when information does not flow, this sclerotic effect diminishes the capacity of the organization to meet patient needs. When practitioners and staff are required to seek permission for decisions, change moves at glacier speed. However, a time of chaos and turbulence is precisely the time when greater speed and flexibility are required. Because speed and flexibility depend on the free flow of information, meaningful, valid, and reliable information must be ubiquitous and available on demand.

SHIFT HAPPENS

It is clear that many HCOs are struggling to meet the demands placed on them by patients, families, communities, state and federal governments, insurers, and its practitioners and staff. We believe that the main impediment to meeting the demands placed on today's HCOs is largely due to how they are designed, operated, and led. Much blame has been placed on the hierarchical structures of yesteryear for an organization's inability to change with the times, and recommendations have been made to flatten organizational structures. Although we believe that organizational structures that are flat, rather than tall, are most appropriate in today's world, being flat in no way guarantees that an organization will be flexible enough to meet the demands of today's fast-paced healthcare world. Although structure is important, behavior is paramount. A flat organizational structure can produce as many impediments to organizational change as a tall one. Although it is rather easy to flatten an organization's structure, it is much more difficult to change an organization's behavior. The astute leader clearly understands that structural changes that are not coupled with behavioral changes will fall short of creating an organization that can evolve and change.

What is clear is that long ago the American healthcare system shifted from being a complicated system to a complex system. Although there are numerous reasons for this transition, such as an aging population, the size of our healthcare system, increased numbers of uninsured and underinsured, complex federal and state reimbursement schemes, technology, pharmaceuticals, and increased specialization, these things are not the cause of all our problems. The problem is that many of our HCOs have not adapted and evolved with these changes and are basically organized and operated much like hospitals in the mid-20th century. Many leaders are discovering that the rigid, hierarchical, industrial, nonadaptive systems that were effective in the past are no longer workable in today's world. These old structures are not workable because they lack the significant formal and informal vertical and horizontal linkages necessary for information to flow freely. Free-flowing information combined with a comprehensive understanding of complexity and empowered and knowledgeable staff and practitioners who are linked in ways that produce new patterns of interaction are requirements for transforming any HCO to meet the ever-changing demands of its environment.

ARE YOU RIGID AND FROZEN IN PLACE?

Most HCOs continue to be organized, operated, and led as rigid mechanistic hierarchies that are overly bureaucratic and very slow to change, much less adapt to environmental changes. According to Leonard (1998), rigid organizations exhibit very distinctive characteristics that are the result of extreme insularity:

- *Limited problem solving:* Rigid organizations, regardless of their structures, exhibit an overdependence on the strategies of the past to solve the problems of today. This type of rigidity is referred to as "path dependence." Organizations select the old path to solve problems even when better alternatives are available (Leonard, 1998). Hammer and Champy (1993) warn us that while the familiar path may be more enticing, "the easy way out leads back in" (p. 62).
- *Inability to innovate:* Rigid organizations become so paralyzed that no amount of energy can bring about meaningful innovation (Leonard, 1998). They suffer from what Barker (1992, p. 155) calls "paradigm paralysis, which is a terminal disease of certainty." These types of organizations are convinced they can continue to do what they have done in the past. In doing so they believe, or hope, that success is just around the corner. The leaders of these organizations deeply believe that what they need to do is to get their practitioners and staff to do more of what they used to do well, and if they can manage to expand and grow, their troubles will go away. This strategy just produces more trouble for the organization because it relies on old strategies to solve new problems (Leonard, 1998). Many of the problems faced by HCOs cannot be overcome by producing more of the same faster. When an organization expands and grows but does not alter its mechanisms of production, it merely produces more of the same thing and in the same way. Producing more of something that an HCO's environment no

longer requires creates greater misalignment between the organization and its environment.

- *Limited experimentation:* All, or most, innovation in rigid organizations is believed to be the exclusive domain of its top executives. The problem with this way of leading is that those at the point-of-service are completely left out of the innovation process. The innovation process is subverted into a top-down command-and-control maneuver. When experimentation is generated from the apex of the organization and is forced down through the system, failure is almost assured (Leonard, 1998; Rogers, 2003).
- *Screening out new knowledge:* Rigid organizations no longer possess the ability to experiment with new methods and processes because the few people who control the flow of external information for internal use literally screen out data and information that does not fit their world view (Leonard, 1998). Barker (1992, p. 153) calls this malady the "paradigm effect." The organization that suffers from this malady has become so invested in the present paradigm that any talk of moving beyond the present paradigm is immediately rejected. "Stay the course" becomes the organization's mantra.

Many HCOs today exhibit the same characteristics of HCOs in the mid-20th century: They are complicated open systems rather than complex adaptive systems. Complicated open HCOs do not possess the necessary adaptive abilities to match the demands of the complex adaptive environment in which they operate. Traditional bureaucratic HCOs must make the transition from complicated open systems to open complex adaptive systems. This transition is impossible without enlisting staff, practitioners, and managers in ways that create ownership and accountability. This transition is an absolute requirement of the 21st century, and many HCOs are getting a very late start.

We believe that transitioning an HCO from a complicated, slow-to-change bureaucratic one to a flexible complex one that has adaptive abilities offers HCOs their best hope for survival. Moreover, complex adaptive HCOs that use WSSG as the platform for identifying and diffusing both externally and internally generated innovations and engaged and empowered staff, practitioners, and managers that have the necessary skills to lead in turbulent times position those HCOs to thrive in our chaotic healthcare world.

Identifying, evaluating, modifying, and diffusing innovations can mean the difference between being a good HCO and a great HCO. The transformation from good to great cannot occur in mechanistic rigid hierarchies. HCOs must be willing to take a journey down a different path to reach their future. This may be a path that is less obvious, less comfortable, and less predictable and, hence, more threatening. An effective way to decrease the threats associated with traveling down new paths is to more clearly understand the new path. It is the accountability of the organization's leadership to guide the rest of the organization in understanding the need for a new path and to make the way forward more understandable and less threatening (Burton & Moran, 1995; Leonard, 1998). When the organization's staff, practitioners, and managers are frozen in fear of the prospect of taking a new and unfamiliar path, they are not likely to design new care processes that meet the changing needs of those they serve.

This may not be a journey that everyone will be eager to take; however, we can say with some confidence that when an HCO is better aligned with its environment, it is more likely to accomplish its core mission of providing exceptional patient care services to everyone who entrusts his or her life to the organization's care. However, care that is departmentalized rather than systematized will fall short of meeting the needs of patients.

We must be committed to building care processes around the patients we serve instead of around the departments and divisions we occupy. Hammer and Champy (1993) posit that successful organizations must change from functional departments to process departments. The process teams that emerge from this new structure are not comprised of "representatives" from various organizational fiefdoms whose purpose for being there is to guard their territory and turf. Instead, we believe that one of the major differences between functional teams and process teams is that the members of process teams are present to advocate for the relationship that the organization has with all it serves. Their focus is the entire care process, not just their part of the process.

Now that we have introduced the reader to the major components of this chapter, we more specifically examine each one. We begin with an overview of complexity science, systems, and complex adaptive systems. We continue with an overview of organization and leadership issues related to managing complex adaptive systems. Finally, we discuss WSSG, DOI in complex adaptive systems, and end with a proposed curriculum for leadership, as well as potential methods for the delivery of the leadership curriculum.

COMPLEXITY SCIENCE, SYSTEMS, AND COMPLEX ADAPTIVE SYSTEMS

Complexity science is a relatively new field of inquiry dedicated to a better understanding of how groups of living things, such as communities, families, groups, and organizations, behave. Much of the foundational knowledge of complexity science is derived from the science of evolution rather than the traditional industrial age view of organizations as machines. The machine metaphor for HCO design and operation has long since outlived its usefulness (Plsek & Greenhalgh, 2001; Rouse, 2008); however, not everyone who leads HCOs has noticed.

Complexity science seeks to more fully comprehend how groups of living things adapt and coevolve over time with the environment they inhabit (Rouse, 2008). An HCO—which is a group of living things—needs to adapt and coevolve with the environment it inhabits, just as any other business is expected to do. HCOs are not exempt from this evolutionary process just because of their special relationship with society. In fact, it is because of our social contract with society that we must remain nimble and flexible and ready to change to meet the complex healthcare needs of those we serve.

If there is anything that complexity science teaches us, it is that the complex problems facing HCOs today cannot be resolved by mechanistic, rigid, top-down, command-and-control hierarchical organizations. The paradigm of health care has changed, but the paradigm of HCOs has not. For example, one cannot meet the complex challenges of space travel in a hot air balloon any more than one can meet the complex challenges of 21st century health care with 20th century structures, thinking, and outdated care processes.

Organizations and environments must coevolve to ensure a goodness of fit between what the organization takes in as inputs and transforms into outputs to match the demands of the evolving environment. For the organization to adapt and evolve over time, it must change its internal structures, patterns, and processes so that its outputs match environmental demands. In this way the organization lives in harmony with its environment and is at the ready to coevolve to the next state when that is required.

SYSTEMS

The basic elements of an open system are inputs, throughputs, outputs, feedback, negative entropy, and homeostasis. Open systems are systems that communicate with and depend on their environments for the energy they require (*inputs*) so they can produce usable *outputs* for their environment. *Throughput* is the process by which a system transforms environmental inputs into useable outputs. To do this the system must be organized so that it is able to anticipate environmental demands and can produce exactly, or approximately, what the environment needs. Open systems are linear and use processes in which small inputs produce small outputs and large inputs produce large outputs. The system is dedicated to maintaining *homeostasis*, or a steady state, where the goal is to preserve the system "as is." The "as is" state is the goal, not adaptation.

Mechanistic open systems are necessary to our way of life. We rely on machines to do much of the work of today. These complicated machines, such as our cars, airplanes, and computers, have become essential to our lives. In fact, our modern HCOs are so reliant on our machines that we go to great lengths to build in redundant systems to ensure that we are never without them. However, they are the machines that assist us in providing safe quality care and, as such, are instruments of care and should not be confused with the system itself.

Systems must be alert to continuous feedback. Feedback is used to keep the system on a steady and unchanging course. To maintain this steady course, open systems do not well tolerate or encourage emergent properties to surface (Schneider & Somers, 2006). The system, in our case the HCO, uses Herculean efforts to keep emergence from occurring. Emergence means that the "machine" is producing variance, and variance threatens the well-established organizational arrangements and, more importantly, those in control of those arrangements. As the system suppresses emergent properties, it can become more-and-more out of synch with its environment. Negative feedback allows the system to perform necessary corrections to its linear processes in an effort to produce usable outputs for its environment. When systems ignore environmental negative feedback long enough, they become so out of synch with their environment that they must be "transformed" to survive. Transformation is much more difficult to lead than leading course corrections over time (Schneider & Somers, 2006).

Feedback, when coded and interpreted properly, allows the system to communicate with its environment to produce goodness of fit. If the feedback is not coded and interpreted properly, the system runs the risk of producing outputs that the environment does not need. If this process is not corrected, the system becomes more and more misaligned with its environment and, over time, entropy sets in. Entropy indicates a high level of internal disorganization (Schneider & Somers, 2006). This state of disorder is a kind of organizational ventricular fibrillation, where large amounts of energy (inputs) are consumed for fewer and fewer outputs. Organizational ventricular fibrillation is just like cardiac ventricular fibrillation in patients: It is a condition that is not compatible with life. This state cannot be maintained by growth and expansion or doing more of the same thing while wishing for a different outcome. Additionally, the system cannot correct itself by following the paths it was so dependent on in the past, such as fragmenting care processes, or by increasing the number of mid-level managers to oversee smaller and smaller segments of the care process.

HCOs have long followed this mechanistic open systems design. However, this organizational design is not one that effectively interacts with its environment in ways that produce a coevolutionary state. These types of HCOs attempt to keep their rigid and highly ordered "machine parts" in their fixed relationships. If they attempt adaptation, and they rarely do, the changes are often superficial and done in an attempt not to adapt but to keep internal and external organizational arrangements "as is." The internal dialogue is focused on "doing what we do now; doing it better and faster; and doing more of it." A more effective dialogue would be, "we had better do something different, and do it better than anyone else."

ORGANIZATIONS, MACHINES, AND PREDICTABILITY

When an organization is perceived and constructed as a "machine," its parts, and their interface with each other, are fixed and must remain so for the machine to operate reliably over time. The machine is organized in a fixed and linear fashion (Plsek, 2003), that is, part 1 must cause part 2 to move in order for part 3 to move, and so on. Plus, all the parts of the machine are of equal value to the functioning of the machine. The machine cannot function if part 2 does not cause part 3 to move.

Why did we use the machine metaphor to design HCOs? We did it because we longed for the predictability that the machine promised us. All humans generally crave predictability (Gardenfors, 2006), and healthcare professionals are keen to seek it out. We are comforted by knowing what comes next.

Today, patient care is not a complicated linear process, yet we now spend billions of dollars annually in an attempt to make it so by departmentalizing and specializing. We attempt to pass the patient from one department or specialty in a linear fashion that lacks iteration. Each department or specialist performs a specific function, often disconnected from the whole; therefore the complex healthcare needs of the patient are often not attended to, and the patient's condition can worsen.

When the complexity level of health care and patient care was low, our mechanistic hierarchical rigid systems were able to meet many of the patient's needs. What we are experiencing today is that the complex demands of patients, and the American healthcare system, has reached a complexity tipping point. As a result HCOs are finding it increasingly difficult, if not impossible, to meet the demands of the environment in which they operate. Something has to change, and it is us!

1 + 1 DOES NOT ALWAYS EQUAL 2

Think about it. As novice professionals we approach patient care hoping for predictability, and rightly so. We want our treatments to act predictably because that is best for the patient. As we are learning our profession, we do "X" and assume that "Y" will happen because we learned it in a textbook. If we do enough "X's" and "Y's" happen as a result, novice practitioners begin to assume that "X" will always cause "Y". However, experienced professionals know that this type of thinking, based on predictability rather than probability, is a trap that can be most harmful to the patients we serve and to the organizations in which we practice. Our experience teaches us that the patient's state of health is a complex and often unpredictable interplay between our treatments and the patient's internal environment of health. We appear to understand the unpredictable nature of patient care, yet we have not applied these principles to organizational design or operation.

Who we are as practitioners also follows an unpredictable path with our organizations. We are interrelated, dependent, and interdependent with the organizations in which we practice. Our relationships with our organizations and our colleagues are far more unpredictable than we sometimes want to admit. We try to control the unpredictable nature of organizational life by having "fixed" organizational charts that Adam Smith, Fredrick Taylor, or Henry Ford would recognize. We have fixed and never-changing job descriptions, fixed ways of relating and interacting that are based on one's position on the organizational chart or job title, and fixed policy and procedure manuals (either electronic or manual). When organizational elements become rigid and fixed, they become scripture, and when something becomes scripture, it becomes sacred as well as unchangeable and, ultimately, frozen in place.

The flaw in this grand machine scheme is that many of us have not realized that health care no longer has a fixed relationship with its environment or consumers; however, that was not always the case. Hammer and Champy (1993) tell us that there was a time when an organization's relationship with its environment was more fixed. They say that the "American people, deprived first by the Great Depression and then by WWII, were more than happy to buy whatever companies offered" (p. 15). Quality was not necessarily the issue; mass production drove the process. Therefore, organizations did not have to pay as much attention to environmental demands.

Henry Ford was rumored to have said, "You can have any color car you wish, as long as it is black." Ford's paradigm worked only until another car manufacturer offered a color other than black; then, suddenly, for Ford to remain viable as a company, it had to change. What business leaders were beginning to understand was that one's environment, and the consumer, had a very strong influence on the products an organization produced and, ultimately, its survival. The process of give-and-take, or coevolution of organization and environment, and particularly the HCO's coevolution with the consumers in its environment, had taken hold, and organizations would never be the same . . . although many tried.

THOSE WERE THE DAYS

The authors of this chapter have a combined practice history of over 60 years. We vividly remember a time when patients, families, and communities were most happy to receive any sort of health care. Patients and their families rarely bucked the system or demanded more input into their care. We generally told the patient what we were going to do, and the patient was expected to defer to us. We were almost completely in charge of the process. It was the horn of plenty. We admitted patients and told them what we were going to do to them. Then we had them sign a consent form. We worked our magic on them, and, after many more days in the hospital than they actually needed, we sent them home. We sent someone else the bill, and someone sent us money. The process seemed like it would go on forever. Nurses and patients rarely questioned physicians or administrators. The hierarchy was firmly in place, and the hierarchy was firmly in charge. Everyone knew their role and limits, and both were set by higher-ups.

What changed is that patients are now much better educated and informed today, and they have access to incredible amounts of information that is not written in "complicated medical speak." We remember when the *Merck Manual* was stamped with "For professional use only." Medical professionals felt like they could go to jail if they shared the sacred text with an outsider. Patients and families are no longer intimidated by our buildings, education, titles, personas, or dress. They insist on being partners in their care. This has not been the easiest transition for many healthcare professionals. The age of healthcare consumerism has arrived. We are no longer completely in charge, and as consumer expectations have soared, we are now being held accountable by patients, families, communities, state and federal governments, and insurers. The world as we knew it no longer exists—shift happened!

Because the American healthcare system is complex and adaptive, we must be too. Otherwise, we will continue to spend astronomical amounts of money, energy, and other resources in a futile effort to ensure predictability. As a result, we will continue to get diminishing returns for the effort. As was mentioned earlier, the currency of the 21st century is goodness of fit, and we must have it to gather the necessary resources from our environment to survive. Goodness of fit means that we are in harmony with our environment rather than doing battle with it.

The healthcare environment we inhabit is evolving and changing. Stability as we knew and experienced it no longer exists. However, many of our hospital machines go on as they did in the past, hoping for a different outcome or a return to the ways of yesteryear. Our paradigm, mental model, ways of thinking, and our world view are out of synch with our environment and reality. What many leaders have not yet comprehended is that our environment has a great deal of power in deciding what survives and what does not. Failure of our leaders to recognize that only complex adaptive systems can meet the demands of complex adaptive environments means they are putting the survival of their organizations in jeopardy. Organizational leaders must thoroughly comprehend that not only practitioners, but all agents in the system, must have the freedom and autonomy to adapt and evolve their relationships within their organization, coworkers, and patients so that the organization can do the same with its environment. Internal goodness of fit is essential to environmental goodness of fit. Adaptation has become essential to survival.

Hammer and Champy (1993) indicate that general industry, in an attempt to deal with increasing complexity, broke work down into smaller and smaller pieces and then hired supervisors to manage the increasingly fragmented work. In an effort to meet increased and more complex needs of patients, families, and communities, many HCOs fragmented care processes into smaller and smaller areas of specialization. They thought that the key to improved performance could be reached by working on smaller and smaller pieces of the overall care process. Hence, one of modern health care's fundamental problems emerged—fragmented care. Care became so fragmented that hardly anyone had the whole picture. Fragmentation ultimately led to uncoordinated care as the patient was passed, sometimes with great difficulty, from one department to another on their journey through the healthcare system.

Fiefdoms helped create the mindset of territory. When someone takes ownership of organizational territory, fragmentation is increased. Over time, the organizational territories of departments and divisions become more important than the whole. This leads to another and equally important crisis. It has become painfully obvious to many that the sum of many HCOs is no longer greater than its parts. We have department and divisional managers who believe that their department, or division, is more important than the organization as a whole. In other words, the organization has become subordinate to the department or division, and the fiefdoms have become institutionalized. Something has to change, and it is us!

One of the most disturbing aspects of fragmented and uncoordinated care was that we began to "empower" the patient and their family. Unfortunately, that often meant the patient, or his or her family member, had to become his or her own case manager. As case managers patients were expected to coordinate a healthcare system that we could not coordinate ourselves. The concept of the empowered patient was, and is, a good thing; however, empowering patients/families to do something we could not do was an unfair transfer of accountability. The problem of fragmentation and uncoordinated care still exists today. For patients to traverse the continuum of care, we must design care pathways that meet the complex needs of the patient without being overly complex. The processes of care need only to be complex enough to produce the desired outcomes yet simple enough to be navigated by the patient and his or her family.

Many HCOs responded to fragmented and uncoordinated care by hiring more midlevel managers, case managers, and, most recently, clinical nurse leaders to watch over and control the processes of care. Unfortunately, this created the current fiefdom structures we see today.

The solution to uncoordinated and fragmented care is counterintuitive. We do not need to hire additional overseers; we need to hire more point-of-service staff and practitioners who are empowered to work across heavily guarded departmental and divisional borders to improve the processes of care. They will need to base their care process improvements on the best available evidence, and when evidence does not exist, leaders must encourage staff to discover and document it. Having more managers to oversee a fragmented process serves only to further fragment it. You defragment a process by making it whole, not by adding more parts and players who act like machine parts or heavily guard their territory.

FROM COMPLICATED TO COMPLEX

The origin of much of our current frustrations in HCOs is because, in the last century, the American healthcare system shifted from being a complicated system to a complex system. However, many of our HCOs did not make the same shift. They are basically organized, structured, and operated much like hospitals in the mid-20th century. Minus our technology, décor, medications, and dress, a nurse from the mid-20th century could recognize and feel comfortable in many of our HCOs today. Our problems are in the 21st century, yet our tools and strategies for solving current problems are of the 20th century. Complexity science teaches us that the complex healthcare problems we face today cannot be adequately resolved by HCOs that are trapped in the traditional mechanistic hierarchical systems of yesteryear. The tools we use to solve today's problems have to be equal to the task. We need many tools in our toolboxes that assist us in managing and leading in this complex healthcare world. When the only tool you have is a hammer, everything looks like a nail. One cannot build a system with a single tool.

COMPLEX ADAPTIVE SYSTEMS

Complex adaptive systems differ from open systems in many ways. For the purposes of this chapter, however, we concentrate on five essential differences: chaos, emergence, coding feedback, path dependence, and adaptation (Schneider & Somers, 2006).

According to Plsek and Greenhalgh (2001, p. 627), "chaos produces insufficient information, making the system's next step less obvious, and by extension less predictable." This unpredictable and uncomfortable situation is the reason many organizations fall back on the old ways and the old paths that worked, only to discover, and often too late, that the old path quickly leads them right back to the place they tried to escape. Being in close proximity to chaos can be a very uncomfortable place to reside, because humans, and especially healthcare professionals, by nature dislike chaos and unpredictability.

A complex adaptive system is capable and, more importantly, willing to reside at the border of chaos and to remain poised there in an effort to discover emerging patterns of behavior that allow it to better meet environmental demands (Schneider & Somers, 2006). It is at the border between now and the future that we learn about the new demands our environment is placing on us (Kouzes & Posner, 2002). The border is where we are offered clues about what internal changes need to occur to meet emerging environmental demands. When one views chaos and rigidity as polarity, the further away from chaos, the more likely the organization is to be rigid and frozen (Schneider & Somers, 2006).

Chaos, much like our sun, provides the heat necessary for the life of the organization. The space between chaos and adaptation is a tricky position to maintain. If an organization moves too close to chaos, it can be incinerated. If an organization gets too far away, the lack of heat can cause the organization to become increasingly rigid, ending in a frozen state. It is much like the Three Bears: The organization's position needs to be just right, not too hot, or not too cold. Maintaining this position takes an organization that is capable of continuous adjustments; one whose goal is never the steady-state. To be in harmony with a complex environment, HCOs must evolve to a more complex state, remaining just close enough to chaos to flourish. This is not an option; it is a requirement for survival.

Emergence and Feedback

Leaders of complex adaptive HCOs understand that when an organization is at the edge of chaos it is time for rapid cycle experimentation, rather than the typical strategy of centralization and control. These leaders understand that it takes novel organizational arrangements, shifting power bases, strengthened internal connections/relationships, and decentralization to allow the organization to survive turbulence. We believe that shared governance is a proven decentralized and flexible organizational arrangement that facilitates the discovery of emergent structures, patterns, and processes that help to secure the new currency of the 21st century—organizational and environmental goodness of fit.

Leaders of complex organizations lead not just with power, or other top-down command-and-control behaviors, but rather with a finely nuanced combination of power and influence. Depending on the situation, they know how to combine power and influence and in what measure to use each. They lead with just enough guidance to keep the organization from descending into total disorder and chaos, while simultaneously encouraging enough experimentation to discover the way forward. Experimentation, or variance, allows the practitioners and leaders to codiscover, and experiment with, emergent properties that create better organizational goodness of fit with the HCO's environment. Variation is an absolute requirement for coevolution.

Discovering, encouraging, and experimenting with the right emergent properties are heavily reliant on reading and coding environmental feedback and having the requisite structures and processes that allow for experimentation. Environmental feedback allows the leader to make mid-course corrections to better align the organization with its environment. These mid-course corrections are not done to reach homeostasis but rather to evolve to the next level, a level compatible with its environment. Competent leaders of complex organizations clearly understand that their environment must be constantly scanned to gather the necessary information to move their organization forward (Burton & Moran, 1995; Leonard, 1998; Schneider & Somers, 2006).

HCOs that secure competent boundary spanners do best in turbulent times. Boundary spanners are those individuals who continually communicate with all elements of their external environment, scanning it to seek out clues to the future (Ferlie, Gabbay, Fitzgerald, Locock, & Dopson, 2001; Tushman, 1977). Organizations that invest this role with only one person are less effective. Boundary spanning should be the work of everyone; after all, the more informed eyes and ears an HCO has, the better it can listen to the feedback and see its way forward. Boundary spanners, and their interactions with each other, assist the HCO in its most important endeavor—adaptation—and hence goodness of fit. WSSG provides the requisite structures for boundary spanners to interact and communicate about future directions.

As an organization adapts to its environment, it does so by a process of self-organization. Self-organization is a response to identifying, encouraging, and experimenting with emergent properties. The wise leader understands that self-organization is facilitated and not designed. Self-organization emerges as an organic process, not as the result of purposeful organizational design (Schneider & Somers, 2006). The process of self-organization can present a threat to long-established territories, fiefdoms, and those who ruled them.

Path Dependence: When You See a Fork in the Road, Take It

Leaders of complex adaptive HCOs (CAHCOs) learned early on that the way forward is not down the worn-out dependable paths of the past. Instead, it is new paths with new challenges that take new skills and organizational arrangements to meet those challenges (Leonard, 1998). Their success depends on many different and sometimes counterintuitive paths. These leaders are willing to put aside much of the received wisdom of the past (Naisbitt, 1984), because they understand that past wisdom, although wise at the time, is now antiquated and based on assumptions that are no longer valid (Barker, 1992). These out-of-date assumptions often lead us down paths that are more like cul-de-sacs than through-ways. Gardnerfors (2006) posits that relying on preprogrammed behaviors makes us less flexible in dealing with novel situations in an effective manner.

When organizations, or people, are overly path dependent, they tend to apply the same decision rules to all situations, regardless of the situation's context. One surprising path-dependent characteristic is that path-dependent behaviors are evoked even when there are better alternatives available (Leonard, 1998; Schneider & Somers, 2006). Path dependence is a form of magical thinking, where a person, or organization, does the same thing over and over again, no matter the situation, hoping for a better outcome. Most healthcare professionals have a great deal of experience with path dependence. We are often surprised when patients ignore our advice and continue on the same ineffective path to health and wellness, all along hoping for a better outcome. We are often very frustrated by these types of patients, because they never seem to be able to change, even when we present them with the very best evidence that change is required. Health care professional . . . heal thyself!

Most of our traditional HCOs are filled with leftover rules, regulations, and processes that act like glue, keeping us stuck to the past. What needs to emerge is the process of discontinuous thinking, a process of thinking that abandons outdated assumptions that are ill fitted to today's world (Hammer & Champy, 1993; Naisbitt, 1984). However, abandoning one's world view is not a simple process. It takes the courage of introspection and the willingness to admit that change needs to occur. Self-actualized, competent, and contemporary leaders understand that changing the world view of an organization begins with them. Additionally, they are willing to follow the cues and clues given to them by anyone in the organization. It has been said that leaders take followers to places where they would otherwise not go. We are suggesting that leadership is also the ability to allow followers to take leaders to places they would otherwise not go: It is both, not either/or.

Most would agree that our leaders must do a better job of leading; however, better leadership is not enough. Practitioners must also be willing to change to new paths as well. We have a long history of changing organizational structures and rearranging departments and divisions on organizational charts without changing practice. To date, this process has produced only marginally effective results. Today's effective HCO leaders understand that the most effective care is care that is organized to meet the needs of the patient. It is designed, implemented, and evaluated by point-of-service staff and practitioners and is evidence based. This care, rather than care that is organized to meet the needs of departments or divisions, will provide the best outcomes and value for all involved.

Most of an organization's problems are not due to its structures alone but are a result of processes used to produce care. HCOs need to redesign their basic service processes, not only their structures. When an HCO redesigns its care processes, a change in structure can be stimulated, as well as a change in behavior. When designing anything, we must remember that form always follows function. The functions embedded in our care processes need to change first, and then we can go about making the necessary, but not fixed, changes in form/structure and behavior.

The key is that both the organization and the people in it must embark, in unison, with the shared goal of discovering their future. Neither management nor staff, as is often the case, can pull the other kicking and screaming into the new world. We can no longer afford the tremendous amounts of energy, time, emotion, money, and other resources it takes to move an organization forward, only to realize minimal improvements in outcomes. Moreover, managers, staff, and practitioners must be willing, and able, to endure the inevitable, and necessary, disagreements that will certainly surface in the pursuit of their desired future. Disagreements about direction are not the problem; the problem is our reaction to the disagreements. While organizations are having this internal battle of the wills, they often take an inordinate amount of time to move forward. When they do arrive at what they believe is the new world, there is no one there to greet them; they have all left for the new new world.

If the organization and the people in it allow disagreements to derail the process of discovering the future, the organization may survive into the future, but in a much diminished state of health. When this occurs, the decision becomes how long to leave it on life support. Practicing or managing in an organization that is on life support creates the feeling that no amount of energy or resources can solve the organization's problems.

In these types of toxic organizations, staff become detached from their work, managers become detached from staff, care suffers, and the organization continues to decline into disorder and chaos.

As an organization descends into disorder and chaos, many managers take the typical action of concentrating power, control, and influence at the organization's apex. The management process becomes, "We at the top think, you at the bottom do, and you at the bottom do what we at the top command you to do. Thanks for coming to the meeting!"

Managers begin to deliver edict after edict that has no input, or input from point-of-service staff is ignored, and staff in turn begin to resent this arrangement. As time goes on, face-to-face communication becomes less and less frequent and increasingly strained, leading to a patina of distrust that forms over the entire organization (Crow, 2006). Distrust is one of the most powerful destroyers of organizations. Centralizing power, control, and influence in turbulent times can create an atmosphere of distance and distrust and is exactly the wrong action to take.

In times of turbulence and uncertainty, as well as in relatively stable times, power and influence should be concentrated at the organization's core. It is at the core of the organization where management, practitioners, and staff act in concert to discover the most productive way to operationalize their mission in a changed and more complex environment. When point-of-service staff and practitioners have no input into direction, it should come as no surprise to managers, but it almost always does, that staff take less and less accountability for outcomes.

Accountability and ownership of outcomes arise from partnerships based on equity and the sharing of power and influence (Porter-O'Grady & Malloch, 2007). Accountability can never arise from top-down command and control processes that attempt to force staff into submission. Managerial reliance on submission can cause some staff to resign, and this can cause great harm to the organization if the most talented staff leave. However, a worse problem can arise. Some staff and managers become disillusioned, disgruntled, and disengaged but remain in their jobs. They become detached from the mission of the HCO. The employee who in essence "quits his job" but remains in his position can become a magnet for others who are discouraged, and before long there is an army of discouraged staff, practitioners, and managers. At this point an organization's ability to innovate, yet alone more forward, is greatly diminished. WSSG offers an organization a path out of this diminished state.

GETTING ORGANIZED FOR SUCCESS

Burton and Moran (1995), when describing what they call the future-focused organization, state that to provide superior customer service and remain focused on the organization's future, the organization must integrate three primary management responsibilities: strategic management, daily management, and lateral management. These three management responsibilities well describe the integrative characteristics of WSSG. Just like the structures and processes in WSSG, these three management responsibilities allow the organization to act on new ideas and potential innovations, to be very focused on satisfying customer needs, to reduce complexity, to provide seamless service, and promote cooperation, integration, and collaboration between all the units of the system. Simultaneously, activities that do not add value to the care processes will be designed out.

Strategic management, or the top executive team of the future-focused HCO, is responsible for developing the organization's strategic goals while also ensuring the strategic goals are well known throughout the organization. The strategic goals are focused on the three primary areas of effectiveness, efficiency, and flexibility (Burton & Moran, 1995).

Strategic managers ensure that both daily and lateral managers have the necessary skills, abilities, capabilities, capacity, and resources to meet strategic goals. Strategic managers ensure that everyone clearly understands what is expected of them and that everyone's actions, including their own, are focused on continuously meeting or exceeding customer expectations (Burton & Moran, 1995).

Daily management, or department managers, form a permanent and routine structure in the organization that primarily focuses on ensuring that inputs are transformed into outputs that add value to products and services. These managers have been delegated responsibility for a specific part of the organization that produces tangible products and services to both internal and external customers (Burton & Moran, 1995). Daily managers are also encouraged to facilitate a seamless approach to producing goods and services.

According to Burton and Moran (1995), daily management has a tremendous impact on, and responsibility for, growing, altering, and sustaining an organization's culture. Because the mission of any organization is operationalized at its core, where its products and services are experienced by the customer, the daily manager must ensure that the organization's culture guides employees to act in ways that satisfy the customer's needs and are aligned with the organization's mission, vision, and values.

It is worth remembering that customers directly interact with an organization's core and remotely interact with the organization's strategic managers. It is for this reason that the skills, abilities, and capabilities of the daily manager are vital to organizational success. When an organization ignores the managerial and leadership growth and development needs of its daily managers, it does so at its own peril, yet many do. Daily managers are the strategic manager's most vital link between themselves and those served by the organization. In health care many, if not most, clinical department managers are promoted to their positions based on how well they performed as practitioners. After they are promoted, they are often left to fend for themselves in gaining the necessary skills of an effective daily manager. This is a huge mistake that many leaders are only now acknowledging. Far more attention must be paid to the daily manager's development because they are accountable on a daily basis for the success of the organization. WSSG offers any organization the perfect platform on which to provide daily managers, staff, and practitioners with the necessary leadership skills to lead today's complex and adaptive HCOs.

Lateral management is the management process that integrates the horizontal with the vertical and is focused on continuous improvement in products and services that are designed, organized, and delivered across an organization (Burton & Moran, 1995). We believe that lateral management in health care can best be facilitated by the structures and processes of WSSG. Lateral management ensures that the continuum for product and service production is linked and integrated so that heavily guarded borders between departments are more permeable.

WHOLE SYSTEMS SHARED GOVERNANCE

Shared governance has been closely associated with nursing systems. Shared governance systems have allowed the registered nurse to fulfill his or her role as part of the primary professional group that links all aspects of the patient care to the HCO's mission, vision, and values. A recent trend in shared governance is the transition from nursing shared governance to WSSG. WSSG is a decentralized and accountability-based system that allows the entire HCO to be linked, interconnected, and, more important, focused on meeting the healthcare needs of all it serves, while simultaneously ensuring internal goodness of fit and external goodness of fit with its environment. A WSSG organization operates from its core where its mission, vision, and values should be most visible. We believe that any system that better integrates care across the continuum and provides multiple interconnections that reinforce the interdependency of all organizational elements will allow the organization to adapt in a timely and effective manner to the complex environment of the American healthcare system.

At the core of WSSG is an infrastructure to support patient care delivery that is intended to enhance outcomes and productivity. Outcomes and productivity realized at the point-of-service define the purpose of the HCO. All workers have both the obligation for accountability and right to contribute to decisions that impact their work (Porter-O'Grady, Hawkins, & Parker, 1997). Horizontal structures must be the dominant model to support effective working relationships and integration of all components and processes involved in delivery of the product, in this case patient care. Establishing and maintaining the integrity of the system requires clear and communicated governance, effective and efficient processes, and a vigilant focus on the organization's service delivery to realize desired outcomes. Because the primary obligation of the HCO is to meet the needs of the community it serves, systems and processes must facilitate and maintain linkages among all elements of the enterprise. Effective systems are those that are open systems, allowing iterative input, throughput, and output to drive the seamless integration or connections among processes, people, the work, and outcomes.

The healthcare team can only develop and sustain high-quality care if the organization's structures and processes are nimble and flexible enough to meet the rapidly changing needs of the patients it serves, yet stable and reliable enough for interdisciplinary collaboration across the continuum. This balance between flexibility and stability is a common feature of complex adaptive systems and takes astute formal and informal leaders to manage and lead. With too much flexibility, disorder and entropy can emerge. With too little flexibility, the organization can become rigid and frozen in place. Either polarity severely diminishes the organization's effectiveness and ultimately its existence.

Governance is about sharing power, influence, control, and authority. In shared governance practitioners and staff are the organization's primary resource for providing care. Therefore they must have influence and control over their professional practice. Structure is vital to shared governance (Hess, 2004). Shared governance provides both a structure and an environment to empower staff, legitimizes control over professional practice, and permanently extends influence to staff and practitioners in areas previously controlled exclusively by managers (Hess, 1994; Westrope, Vaughn, Bott, & Taunton, 1995).

WSSG is a professional practice and governance model of empowerment that is based on the principles of equity, partnership, ownership, and accountability (Box 8-1). These principles are as follows:

- Decentralize power and authority to practitioners for their practice, and establish ownership and accountability for the outcomes of their practice.
- Delineate performance expectations.
- Extend influence to areas of administration previously considered the exclusive domain of management, such as their legitimate professional accountability for practice, quality, and competence.
- Promote effective and efficient interdisciplinary evidence-based care processes that are consistent with national standards and the mission, vision, and values of the organization (Hess, 1994; Porter-O'Grady et al., 1997; Westrope et al., 1995).

The whole-systems framework on which shared governance is based affords many benefits. Box 8-2 summarizes the characteristics and features of a whole systems orientation.

WSSG council members, and specifically chairs and cochairs of the councils, are composed of staff, practitioners, and managers from across the HCO. Their primary focus is to ensure that the HCO provides barrier-free gold standard care to patients and families. Because council members are present to build care processes around the needs of the patient, rather than their departments, the council experience can create that

---

Box 8-1 Principles of Leadership in Whole Systems Shared Governance

Partnership
    Expectations negotiated, clearly defined, and communicated
    Equality among individuals
    Relationships based on shared risk
    Measures for contributions established
    Horizontal links, practices, processes well defined
Equity
    Each contribution understood by all
    Payment for contribution reflects value to outcomes
    Role based on relationships not status, given title/position
    Team defines service roles, relationships, outcomes
    Methodology defined, established to manage conflict and service issues
    Assessment/evaluation of team outcomes and contributions conducted
Accountability
    Internally defined by the person in the role
    Role defines, not job or task
    Based on outcomes, not processes
    Defined in advance of performance
    Linked, leads to defined and desired results
    Processes are overt, observable, evident
Ownership
    All invested in enterprise
    Every role is stakeholder in outcomes
    All members associated with a team
    Processes support relationships not limited to supporting tasks
    Opportunities based on demonstrated competence

Source: From Porter-O'Grady, Hawkins, & Parker (1997, p. 49).

---

much-needed sense of ownership for the entire care processes rather than the part their individual department plays in a care process. WSSG councils come together in an alliance to develop, maintain, and evaluate seamless care processes that deliver effective, efficient, timely, and value-added services and products to patients and their families.

Porter-O'Grady et al. (1997, p. 48) state that "90% of decisions made in the organization should be made within the context of service pathways." Within HCOs a service pathway is where patients and care providers meet (i.e., the point at which the work is done). Decisions made at the point-of-service involve the stakeholders with vested interest and accountability for outcomes. Locating accountability and the authority for

---

Box 8-2 Characteristics and Features of Whole Systems

- Whole always defines parts
- Each element/component supports whole system
- Problem, failure in performance/outcomes impacts whole system
- Heart of system (where it "lives") is at level where service is provided
- All roles/functions serve customer or support someone who does
- Design and structure must be centered on point-of-service
- Form must always follow function
- All members of the system are stakeholders, invested in outcomes
- Managers are facilitators, integrators, coordinators of processes to support work or providers; they do *not* control, decide
- Outcomes always define the value of the processes and performance (function is subordinate to purpose)

Source: From Porter-O'Grady, Hawkins, & Parker (1997, p. 38).

---

making decisions to the point-of-service requires a value for, and commitment to, shared decision making by staff, practitioners, and managers. Shared decision making supports the empowerment of those who do the work. Decentralized authority for decision making empowers and engages each member of the healthcare team to partner in interactive and iterative processes that support planning, implementation, and evaluation of care processes that are designed around the needs of the patient (Porter-O'Grady et al., 1997).

The skills and abilities required of both formal leaders (managers) and informal leaders (staff and practitioners) in WSSG require a new mindset. The principles of partnership, equity, accountability, and ownership (Porter-O'Grady et al., 1997) among staff, practitioners, and managers takes on new meaning and heightened impact in environments in which governance models are implemented. "Work environments that are structurally empowering are apt to have management practices that enhance mutual respect, communication, trust, information sharing, and inclusive decision making" (Moore & Hutchison, 2007, p. 565).

In WSSG, decision-making authority is decentralized throughout the organization. If stakeholders are located everywhere in the HCO and are supported in making decisions at the point-of-service, a mechanism must be in place that enables them to interact, to ensure that their decisions are mutually supportive, and to facilitate achievement of desired outcomes. This is a critical function served by the infrastructure of WSSG. Interdependent, interactive councils honor the principle of no single authority or locus of control (Porter-O'Grady et al., 1997). In nonlinear, horizontally linked organizational structures, emphasis is placed on relationships and integration of processes across the organization to support desirable patient outcomes.

In a top-down, vertical hierarchy, which is historically a characteristic of traditional HCO structures, administrators define the direction, make decisions, and design systems and operational policies and send them down the chain of command to subordinates as a mandate for implementation. This process creates a misfit of both form and function. Not only is the decision-making process and authority far removed from the point-of-service, and therefore out of context, but often those promoted to positions of authority have not developed the knowledge, skills, and experience to expertly lead and manage. "It can no longer be assumed that one's competence increases as one climbs the organization ladder" (Porter-O'Grady et al., 1997, p. 102). Described as "The Peter Principle" (Peter & Hull, 1969), promotions are successively granted for competent performance in a given role, until eventually a promotion leads to a position for which the individual is no longer competent. Far too often, little or no education or mentorship is provided to prepare the newly promoted individual. As a result, his or her leadership and management performance is ineffective at best and destructive at worst.

When form follows function, decision authority is moved to those who are providing care at the point-of-service; those who are most directly engaged with the complexity, context, content, and reality of the situation. When these direct-care providers possess the necessary knowledge and competencies, they are ideally positioned and best suited to partner with patients, other staff, and other clinicians to make decisions related to the design and management of care delivery (Porter-O'Grady et al., 1997).

Traditionally, true partnerships in HCOs are often limited to the practice of physicians and consultants (Hendel, Fish, & Berger, 2007; Kramer & Schmalenberg, 2003; Patterson & McMurray, 2003). Patient care staff and those who provide support services are often excluded from these partnerships. When point-of-service staff members are limited in establishing partnerships and are not empowered to make decisions related to the care they provide, they are limited in directing their own discipline-specific work, and patient outcomes are potentially compromised. Engagement and empowerment in one's work and the outcome of that work are critical to taking responsibility and accountability for that performance (Kramer & Schmalenberg, 2003; Patterson & McMurray, 2003).

Because the infrastructure in WSSG is nonhierarchical and is built on shared decision making, there are increased opportunities for input and decisions to modify operations, standards, and services, which also benefits any DOI process. Because decision making is decentralized and distributed among the various councils in WSSG, the governance structure itself provides a series of checks and balances to manage potential conflict and to limit the power and influence of any one person or group. WSSG as an organizing infrastructure facilitates the active participation and investment by all council members as stakeholders in process, decision making, and outcomes. The stakeholder concept increases the likelihood that decisions will be implemented and outcomes realized without confusion about the locus of control and decision-making authority. When accountability is clearly delineated, determination of expectations for and measurement of performance are facilitated within each context wherein decisions are made (Porter-O'Grady et al., 1997).

When those who provide the care are partners in problem identification, solution creation, decisions, and evaluation of outcomes and processes, higher levels of care quality are realized and both patient and staff satisfaction are enhanced (Laschinger & Wong, 1999). "Quality is about achieving sustainable outcomes. Outcomes are what we use to measure the value of processes. Our actions have no meaning separated from the ends to which they are directed" (Porter-O'Grady et al., 1997, p. 17). Individual expertise and performance alone cannot get the job done; effective partnerships are required for success in contemporary, complex, evolving HCOs.

Because WSSG council members rotate on and off councils, staff, practitioners, and managers gain a much broader perspective of their organization. Any process that facilitates employees in gaining the big picture of their organization allows the organization to more effectively deploy their core competencies in ways that maximize customer service and quality. Moreover, because WSSG councils are composed of practitioners and staff who are in constant contact with patients and families, they can keep the organization aligned with its customers and environment.

Everyone who participates on WSSG councils must be constantly on the lookout for ways to alter both structures and processes to meet the challenges of unrelenting change. Moreover, everyone must understand and be comfortable with the fact that both structure and process will continually evolve as the WSSG system seeks out emerging patterns and self-organizing structures and processes that more effectively align the HCO with the needs of the patients it serves and the environment in which it operates. The CAHCO's troika of organization–patient–environment continually seeks out new levels of harmony and goodness of fit, and WSSG facilitates an organization's ability to achieve goodness of fit.

Accountability and Responsibility

"Accountability abhors ambiguity, and therefore clarity of accountability and contribution must be one of the attributes of every single role that makes up the system" (Porter-O'Grady et al., 1997, p. 54) Accountability is the obligation to bear the consequences for failure to perform as expected, to be answerable, compelled, and obligated (*Merriam-Webster Online Dictionary,* 2008). Responsibility is a duty or obligation that is demanded of one by position, custom, law, or belief (*Merriam-Webster Online Dictionary,* 2008). To be responsible is to be effective, efficient, and accountable for one's actions.

The WSSG framework is based on shared function, shared obligation, shared decision making, and therefore shared responsibility and accountability among stakeholders throughout the system (Porter-O'Grady et al., 1997). It is not an option for stakeholders to decline accountability for performance of their role and the outcomes resulting from their actions. "It is as important to know the result of a team's work as to know its processes. Work has no value if there is no desired outcome" (p. 111).

In vertical, hierarchical systems the ultimate responsibility is located "at the top." In horizontal, complex adaptive systems that are supported by the WSSG paradigm, accountability is located where care occurs and decisions are made. Accountability results not from a structural or functional model, but from the interdependent decisions made within various councils and teams who are doing the work. Accountability is generated from within a role and is defined by the associated scope of practice. Accountability cannot be delegated (Porter-O'Grady et al., 1997). Lack of accountability in any part of the system negatively impacts all parts of the system and, therefore, the enterprise.

Two types of accountability are represented within the WSSG paradigm: system accountability and service accountability. System accountability involves activities and operations concerned with process and outcome effectiveness and ensures the integrity of the system and all its parts (Porter-O'Grady et al., 1997). Service accountability is concerned with the shared obligations of everyone in the HCO to perform those duties and activities that enable the organization to meet its purposes (Porter-O'Grady et al., 1997). In HCOs this purpose is clearly the provision of patient care, requiring multiple teams of individuals to carry out this mission and to demonstrate safe, effective, efficient, cost-effective, population-sensitive patient care outcomes.

In WSSG the focus is on mutual goal setting, shared decision making, support for synergistic functions and roles, and the promotion of shared accountabilities. Expectations for quality outcomes are achieved by consistent demonstrated performance against established standards. Efficiency outcomes are met by balancing the shared accountabilities between system and service roles as a result of the interactive, iterative nature of this model. The design places all members of the enterprise within the same system; therefore the impact of decisions, influence, leadership, and actual performance impact all aspects of the system. Managing the challenge to balance system and service accountability is a shared responsibility in WSSG.

Engagement and synergism, both hallmarks of WSSG, among all members of the healthcare team facilitate sustainable quality outcomes because they integrate the concepts and behaviors of continuous quality improvement into the expected performance behaviors of everyone in the organization. According to Senge (1990), a system's structure influences behavior patterns. Changing structure can motivate change in behaviors. A structure that empowers staff enhances individual and group influence within the system. Facilitating individual and team accountability for the concepts of continuous quality improvement through the structures of WSSG promotes an outcomes and value-added focus among healthcare team members that involves all stakeholders in a continuous effort to improve the quality of care, manage costs, and enhance the level of services provided by the HCO (Gardner & Cummings, 1994).

Organizational effectiveness is improved in organizations wherein employees self-manage and self-improve their performance in highly flexible teams (Kim, 1992). The WSSG structure provides a focus on the organization's mission, purpose, and operations that creates a shared mental model that aligns team priorities and outcomes with those of the organization. Organizations that embrace structures and procedures that are flexible and responsive to both external and internal change realize the greatest organizational success (Gardner & Cummings, 1994). Integrating continuous quality improvement provides the tools for problem solving; it also supports systems thinking and continuous learning.

Councils: Structure, Membership, and Function

In WSSG a "council" is the location for consultation, deliberation, advice, authority, and decision making. It is the venue for gathering practitioners, staff, and managers together to make decisions. Mitchell, Brooks, and Pugh (1999) state that the council structure enables staff, practitioners, and managers to jointly question policies, procedures, and practices regarding patient care. Mitchell et al. also report that members of the council can "ask questions they previously dared not ask," feel they are equals, and through the council structure of shared governance, "have greater access to information from senior staff" (p. 198).

Although each HCO must design a WSSG framework specific to its needs, there are some general councils that appear with great regularity:

- *Coordinating Council:* The purpose of the Coordinating Council is to oversee coordination and integration of the work of the other councils. Additionally, the Coordinating Council provides a portal of entry for all entities to access individual councils. Other functions of the Coordinating Council are to provide a forum for communication, collaboration, and conflict resolution between all the councils. In addition, the Coordinating Council links and integrates the administrative structure with the structures and processes of WSSG. The Coordinating Council, in conjunction with the top executive team, "translates and interprets the board's mission, purpose, goals, and strategy for the HCO" (Porter-O'Grady, 1995, p. 172). In many HCOs the chair and cochair of the Coordinating Council, who are always practitioners or staff and not managers, are members of the top executive team of the HCO. This vital link serves as one of the vertical and horizontal links that create the partnership that is paramount to the success of WSSG.
- *Quality and Safety Council:* The Quality and Safety Council has the overall accountability to ensure that national, state, local, and organizational quality and safety standards are integrated throughout the HCO. This includes using evidence-based

research and other sources of best evidence to guide the quality and safety processes of the HCO. Other sources of information for the Quality and Safety Council are derived from the HCO's patient satisfaction surveys and by using the national patient safety goals. These resources guide the metrics and processes linked to quality and safety. The Quality and Safety Council ensures the existence of a continuum-based quality plan that is vertically and horizontally integrated and linked with all patient care activities.

- *Education Council:* The Education Council ensures that the existence of ongoing education and development of all employees is consistent with the mission, vision, values, and strategic plan of the HCO. It is also responsible for providing educational activities that have a particular focus (i.e., leadership and management development programs that support the WSSG process). This council establishes and maintains a system-wide educational framework that inculcates the need for continuous learning to every corner of the HCO. The Education Council should ensure that its educational methods and practices are developed using the best available evidence regarding instruction and that the content of all educational offerings is evidence based. This is the council that ensures that staff, practitioners, and managers have the requisite skills, abilities, and capacity to ensure current and future organizational success.

- *Resource Council:* The Resource Council ensures the optimal deployment and use of human, physical, fiscal, and material resources that directly support the staff, practitioners, and managers in operationalizing the mission, vision, values, and strategic plan of the HCO. The Resource Council "creates a broad-based framework for ensuring the integrity of the system and the effectiveness of resource decisions throughout the system" (Porter-O'Grady et al., 1997, p. 138). The council ensures that adequate resources are in the hands of the right people, in the right amount, and at the right time so they can deliver exceptional patient care. The Resource Council "anticipates future resource issues and circumstances impacting the service areas" (Porter-O'Grady, 1995, p. 169). This is done to ensure a steady supply of resources year-to-year so that there are no service delays or interruptions.

- *Patient Care Council:* The Patient Care Council defines and integrates a comprehensive approach to patient care services that span the continuum and is designed to meet the needs of everyone the HCO serves. The Patient Care Council is the "final locus of control for point-of-service decisions" (Porter-O'Grady, 1995, p. 164). It must ensure that the standards on which care is developed are contemporary and evidence based. The Patient Care Council ensures that patients can traverse the entire HCO in a seamless manner and that the care they receive is consistent, regardless of where patients enter the HCO. The Patient Care Council evaluates care processes to ensure they meet preestablished standards for quality and satisfaction.

• *Innovation Council:* A new council we are beginning to see is the Innovation Council. The Innovation Council is accountable for identifying, investigating, evaluating, and recommending new ideas, technologies, and processes for improving patient care and organizational effectiveness. The Innovation Council serves as the organization's think tank, where organizational boundary spanners seek out new ways to provide patient care that helps the organization remain ahead of the curve. This council resides at the border, between now and the future, and is the catalyst for keeping the HCO nimble and flexible in how it designs, implements, and evaluates innovations in patient care delivery. WSSG provides an excellent vehicle for diffusing any innovation because it is vertically and horizontally integrated. An additional advantage of WSSG in the DOI process is that councils are populated with staff, managers, and practitioners, thereby ensuring that important stakeholders are at the table.

WSSG Fosters Healthy Work Environments

Numerous studies have identified the components of positive work environments. Two key findings are that employees desire the need for collaboration and empowerment. Kanter (as cited in Laschinger & Wong, 1999; Moore & Hutchison, 2007) posits a theory for empowerment that suggests social structures in the workplace influence attitudes and behaviors to a greater degree than do individual personality predispositions. Formal pathways to power are facilitated by the structures within an organization. Laschinger and Wong (1999), in a study of staff nurse empowerment and accountability, report the following as associated factors: "access to information, resources, support, and opportunity in their work environment are important determinants of collective accountability and their ability to be effective in their work" (p. 315). Laschinger and Wong also cite the importance of informal power by suggesting that "Informal power is strongly related to accountability, productivity, and work effectiveness highlighting the importance of alliances with peers, sponsors, and subordinates within the organization in fostering a sense of collective accountability for practice and work effectiveness" (p. 315). Moore and Hutchison (2007) report similar findings that access to various "avenues of power" and workplace alliances are correlated with empowerment and satisfaction.

The literature reports strong correlations among perceived work empowerment, work satisfaction, and control (autonomy) over one's professional practice (Anderson, 2000; Laschinger & Finegan, 2005; Laschinger & Havens, 1996; Schmalenberg & Kramer, 2008; Scott, Sochalski, & Aiken, 1999). In a study of nurses, Schmalenberg and Kramer (2008) indicate that "collegial and collaborative nurse-physician and interdisciplinary relationships" (p. 66) are attributes of satisfying and productive work environments. Laschinger and Havens (1996) report perceived empowerment relates strongly to perceptions of control over clinical practice ($r = 0.625$, $P = 0.000$), control over practice correlates with informal power ($r = 0.65$, $P = 0.000$), and "formal and informal power and overall empowerment were found to explain 48.5% of the variance in control over practice ($R^2 = 0.485$, $F(3, 122) = 38.3$, $P = 0.000$)" (p. 8). A review of magnet hospital research by Scott and colleagues (1999) reveals that the two most important factors that foster collaborative relationships are mutual respect for one another's knowledge and competence and a mutual concern for the provision of quality patient care. This collaboration must occur at the point-of-care.

Pearson et al. (2007) conducted a systematic review of 48 studies that identified factors that foster healthy work environments in health care. They reported that work environments in which meaningful collaboration is actively supported impact satisfaction for both healthcare staff and their patients. Social and transformational leadership styles were also positively associated with job satisfaction. When leaders encourage and support staff involvement in professional development activities, higher levels of job satisfaction are reported.

The knowledge, skills, and abilities required of both formal leaders (managers) and informal leaders (staff and practitioners) within the paradigm of WSSG require a new mindset. The principles of partnership, equity, accountability, and ownership take on new meaning and heightened impact in environments in which governance models are implemented (Porter-O'Grady et al., 1997). The decentralization of power, authority, influence, and decision making requires new abilities and new behaviors and therefore new learning. Embracing a structure that identifies the required abilities and supports the change by implementing a continuous educational program creates a healthy and productive work environment. "Work environments that are structurally empowering are apt to have management practices that enhance mutual respect, communication, trust, information sharing, and inclusive decision making" (Moore & Hutchison, 2007, p. 565).

Shared governance models provide the platform that supports all these factors. Managers in WSSG share power, stimulate enthusiasm among staff, listen to new ideas, encourage risk taking and innovation, and mentor staff to develop new skills and competencies in response to the changing dynamics and demands of the workplace. They continue to set and maintain high expectations for performance but involve staff at all levels in identifying the competencies required of their work and point out the barriers and constraints that impede their ability to perform at target levels. Managers are challenged to relinquish control and commit to the empowerment process, which includes decentralizing decision making for those functions directly related to staff work.

Empowerment in WSSG requires all leaders to develop and practice "facilitative leadership." Moore and Hutchison (2007) identify seven practices consistent with facilitative leadership: "(1) sharing an inspiring vision, (2) focusing on results, processes, and relationships, (3) seeking maximum appropriate involvement, (4) designing pathways to action, (5) facilitating agreement, (6) coaching for performance, and (7) celebrating achievement" (p. 565). All these leadership behaviors are essential to implement and sustain WSSG. Managers are challenged to transform their own leadership behaviors from a focus on controlling and monitoring to a transformational model that is facilitative, participative, and directed at developing successful leadership skills among individuals and groups at all levels of the service line. This change in focus serves to inspire and empower team members to commit to achievement of mutually developed and mutually achieved goals and outcomes. Most importantly, these leadership behaviors support the HCO as a complex system to remain adaptable to dynamic variables and facilitate DOI. The participative design of WSSG provides the structure for such changes in leadership behaviors among managers, staff, and practitioners with the HCO.

Teams in WSSG

Self-directed work teams, empowered and supported by the principles and practices of WSSG, collaborate to make essential decisions concerning their care and service accountabilities. They manage their own relationships between and among the various teams along the service-line pathway to ensure that care delivery is consistent with clinical standards. Self-directed work teams facilitate activities that are fundamental to their work (Porter-O'Grady et al., 1997). They manage barriers, constraints, problems, issues, and concerns that threaten achievement of performance targets and thresholds.

There are two types of teams within WSSG: care teams, which have a clinical focus, and service teams, which have a systems focus (Porter-O'Grady et al., 1997). Care teams concentrate on standards of care, functions, and activities that are specific to patient care delivery. This focus includes essential support services. Care teams, through collaboration, self-direction, and shared decision making, monitor and evaluate the care they provide to confirm that delivered care reflects established standards and that intended outcomes are actually achieved.

Service teams focus on systems aspects; relationships among teams; the design, structure, and components of the system itself; and the linkages or connections among those elements (Porter-O'Grady et al., 1997). Service teams also focus on team support and effectiveness. Both types of teams are challenged to develop new competencies as self-directed teams. These competencies include (1) self-organizing to plan and schedule team conferences and meetings, (2) defining standards and measures of team performance, (3) conducting peer review, (4) self-assignment of workload and team activities, (5) managing professional interpersonal interactions among team members and with others who integrate with patients and the care delivery process, and (6) managing the conflict that is inherent in team activities.

The impact of self-directed teams within WSSG emerges not only from the authority and accountability sanctioned by the structure itself, but from the diversity of the different disciplines represented. Each discipline brings its professional "point of view" to a given situation, problem, issue, or concern related to the provision of patient care

(Ashmos, Huonker, & McDaniel, 1998). This internal perspective represents discipline-specific expertise but may reflect opinion rather than a comprehensive understanding of the service continuum. The council design of WSSG mitigates the potential for isolated discipline-specific thinking and the limitations of superficial knowledge of other disciplines.

Organizations learn through the individuals who learn (Senge, 1990). In contemporary HCOs problems are complex and the solutions are not always readily apparent to an individual or discipline. The design and structure of WSSG promotes an integrated, interactive environment to conduct the business of healthcare delivery. It is here where individuals and teams learn to deepen and broaden their understanding to include multidisciplinary perspectives to effectively and efficiently create meaningful change and to respond to clinical challenges.

People are an organization's most valuable and critical resource (Gardner & Cummings, 1994). When an organization is designed as a "learning organization" (Senge, 1990) where continuing education, exploration, and the quest for new knowledge and understanding are not only encouraged but supported and funded, employees in that organization become valuable resources. The value added to the system is not generated merely by the enhanced performance of an individual or group (team) but results from the synergism of interactive, collective experience and action. In a learning organization contributions emerge from the processes of learning to think in new ways, by reframing past approaches and behaviors, by abandoning path-dependent thinking, and by collaboratively creating solutions and direction for the way forward.

DIFFUSION OF INNOVATION

DOI is a nonlinear and often complex process by which a few early adopters within a social network identify, refine, and accept an innovation and over time influence others to accept the innovation as well (Geibert, 2006; Meyer & Goes, 1988; Plsek, 2003; Rogers, 2003; Valente, 1996; West, Barron, Dowsett, & Newton, 1999). West et al. (1999) make one of the most important statements found in our literature review when they posit that "adoption is a process rather than an event" (p. 634). They go on to say that without allowing the end user of the innovation sufficient time, autonomy, and support to discuss, challenge, reframe, and refine the innovation, the innovation is likely to fail.

This nonlinear complex process of diffusing innovation is very difficult to execute in mechanistic rigid hierarchies. Forcing a nonlinear organic process to be operationalized in a mechanistic rigid linear system is like forcing a square peg into a round hole; it can be done, but in the process both the peg and hole are damaged. Although authoritative decisions may increase the initial acceptance of an innovation, they can also reduce the likelihood of the innovation being ultimately accepted by most of the organization (Rogers, 2003).

Because most HCOs are operated as hierarchical, linear, mechanistic systems (Crow, 2006), the innovation "process" is often truncated, or outright omitted, in favor of the "event" that management uses to introduce the innovation to the staff. Because of this truncation, many innovations fail. Without the engagement of those who are impacted by the innovation, the innovation is likely to be rejected, regardless of its usefulness. When the DOI process is subverted into an authoritative forced-decision process, it can further separate management from staff. When management and staff are estranged from each other, organizational effectiveness decreases.

In contrast, a system that is more organic, with a high degree of management and staff interaction that is based on trust, partnership, and equity, allows innovations to arise from anywhere in the system. DOI, when done properly, is an organic process that allows sufficient time for the organization, and its end users, to adapt to the innovation while simultaneously allowing the innovation to adapt to the organization (Valente, 1996; West et al., 1999). These types of organizations are more likely to be successful in adapting to the ever-changing and complex American healthcare system. However, there must be an adequate number of formal and informal leaders who can facilitate the identification and implementation of innovations. Organizations that are rich in both formal and informal leaders, who are capable of identifying innovations that create better goodness of fit between the organization and its environment, are likely to be successful. An additional advantage to coupling DOI with WSSG is that WSSG provides the vertical and horizontal linkages between management and staff and the necessary time to clarify the meaning of any innovation. Organizational structures and processes that facilitate sustained interactions between management and staff, such as WSSG, can mean the difference between acceptance or rejection of the innovation.

Rogers (2003) identifies five main characteristics of the DOI process: (1) relative advantage, (2) compatibility, (3) complexity, (4) trialability, and (5) observability of the proposed innovation. These five characteristics, although presented in a linear fashion, are anything but linear. The DOI process is an iterative one where each new piece of information informs and reinforms the entire process (Rogers, 2003). The DOI process is truly greater than the sum of its parts; however, any single characteristic can derail the entire DOI process. Equal attention must be paid to every step and characteristic; failure to do so will certainly place the innovation at risk.

We believe that WSSG can strengthen any DOI process because it brings together process teams from across the organization to a forum where the focus is not their department or division but rather on providing better patient care across the continuum. WSSG can help to decrease an organization's over-reliance on the traditional overly structured and tightly controlled approaches to managing a HCO by developing the leadership skills and abilities of everyone serving on WSSG councils.

The relative advantage of the innovation is its perceived value to the end user. Simply said, perception *is* reality. The innovation must be perceived as a better fit with the end user's practice than the practice it supersedes. It does not matter if the proposed innovation has a great deal of objective advantage or is based on the best available evidence; the adopter must perceive that the innovation is better. Because an individual's perception about an innovation *is* their reality, they must be allowed time to evaluate its usefulness (Rogers, 2003). One must remember that an organization's time line for DOI is not always shared by a department or individual (Geibert, 2006). This is why we recommend the platform of WSSG as one of the ways to lead the DOI process. WSSG brings together management and staff in a forum uniquely designed to provide the give-and-take required to identify an innovation's relative value.

An innovation's *compatibility* with the adopter's needs, professional norms and values, and past experience must be evident before the potential adopter will accept the innovation (Denis, Herbert, Langley, Lozeau, & Trottier, 2002; Ferlie et al., 2001; Rogers, 2003). Rogers (2003) indicates that the intended adopters must have the necessary time and autonomy to refine the proposed innovation to increase its goodness of fit with the people who will use it. The process takes time. Determining compatibility cannot occur in one "event" or one "process" meeting where the innovation is announced. Not even the later adopters are likely to fall for this ruse. Again, WSSG provides the crucial vertical and horizontal linkages between management and staff where an innovation's compatibility with the organization, and the end user, can be jointly ascertained.

The *complexity* of the innovation is concerned with how difficult the proposed innovation is to understand. Innovations that are overly complex or require a great deal of learning are slower to be accepted. If a proposed innovation is labeled as overly complex by early adopters, its chance for acceptance is harmed or outright killed (Rogers, 2003). Maeda (2006, p. 1) informs us that "reaching a balance between how simple you can make an innovation with how complex it has to be to be effective, is not a simple process. The goal of innovation is to develop a process or product that is easy to use, while ensuring that it will do everything that a user might want it to do." We believe that WSSG is an excellent platform in which the best balance between complexity and simplicity can be negotiated.

The *trialability* of the proposed innovation is concerned with whether or not the intended end users have the opportunity to experience what the innovation means to them (Geibert, 2006; Rogers, 2003; Yetton, Sharma, & Southon, 1999). Crow (2006, p. 239) states that "all change is experienced locally, and through this experience the end user gets to identify WIIFM (what's in it for me)." The WIIFM test for goodness of fit is paramount to acceptance of any innovation. Perhaps Lewin's (1935) change model best explains this characteristic. He identifies three stages of movement during change: unfreezing, moving, and refreezing. In the moving phase the end user is afforded the opportunity to actually experience what the change means to him or her. Because all change is experienced locally (Crow, 2006), this step is vital to the entire process. A user's ability to experience what the change means to him or her will impact the innovation's relative advantage and compatibility, as well as its trialability. Again, the DOI process is iterative, not linear.

Trialability is about the "experience" of the innovation as well as how the usefulness of the innovation is communicated throughout the organization (Rogers, 2003). One negative comment indicating that the innovation is not helpful can derail the DOI process. Organizations that lack ongoing vertical and horizontal linkages between management and staff can more easily fall prey to the rumor mill. Bad news travels at the speed of light, whereas good news travels at the speed of sound. The difference in the speeds can be potentially overcome when the organization has robust horizontal and vertical linkages that are composed of well-respected peers to whom others turn to for information, guidance, and advice and have the leadership skills to effectively communicate and manage the message concerning innovation. We believe that WSSG provides the much-needed opportunity for the clinical leaders and early adopters, in the presence of later adopters, to discuss the good and bad of the proposed innovation, thereby increasing the likelihood that the effects of one negative comment can be overcome.

The *observability* associated with the innovation is concerned with how visible the advantages of the innovation are to the potential adopter. When potential adopters can actually "see" the results of the innovation and those results clearly lead to increased value and performance, the innovation is more likely to be adopted (Geibert, 2006; Rogers, 2003; Yetton et al., 1999). The need to see how an innovation will aid the practitioner to improve patient care, increase patient satisfaction, and control costs is a powerful way to increase the likelihood that the innovation will be adopted. The observability characteristic of the DOI process provides the late adopters an opportunity to observe how the early adopters demonstrate the innovation's advantages (Rogers, 2003). The observability and the advantages of the innovation can be facilitated by the highly interconnected and interactional structures that make up WSSG.

The DOI process is a vital element in organizational success. When done properly, it can put tools in the hands of practitioners that can decrease the cost of care, while simultaneously increasing the effectiveness and quality of that care. WSSG can aid the leader and early adopters of potential innovations in convincing others of an innovation's usefulness. DOI is not a top-down command-and-control process but rather a horizontal practitioner-to-practitioner influencing process that takes time as well as astute informal and formal leaders to facilitate. HCOs, like all organizations, cannot assume staff or managers have the necessary skills to position the organization for goodness of fit. We believe that WSSG is the perfect structure to educate and develop staff, practitioners, and managers who courageously step forward to meet the complex challenges of the American healthcare system. We also believe that the DOI process, coupled with WSSG, is a powerful and effective way to diffuse one of the most important innovations of the 21st century: managers and staff who have the capacity to successfully lead complex adaptive HCOs. We believe that in an effort to deal with the increasingly complex American healthcare system, leaders must decentralize power, influence, and control over care processes and resources to point-of-service staff and practitioners and, in turn, have the added obligation to ensure they use this new-found power and influence to benefit the patients and organization rather than themselves. For this to occur, executives must ensure that staff, practitioners, and managers have the necessary skills, abilities, capabilities, and capacity to lead in complex organizations.

GETTING THERE: ALCHEMY FOR THE 21ST CENTURY

According to *Webster's Dictionary* (1994), the word "alchemy" has two meanings: (1) "an art practiced in the middle ages and the Renaissance, concerned principally with discovering methods for transmuting base metals into gold, and with finding an elixir of life, and (2) any magical power or process of transmuting a common substance into a substance of greater value" (p. 35). The base elements for the elixir required for transmuting slow-to-change rigid complicated HCOs (CHCOs) into nimble and flexible CAHCOs that are better equipped to meet patient needs are WSSG and the process of DOI. The formula is

$$CHCO + WSSG + DOI = CAHCO$$

For HCOs to adequately meet the growing and complex needs of everyone they serve, the HCO must transmute the "common substance of health care services" into a substance of greater value to those it serves. HCOs have the obligation to provide care to everyone that is based on the gold standard, for example, care that is culturally sensitive, seamless across the continuum, outcomes based, value added, practitioner driven and in partnership with the patient/family, based on the best available evidence, and maximizes and optimizes the use of all resources.

We believe that shared governance, and specifically WSSG, is a particularly effective way for HCOs to more closely reflect their mission statements which frequently contain the following goals:

> To serve our community by providing high quality, cost effective health care services in a compassionate and respectful environment which is supported and stimulated by education and research . . . deliver humanistic, cost effective and culturally competent care . . . to care, to serve, and to heal by providing world class care in our community.

It is a given that in today's complex healthcare world that HCOs need a participatory management practice and process that successfully integrates vertical and horizontal organizational elements. Participatory management structures and processes, when implemented properly, lead to the creation of lateral management structures and processes that empower and engage staff, managers, and practitioners in a cooperative effort to improve all aspects of the patient care services they provide.

WSSG creates the structures and processes by which an HCO can realize its mission; however, without adequate numbers of well-prepared staff, managers, and practitioner leaders, the effort is likely to fail. Without adequate WSSG leadership, the HCO is more likely to become engulfed in chaos and disorder, more complicated, more territorial, and more likely to return to the old familiar paths for comfort.

To accomplish the transmutation from good to great, leadership skills and abilities must be diffused to the entire WSSG structure and specifically to every council member, regardless of their position in the organization. To empower council members who lack the requisite skills to lead in these complex times will not solve any significant problems for which WSSG was implemented to solve. If empowerment is not coupled with leadership knowledge, skill, and ability, an organization's problems are likely to get worse. The principles of DOI are a proven effective and efficient process by which any innovation, including management and leadership development programs, can be diffused.

Developing Leadership and Management Skills in Complex Adaptive Systems

The diversity of knowledge, skills, and abilities in an HCO creates both a challenge and an opportunity for educating an organization. "Because shared governance is a continuum, people need to be met where they are on their journey and coached to progress to the next point" (Moore & Hutchison, 2007, p. 566). A robust continuing education program that is integrated into all departments and service lines throughout the organization can provide the mechanism for continuous learning and performance improvement. The educational process is designed to develop the knowledge, skills, and abilities of the organization's informal and formal leaders to prepare them for a leadership role in the accountability-based governance environment. A key desired outcome of the educational program is for participants to apply their new leadership skills to assist the organization in developing its adaptive capacity.

"Shared governance is a journey, not a destination. Organizations that pursue shared governance move incrementally from past orientations where the few rule, to an orientation where many learn to make consensual decisions" (Hess, 2004, para. 22). WSSG requires significant changes in values, philosophy, structures, and systems. If an organization does not make these changes, the transition to WSSG is impossible. A comprehensive learner-focused educational initiative is a critical component that helps organizations manage the major changes that must occur to successfully implement and sustain WSSG.

Expectations for demonstrating leadership behavior, commitment and contribution, and accountabilities for individual and group outcomes are made explicit by the WSSG model and the various council charter documents. Participation by all council members (staff, practitioners, and managers) in educational activities must also be an expectation rather than an invitation. The interaction that occurs during the education process builds relationships, enhances understanding of diversity in opinions and perspectives, and builds supportive team behaviors. Serving on WSSG councils, and participating in service team projects, enables everyone to see the big picture of the organization and to understand how their contributions directly and indirectly support the mission and services of the organization. If active and consistent participation in professional development activities is not an expected part of everyone's job, inconsistent participation will become a barrier to successful implementation of WSSG (Caramanica, 2004).

The design and delivery of the education program for leadership and management development cannot be produced and delivered by those in formal positions of authority (e.g., senior leadership or managers). When the organization defers to those in formal leadership roles, assuming they have either the competence or the influence to diffuse leadership skills, this practice violates the principles and desired practices of shared leadership and accountability. Along the same line, assigning development of the WSSG educational program to the organization's education department should be avoided because the department's internal perspective reinforces path dependence (Schneider & Somers, 2006), fosters paradigm paralysis (Barker, 1992), and limits creativity and innovation. If the organization was capable of seeing and acting differently, it would have already done so. Therefore changing the culture and its methods for leading and managing the organization requires knowledge, guidance, and direction from outside resources.

Seeking direction from an external consultant who holds expertise in leadership and management development, DOI, WSSG, and complex adaptive systems prevent the "old way" from being repackaged and taught as the "new way." A consultant who is external to the environment is free of the organization's history of hierarchies, roles, and management practices; can provide a fresh perspective to the process; and brings expertise in curricular development, instructional design, and teaching methods.

The consultant works with the Education Council to identify competent individuals to assist with the design and delivery of education programs. This includes those within the organization who have demonstrated expertise in leadership and management skills. It is also beneficial to include external experts from non–healthcare agencies because we have a lot to learn from how other organizations conduct their business. Their input often results in new insights regarding strategies and techniques that were not apparent or thought to not apply to HCOs.

The educational plan is aligned with the organization's mission and goals and is designed to facilitate the necessary changes in the organization's mindset. Managers, administrators, representatives from the service lines (staff and practitioners, including physicians), and WSSG council members should all participate in educational activities identified in the plan. The multidisciplinary representation of the participants contributes to parity in representation of opinions, perspectives, contribution of data, and perceptions of equity and power. Leadership in complex adaptive systems includes everyone. The educational challenge is to teach and develop leadership skills that are critical to adaptive complex systems while honoring the principles of shared governance.

The content of the curriculum is informed by the principles of leadership in WSSG. Broad topics include partnership, equity, accountability, and ownership (Box 8-1). Initial education sessions are designed to prepare council members for implementing WSSG. Didactic and experiential learning activities are focused both on content specific to the WSSG model and on those foundational leadership capabilities that promote DOI and facilitate success in complex adaptive systems.

Enrichment and support workshops are scheduled monthly and supplemented with online education offerings and other learning resources (reference and resources lists, self-study modules, audiovisual programs). It is important to provide educational opportunities for both current and new employees. To ensure that new employees are prepared to fully participate in WSSG, it is essential to initiate their exposure to WSSG during their new employee orientation. Ideally, a practice partner or mentor is assigned to new employees during their first year of employment. Managers, staff, and practitioners are equal partners in applying what they have learned and in coaching each other to improve over time.

Transformation in thinking and behaviors is critical to make the changes required for WSSG. It is imperative for everyone involved to commit to moving from an authority-based leadership model to one of shared accountability. Without this emphasis, instruction that is limited to operational aspects and roles can become a barrier to the implementation and ongoing success of WSSG (Caramanica, 2004).

Providing leadership and management development training requires a significant investment in time and money. Financial resources must be designated for costs related to developing the educational plan, preparing instruction, software and technology support, and employee release time to attend educational sessions. The Education Council works in conjunction with the Resource Council to develop a centralized cost center and budget for initial and ongoing education costs for human and material resources. Senior leadership commitment to provide financial and human resources to fund continuous learning throughout the HCO is essential to the success of WSSG.

To be most effective, the curriculum for developing leadership and management skills must conform to the concepts of DOI. Because the DOI process is being used as a framework for disseminating the learning content, the program must be supported by the five main features of the DOI process as described by Rogers (2003): (1) relative advantage, (2) compatibility, (3) complexity, (4) trialability, and (5) observability. If those who are expected to participate in the leadership development program and then to use the new skills do not see the relative advantage of both the program and the outcomes, the educational process will be doomed from the start. Participants must see that the new skills for leading and managing are appropriate for the new age. It is only then that they will likely support the structures and processes of WSSG.

As the educational program is developed, the Education Council must consider its compatibility with the culture, values, and norms of the HCO as well as the adopter's needs, professional norms, and values (Rogers, 2003). It is well known that many registered nurses are very surprised when they enter the profession to find out that in the typical HCO, it is their manager or other entities in the organization that control most, if not all, of their practice. Practitioners will very likely find WSSG to be compatible with their professional norms and values that support the belief that professionals should be in control of their own practice.

When considering the culture, norms, and values of an HCO, it isn't a stretch to say that the implementation of WSSG within an organization can represent a significant threat to those who previously, and firmly, were in charge of the system. As stated earlier in this chapter, most HCOs are operated and governed from the apex of the organization rather than its core; therefore the leadership development curriculum must take into account that unfreezing the old ways takes significant time. If the program asks too much too soon, the push-back is likely to doom the program. Cultural change does not proceed at the same rate as learning; lag time is always involved. What the Education Council, along with senior leadership, will need to decide is just how much change is required and the pace necessary to move the culture along without destroying the likelihood that the transition will take place.

It is important to be aware of the education program's complexity. As was stated earlier, Maeda (2006, p. 1) informs us that "reaching a balance between how simple you can make an innovation with how complex it has to be to be effective, is not a simple process." The complexity of the leadership program needs to be addressed in several aspects. If the design of the program is either too complex or not compatible with the learner's style or preference for learning, the educational outcomes will be less successful. For example, using only classroom-based lectures or workshops (known as face-to-face learning sessions) or using only technology-mediated methods such as self-study CDs, DVDs, or Web-based learning modules will not appeal to all learners. Because learners learn in different ways, a single method or strategy will not meet the needs of all participants; therefore multiple approaches should be part of the instructional design. When using technology-based instruction, it is important to understand that not all participants have the prerequisite skills to use this form of instruction. They either need to be taught how to use the technology or other methods should be used.

The complexity of teaching materials should also be evaluated. If educational materials are written at a level that does not allow all participants to comprehend the content, learning among group members will be inconsistent. Learning materials need to be simple enough to keep everyone involved yet complex enough to keep everyone interested and engaged in the learning process. Recommended core curriculum content areas to support a program of continuous leadership and management development are identified in Box 8-3.

Rogers' (2003) concept of "trialability" of the learning partnership is concerned with how the participants experience the program and how they will apply what they have learned. The participants' learning experiences must lead them to believe that, as a result of their instruction, they are better leaders. They need opportunities to practice and refine new skills as they learn them and to experience the impact of their new knowledge. Knowing something is very different from actually doing something. Adult learners want to see the immediate utility of new knowledge and learn best through experience (Knowles, 1980).

Box 8-3 Core Curriculum for Diffusion of Leadership and Management Skills in Complex Adaptive Systems

- Systems theory
- Complexity science, social networks, chaos theory
- Paradigm effects and paralysis
- Complex adaptive systems
- Social networks
- Diffusion of innovation, creativity
- Change theory and successful adaptation
- Organizational dynamics and culture
- Human dynamics
- Continuous quality improvement
- Facilitative leadership
- Delegation and empowerment
- Communication, collaboration, negotiation, conflict management
- Working in teams: partnerships, equity, accountability, ownership
- Facilitating effective meetings
- Performance assessment and coaching for improved performance
- Diversity
- Evidence-based practice
- Whole systems shared governance: structure, principles, processes
- Financial management (capital, operating budgets and monitoring)
- Information technology for learning and communication

The immediate application of new learning is critical to ongoing skills development and change in behaviors. As new knowledge is acquired and applied the sudden gain in power, whether real or imagined, can be an intoxicating experience and can lead to abuses of that power. It is often said the knowledge is power, and therefore the empowerment new knowledge brings can lead to behaviors that reflect a return to the vertical hierarchies that are counterproductive to participative, distributed leadership, and decision making. The power and influence that acquisition of new knowledge and skills in leadership and management brings are experienced not only by those in formal management roles but also by WSSG council chairpersons and emerging informal leaders throughout the organization. The "observability" of the outcomes of the management and leadership training program are likely to be immediate and dynamic. Because it is expected that distributed leadership emerges throughout the organization and because of the potential for abuses of new-found power and influence, ongoing coaching and feedback must be an integral component of the educational program. It is important to elicit feedback from both providers and recipients of the leadership. Based on this input, modifications to the education program can be made to conduct additional training to update and extend the knowledge, skills, and abilities necessary to enhance the adaptability of the organization. An example of such "follow-up" and reinforcing education might be workshops in conflict management and human dynamics training.

Designing for Success

The educational consultant works with the Education Council to design the structural and operational aspects of a comprehensive educational program. Structural elements include the core curriculum, with specified knowledge, skills, abilities, and learning outcomes for each topic; instructional design and delivery strategies; and specified methods for assessment of learning outcomes. Operational elements include methods for initial and ongoing surveys of learning needs, identification of target audiences, recruiting course developers and instructors with appropriate teaching and learning assessment skills, clearly identified and tested methods to disseminate content and ensure accessibility to learning resources and activities, technology support for design and maintenance of online components, organization and scheduling of face-to-face meetings and workshops, methods to evaluate participant satisfaction and effectiveness of all educational offerings, and financial and human resources to design, deliver, and evaluate the program.

Because release of staff, practitioners, and mangers from their work duties to attend continuing education activities is frequently cited as a barrier to implementation and maintenance of shared governance models (Caramanica, 2004), it is essential that the instructional design accommodates this constraint. Designing a flexible, yet comprehensive leadership and management development program that is widely accessible to all is clearly an essential outcome of instructional design. Equally important is to incorporate innovation, creativity, and the principles of adult learning theory (Box 8-4).

Box 8-4 Characteristics of Adult Learners

- Autonomous and self-directed in learning
- Need to connect learning to accumulated life experiences and knowledge
- Goal oriented and seek links between learning and goal achievement
- Relevancy oriented; seek the reason and applicability for learning that reflect their own interests
- Practical and focus on learning that is most useful to them
- Expect to be respected; acknowledged for knowledge and experience, and allowed to express opinions freely

Source: From Lieb (1991).

Forward-thinking organizations that embrace the concepts of complex adaptive systems and DOI demonstrate value and commitment to the need for ongoing, accessible education and professional development for all employees in the organization. Successful educational programs are those that accommodate the diversity of learners, provide multiple methods to access learning activities, and enhance the impact of teaching and learning by use of contemporary multimedia technologies. It is important to include a variety of learning modalities and instructional methods that acknowledge and accommodate individual learning preferences, promote the principles of adult learning (Box 8-4), and consider factors that motivate adult learners (Box 8-5). Operational aspects of the education program design must ensure convenient accessibility to learning activities and a commitment to adequate release time from usual duties to participate in learning activities.

Box 8-5 Six Factors That Motivate Adult Learners

1. **Social relationships:** meet the need for associations and friendships
2. **External expectations:** comply with instructions from others; fulfill expectations or recommendations of those with formal authority
3. **Social welfare:** improve ability to serve mankind; service to the community; participate in community work
4. **Personal advancement:** achieve higher status in a job; secure professional advancement; stay abreast of competitors
5. **Escape/Stimulation:** relieve boredom; break in routines; provide contrast to exacting details of life
6. **Cognitive interest:** learn for the sake of learning; seek knowledge for its own sake; satisfy inquiring mind

Source: From Lieb (1991).

Core foundational content from the curriculum can be "modularized" into self-paced, instructional units that are completed as the primary learning activity itself or as preparation for a face-to-face, classroom-style workshop or seminar. The modules can be produced as paper and pencil products or distributed as hard-copy documents or electronic copies disseminated via e-mail or downloaded from a Web site. To provide variety, interest, and engagement in learning, self-study materials should take advantage of technologies that amplify instructional impact and involve individuals in active learning. This engagement is especially important for solitary learning activities. Multimedia such as narrated PowerPoint presentations, audio programs (podcasts), and on-demand video learning programs (vodcasts) can be used to stimulate interest and involvement in learning.

An essential element in any self-paced learning activity is the opportunity for immediate application of new knowledge and skills. Application is accomplished through use of text-based case studies or video clip scenarios that require an active response by the learner. These application opportunities are embedded in the learning modules. After each major content area in the module, the learner completes a brief application exercise that provides feedback about what was just learned (formative assessment). At the conclusion of each learning module, a culminating exercise enables the learner to synthesize and apply new knowledge (summative assessment). Feedback for performance (ideal responses for the exercise) is provided immediately after completion of the learning module.

Although the availability of self-study learning modules provides opportunities to acquire foundational knowledge of the leadership and management development curriculum, it is critical that this solitary study be followed by multiple opportunities for collaborative, interactive learning. Collaborative learning is facilitated by using a combination of online and classroom-based face-to-face forums. Online collaboration during learning is facilitated by "meeting online" to participate in asynchronous (any time, any place) interactive discussion forums wherein participants post and respond to questions and case studies and participation in synchronous (scheduled same time, any place), live, "chat" sessions that are conducted using either text-based (keyboard entries) or interactive video teleconferencing. Although collaborative learning can be accomplished online, it is essential that there are also opportunities for face-to-face or classroom-based gatherings. Once learners have obtained the prerequisite content knowledge through self-study, they need multiple opportunities to develop process knowledge as a group, refining communication skills, establishing interpersonal and functional work networks, building team cohesiveness, and practicing new leadership behaviors.

The teaching–learning approach that uses a combination of online and face-to-face instruction is known as "blended" or "hybrid" instruction. A blended design can enhance learner engagement, participation, and satisfaction with the experience, lower costs of instruction, and positively impact learning outcomes (Dziuban, Hartman, & Moskal,

2004; Lamoureux, 2006; Vignare et al., 2005). Collaborative, social learning designs (compared with solitary, individual learning) provide opportunities for knowledge and collective understanding to emerge from the interactive process within and among groups. The emergence of "collective intelligence" promotes networking, DOI, and a focus on people and performance rather than on content (Horizon Report, 2008).

Critical to the success of any educational program is the opportunity to immediately apply new learning in the context in which those skills are used and with members of their work team. Collaboration during learning and the opportunities to create shared meaning within a work group are valued by adult learners (Horizon Report, 2008). Blended-learning designs that use a variety of instructional modalities and mobile technologies (wireless access to Web sites, study modules, interactive video conferences and discussion forums) facilitate group learning and afford adult learners choices for interaction and engagement. The blended designs for learning promote the iterative, interactive learning environments that are consistent with the philosophy and structure of WSSG and the principles of DOI. The highly participative structure and processes of WSSG provide both the mechanism for collaborative learning and the opportunities for immediate application of new learning and leadership behaviors in a group setting. The integration of WSSG with a comprehensive, continuous education program that supports the principles of adult learning (Knowles, 1980) and is based on an effective instructional design establishes a successful paradigm for DOI and the potential for adaptability within the complex system.

Assessment of Learning Outcomes and Behavior Change

The measure of new learning is behavior change. The acquisition and application of new knowledge, skills, and abilities are evaluated after each learning activity and by assessment of performance within the organization. Each learning activity concludes with a summative assessment of new knowledge acquired and may include posttests, case study responses, dynamic situation role play or simulation assessments, and reports or projects that demonstrate applied skills. Debriefing sessions serve as both a tool for learning and for assessment of learning achievement. Debriefing sessions conducted immediately after a face-to-face workshop or meeting are useful to confirm that participants understand the learning content before applying new knowledge and skills on the job. It is in these debriefing sessions that participants interact to reflect on new information, clarify understanding and seek additional information, practice new leadership skills, construct shared meanings, and build individual confidence in leadership abilities. Debriefing for individual and team performance at the point-of-service should also be conducted by supervisors of the various service lines at regular intervals to provide specific and timely feedback about the effectiveness of performance and the achievement of care outcomes.

Supervisors traditionally conduct an annual employee review that is designed to reflect observed performance evaluated against their job description. These job descriptions are often out of date, reflect the minimum competencies required for the job, and frequently do not reflect the true scope of the position or clearly identify expectations for leadership and management skills in contemporary HCOs. The demand for adaptive performance in these complex environments creates a constant need for new knowledge and skills and therefore continuous learning. Job descriptions should evolve as learning evolves, and performance assessments should be iterative and formative to reflect the true nature of the work environment. As new knowledge, skills, and abilities are acquired, learned, and applied, performance evaluation metrics and documentation should be updated. Managers and supervisors are challenged to develop iterative, formative methods to accurately evaluate staff performance. In WSSG the Education Council, by virtue of its charge to ensure an organization-wide mechanism for continuous learning that reflects current evidence, safety, and quality standards, provides input to frequent revisions of job descriptions and performance appraisals. Job descriptions and performance appraisal tools are living documents and, as such, need to evolve with learning.

As part of the comprehensive education program for leadership and development, the Education Council designs tools and methods to identify emerging learning needs and to collect data reflecting overall participant satisfaction and program effectiveness. Continuous quality improvement is facilitated by conducting formal evaluation after each educational activity. Criteria for evaluation include measures of design, accessibility, ease-of-use, appropriateness of instructional modality to the content and learning task, and the effectiveness of instructional delivery (teaching) for face-to-face sessions. Data from these assessments and other sources (such as input from administrators, managers, supervisors, and the WSSG councils about unmet quality thresholds, sentinel events for safety, error, and complications, and observed leadership performance deficits) are used to continuously modify and update both content and process of the educational offerings. Learning outcomes are evaluated by the formative and summative measures that are embedded into each learning activity. Behavior change is assessed by peer review within councils and teams and by supervisors using established employee performance review tools and methods. The Education Council prepares an annual written report that summarizes findings reflecting the three measures (emerging learning needs, participant satisfaction, and overall program effectiveness), and this report is distributed to all WSSG councils for communication throughout the organization.

CONCLUSION

A renaissance in health care is not likely to occur if leaders are not willing to significantly change the way they lead, design, and operate HCOs. Leaders of 21st century HCOs must continuously seek goodness of fit between the HCO and its environment, as well as internal goodness of fit between the staff, managers, and practitioners and the HCOs in which they work and practice. For this to occur, staff, practitioners and daily managers must decentralize power, authority, autonomy, and accountability for what happens at the point-of-service. Moreover, power, autonomy, authority, and accountability must be codified into a workable participatory management structure such as WSSG. Care processes must be embedded with the best available valid and reliable evidence and put the patient's needs ahead of the department's needs. Moreover, care processes must be designed so that they can be easily navigated and accessed. Practitioners, staff, and managers must develop care processes that continuously balance the cost and quality of care. Care that is of high quality but too expensive will not allow the HCO to sustain itself anymore than care that is of poor quality. When care is of poor quality, it is always too expensive. Care must be value added and sensitive to the needs and requirements of the patients as well as the payers.

REFERENCES

Anderson, E. F. F. (2000). Empowerment, job satisfaction, and professional governance of nurses in hospitals with and without shared governance: A descriptive correlational and comparative study. *Dissertation Abstracts International, B61*(04) (UMI No. AAI9968766).

Ashmos, D. P., Huonker, J. W., & McDaniel, R. R. (1998). Participation as a complicating mechanism: The effect of clinical professional and middle manager participation on hospital performance. *Health Care Management Review, 23*(4), 7–20.

Barker, J. A. (1992). *Paradigms: The business of discovering the future.* New York: Harper Press.

Burton, T. T., & Moran, J. W. (1995). *The future focused organization: Complete organizational alignment for breakthrough results.* Englewood Cliffs, NJ: Prentice Hall.

Caramanica, L. (2004). Shared governance: Hartford hospital's experience. *Online Journal of Issues in Nursing, 9*(1). Retrieved October 10, 2008, from www.nursingworld.org/MainMenuCategories/ANAMarketplace/ANAPeriodicals/OJIN/TableofContents/Volume92004/No1Jan04/HartfordHospitalsExperience.aspx

Crow, G. L. (2006). Diffusion of innovation: The leader's role in creating the organizational context for evidence-based practice. *Nursing Administration Quarterly, 30*(3), 236–241.

Denis, J. L., Herbert, Y., Langley, A., Lozeau, D., & Trottier, L. H. (2002). Explaining diffusion patterns for complex health care innovations. *Health Care Management Review, 27*(3), 60–73.

Dziuban, C. D., Hartman, J. L., & Moskal, P. D. (2004). *Blended learning: Research bulletin.* Educause Center for Applied Research, 7, 1–12. Retrieved October 25, 2008, from http://net.educause.edu/ir/library/pdf/erb0407.pdf

Ferlie, E., Gabbay, J., Fitzgerald, L., Locock, L., & Dopson, S. (2001). Evidence-based medicine and organizational change: An overview of some recent qualitative research. In L. Ashburner (Ed.), *Organizational behavior and organizational studies in health care: Reflections on the future.* Basingstoke, England: Palgave.

Gardenfors, P. (2006). *How homo became sapiens: On the evolution of thinking.* London: Oxford University Press.

Gardner, D. B., & Cummings, C. (1994). Total quality management and shared governance: Synergistic processes. *Nursing Administration Quarterly, 18*(4), 56–64.

Geibert, R. C. (2006). Using diffusion of innovation concepts to enhance implementation of an electronic health record to support evidence-based practice. *Nursing Administration Quarterly, 30*(3), 203–210.

Hammer, M., & Champy, J. (1993). *Reengineering the corporation: A manifesto for business revolution.* New York: Harper Business Essentials.

Hendel, T., Fish, M., & Berger, O. (2007). Nurse/physician conflict management mode choices: Implications for improved collaborative practice. *Nursing Administration Quarterly, 31*(3), 244–253.

Hess, R. G. (1994). Shared governance: Innovation or imitation? *Nursing Economics, 12*(1), 28–34.

Hess, R. G. (2004). From bedside to boardroom: Nursing shared governance. *Online Journal of Issues in Nursing, 9*(1). Retrieved October 5, 2008, from http://www.cinahl.com/cgi-bin/refsvc?jid=1331&accno=2004169234

Horizon Report. (2008). The New Media Consortium and Educause Learning Initiative. Retrieved October 25, 2008, from http://www.nmc.org/publications/2008-horizon-report

Kim, D. H. (1992). *Toward learning organizations: Integrating total quality control and systems thinking.* Cambridge, MA: Pegasus Communication.

Knowles, M. S. (1980). *The modern practice of adult education: From pedagogy to andragogy.* Englewood Cliffs, NJ: Prentice Hall/Cambridge.

Kouzes, J. M., & Posner, B. Z. (2002). *The leadership challenge* (3rd ed.). San Francisco: Jossey-Bass.

Kramer, M., & Schmalenberg, C. (2003). Securing good nurse physician relationships. *Nursing Management, 34*(7), 34–38.

Lamoureux, K. (2006). High-impact leadership development: Essential components, best practices and case studies. Retrieved October 22, 2008, from http://www.bersin.com/Lib/Rs/Details.aspx?docid=10333554&id

Laschinger, H. K. S., & Finegan, J. (2005). Using empowerment to build trust and respect in the workplace: A strategy for addressing the nursing shortage. *Nursing Economics, 23*(1), 6–13.

Laschinger, H. K. S., & Havens, D. S. (1996). Staff nurse work empowerment and perceived control over nursing practice: Conditions for work effectiveness. *Journal of Nursing Administration, 26*(9), 27–35.

Laschinger, H. K. S., & Wong, C. (1999). Staff nurse empowerment and collective accountability: Effect on perceived productivity and self-rated work effectiveness. *Nursing Economics, 17*(6), 308–316, 351.

Leonard, D. (1998). *Wellsprings of knowledge: Building and sustaining the sources of innovation.* Boston: Harvard Business School Press.

Lewin, K. (1935). *A dynamic theory of personality.* New York: McGraw-Hill.

Lieb, S. (1991). Adult learning principles. Retrieved October 26, 2008, from http://honolulu.hawaii.edu/intranet/committees/FacDevCom/guidebk/teachtip/adults–2.htm

Maeda, J. (2006). *The laws of simplicity.* Cambridge, MA: MIT Press.

McClellan, M. B., McGinnis, J. M., Nabel, E. G., & Olsen, L. M. (2008). *Evidence-based medicine and the changing nature of health care: Workshop summary,* IOM roundtable on evidence-based medicine (October 8, 2007). Washington DC: National Academies Press.

Merriam-Webster Online Dictionary. (2008). Retrieved October 11, 2008, from http://www.merriam-webster.com/dictionary/accountability

Meyer, A. D., & Goes, J. B. (1988). Organizational assimilation of innovations: A multilevel contextual analysis. *Academy of Management Journal, 31*(4), 897–923.

Mitchell, M., Brooks, F., & Pugh, J. (1999). Balancing nurse empowerment with improved practice and care: An evaluation of the impact of shared governance. *NT Research, 4*(3), 192–200.

Moore, S. C., & Hutchison, S. A. (2007). Developing leaders at every level: Accountability and empowerment actualized through shared governance. *Journal of Nursing Administration, 37*(12), 564–568.

Naisbitt, D. (1984). *Megatrends: Ten new directions transforming our lives.* New York: Warner Books.

Patterson, E., & McMurray, A. (2003). Collaborative practice between registered nurses and medical practitioners in Australian general practice: Moving from rhetoric to reality. *Australian Journal of Advanced Nursing, 20*(4), 43–48.

Pearson, A., Laschinger, H., Porritt, K, Jordan, Z., Tucker, D., & Long, L. (2007). Comprehensive systematic review of evidence on developing and sustaining nursing leadership that fosters a healthy work environment in healthcare. *International Journal of Evidence-Based Healthcare, 5*(2), 208–253.

Peter, L. J., & Hull, R. (1969). *The Peter Principle: Why things always go wrong.* New York: William Morrow.

Plsek, P. (2003). Complexity and the adoption of innovation in health care. Paper presented at Accelerating Quality Improvement in Health Care: Strategies to Accelerate the Diffusion of Evidence-based Innovations.

Washington, DC: National Institute for Healthcare Management Foundation and National Committee for Quality in Health Care. Retrieved October 16, 2008, from http://www.nihcm.org/~nihcmor/pdf/Plsek.pdf

Plsek, P. E., & Greenhalgh, T. (2001). The challenge of complexity in health care. *British Medical Journal, 323*(7313), 625–628.

Porter, M. E., & Teisberg, E. O. (2006). *Redefining health care.* Boston: Harvard Business School Press.

Porter-O'Grady, T. (1995). *The leadership revolution in health care: Altering systems, changing behaviors.* Gaithersburg, MD: Aspen.

Porter-O'Grady, T., Hawkins, M. A., & Parker, M. L. (1997). *Whole-systems shared governance: Architecture for integration.* Gaithersburg, MD: Aspen.

Porter-O'Grady, T., & Malloch, K. (2007). *Managing for success in health care.* St. Louis, MO: Mosby.

Rogers, E. M. (2003). *Diffusion of innovations* (5th ed.). New York: Free Press.

Rouse, W. (2008). Healthcare is a complex adaptive system: Implications for design and management. *The Bridge, 38,* 1–10. Retrieved September 9, 2008, from http://www.nae.edu/nae/bridgecom.nsf/weblinks/MKEZ-7CLKRV?OpenDocument

Schmalenberg, C., & Kramer, M. (2008). Clinical units with the healthiest work environments. *Critical Care Nurse, 28*(3), 65–77.

Schneider, M., & Somers, M. (2006). Organizations as complex adaptive systems: Implications of complexity theory for leadership research. *Leadership Quarterly, 17,* 351–365.

Scott, J. G., Sochalski, J., & Aiken, L. H. (1999). Review of magnet hospital research: findings and implications for nursing practice. *Journal of Nursing Administration, 29*(1), 9–18.

Senge, P. M. (1990). *The fifth discipline: The art and practice of the learning organization.* New York: Doubleday.

Tushman, M. (1977). Special boundary roles in the innovation process. *Administrative Sciences Quarterly, 22,* 587–605.

Valente, T. W. (1996). Social networks thresholds in the diffusion of innovation. *Social Networks, 18*(1), 69–89.

Vignare, K., Dziuban, C., Moskal, P., Luby, R., Serra-Roldan, R., & Wood, S. (2005). *Blended learning review of research: An annotative bibliography.* Retrieved October 26, 2008, from http://www.uic.edu/depts/oee/blended/workshop/bibliography.pdf

Webster's Encyclopedic Unabridged Dictionary of the English Language. (1994). New York: Random House.

West, E., Barron, D. N., Dowsett, J., & Newton, J. N. (1999). Hierarchies and cliques in the social networks of health care professional: Implications for the design of dissemination strategies. *Social Science and Medicine, 48*(3), 633–646.

Westrope, R. A., Vaughn, L., Bott, M., & Taunton, R. L. (1995). Shared governance: From vision to reality. *Journal of Nursing Administration, 25*(12), 45–54.

Yetton, P., Sharma, R., & Southon, G. (1999). Successful IS innovation: The contingent contributions of innovation characteristics and implementation. *Journal of Information Technology, 14,* 53–68.

CHAPTER 9

Leadership, Innovation, and Healing Spaces

Jaynelle F. Stichler, with Sandra Davidson
and Jamil AlShraiky

The world is suddenly focused on the need for change, and we want it right now! Presidential candidates promised radical change; other politicians attested to changes they had already implemented in their term of office; books on change fill our bookshelves; popular magazines and professional journals feature articles assailing the need for change; newspapers and Internet Web casts prescribe the need for radical changes to save our threatened environment; and health care as an industry and service is witnessing the greatest demand for change in a century of care delivery. It would seem that as a global neighborhood we are no longer tolerant of the status quo. The paradox about change is that as humans we are generally quite resistant to change when it actually occurs, and we can find many great reasons to explain our resistance to minimal or radical change: "it costs too much", "it's not fair and equitable to all", "it doesn't meet the actual needs that we expressed", or "we didn't understand the consequences of the decision." The real bottom line to change resistance is that it moves us from a comfort zone to uncharted territory and that makes us uncomfortable, even when we specifically asked for the change to occur.

Perhaps this explains why many nurses and other providers are unhappy when they first move into a newly built environment, whether it is a new hospital, outpatient setting, or renovated unit. There seems to be more to the story than the completed design, and moving to the new environment creates a period of chaos and disruption of the familiar while we try to re-create everyday realities in a new setting. Even when nurses are involved in the design process, there is still significant unrest that occurs when moving in and adjusting to the new environment: "Who decided to design it like this?" or "What were they thinking?" or "Why didn't they ask us?" Something seems to be lost in the translation from conceptual thinking or conceptual design or the reality of the built environment. Could it be that even though nurses were involved, they may not have been actually engaged in the process? Could it be that they were not armed with the knowledge and competencies about design, the evidence, or even best practice examples before they met with the architects and designers? Perhaps they weren't even involved at all in the process. There are many very logical reasons why the built environment does not meet expectations of the providers, or even the patients, and yet a new building affects patient care delivery for the next 30 to 50 years. A new building is the most concrete influence on how patient care is delivered: Design decisions are encased in steel, and they do create change in our practice environment and influence the patient and family experience.

This chapter focuses on leadership to inspire innovative thinking in the creation of healing spaces, and in the midst of the largest healthcare construction boom in the history of the United States and the world, innovative designs are clearly needed. It is estimated that more than $200 billion dollars will be spent in the United States on new hospital construction before the year 2020, excluding what is currently spent and planned for new medical office buildings and outpatient centers. The United States is not alone in this quest for new healthcare environments. There seems to be a world focus on building new or renovating old healthcare settings, largely the result of a need for new capacity, new configurations to support new diagnostic and interventional technology or the merging of existing technologies, and the need to replace old, crumbling facilities. The challenge is to think futuristically about healthcare delivery because the new building will last 30 to 50 or more years, and it must adapt to changes in healthcare delivery models and flex with variations in patient volumes, diagnoses, and care trends over the life span of the building. But, current realities in bioterrorism, worldwide epidemics, and global economic and climate changes are serious challenges that are also affecting healthcare design considerations today. Designing a new facility is an awesome responsibility and likely one of the largest capital decisions that any healthcare executive will ever make.

So how do we think innovatively about healthcare design? What can we do as transformational leaders to ensure that nurses, physicians, and other healthcare providers are empowered, engaged, and recognized for their leadership competencies in healthcare design? How can innovations be tested before they are built in concrete and steel, leaving us with "built experiments" that may yield less than optimal environments to work or for patients to heal? As leaders how can we ensure that our professional colleagues are prepared for changes in their everyday realities when they move into a new facility? These are but a few of the challenging questions faced by healthcare executives and leaders who look future in the face when they sit down at the table with a team of architects, designers, and engineers and envision the future of patient care delivery and nursing practice. These are concrete changes encased in steel, and the decisions made today affect everything: organizational culture and climate, care delivery, communication patterns among disciplines, costs, patient outcomes, employee and patient safety, market share, community image, perceptions of quality, staff efficiencies, and just about everything we know to be true in our everyday "reality." The usual attitudes and comments that "we've always done it this way" or "we are different here from other hospitals" will not work anymore in solving current and the future's complex problems in a chaotic healthcare system. New innovative thinking about the future of nursing and patient care delivery is required when designing healthcare environments for the future.

LEADERSHIP IN TRANSFORMING HEALTHCARE DESIGN

Transformation is as the root of this word implies—a change that cuts across (trans) the form of the current reality. Leaders demonstrate the courage and tenacity to change the focus of healthcare design. Transformational leaders have been described as risk takers, innovators, collaborators, and visionaries who are driven by a passionate belief in a purpose or cause they believe will make a significant difference (Bass, 1985; Somerville & Mroz, 1997). Many of the leaders who radically changed the design of hospitals and other health facilities were driven by a higher purpose than obtaining credit for themselves, and they often achieved the transformation by being vulnerable, courageous, and tenacious.

Until the last two decades, not much changed in healthcare design for nearly a century. Imagine all the changes in science, increasing knowledge in infectious disease processes, emerging surgical interventions resulting from new anesthetic methods, diagnostic and interventional technologies, and even new pharmacological interventions for the treatment of pain for acute and chronic conditions. The thought that the physical environment made any difference at all in the healing process was lost since the days of Florence Nightingale. As a visionary and tenacious leader, Florence Nightingale radically transformed health care in the 19th century with her innovative thinking that natural light, proper ventilation, clean and orderly surroundings, quietness, diversion (variety), and clean water and nutrition were essential to the healing process. She also espoused the belief that patients needed to be observed at all times by the providers and designed open ward units with a clear line of sight from the nurse to the patient (Nightingale & Barnum, 1992). The open ward with varying numbers of patients was the design of choice until the 1950s and 1960s when newer units were built with smaller four-bed wards or two-bed rooms with Hill-Burton monies appropriated by the government for the construction of new hospitals after World War II.

Consumers drove the next radical change in healthcare design in the 1960s and 1970s with the help of a few courageous leaders who cut across the grain of mainstream medicine and the very controlling attitudes of medical and nursing providers who dictated how births would happen, separated infants from their mothers and mothers from the fathers during and after the birth, and initiated policies and procedures that limited who and how many could visit the patients while they were in the hospital. In response, women demanded that they labor, deliver, and stay in the same room, which was referred to as the "alternative birth room" or "alternative birth center" (ABC room). The ABC room was the consumer's way of regaining control of the childbirth experience and having a voice in how the experience would unfold.

Nearly every labor and delivery unit created at least one of the token ABC rooms, and the physicians' and staff's eyes often rolled when the woman and her husband were cared for in this one room without being transferred to the delivery room, recovery room, or postpartum room and without infants being whisked off to a nursery. It was never quite clear to some providers if the room was alternative or if the patient was "alternative," because many providers had strong biases that these "demanding" women were clearly not representative of mainstream America. Only these women were very mainstream and were encouraged by transformational leaders who had a vision that birth should be "family centered" and "patient directed." Amidst many accusations from the medical establishment that nurses or physicians who encouraged or participated in this alternative practice were subquality providers, these courageous and transformational leaders continued on their quest to ensure that every woman was empowered to direct the birth experience as she wished through birth plans and in an environment conducive to an intimate, family-centered experience. The consumer movement for a more homelike environment for birthing radically changed the design of birthing centers nationwide, as well as in many other countries. These ABC rooms were market drivers, and hospitals that did not create such birthing facilities soon realized their market share was challenged by those who built one or more ABC rooms.

In the 1980s the ABC rooms became the LDRs (labor-delivery-recovery) or the LDRPs (labor-delivery-recovery-postpartum, also known as single-room maternity care) of maternity centers, and nearly every hospital began building new or renovated existing space to create entire units of the new LDRs or LDRPs. For some hospitals the LDR or LDRP was simply a marketing initiative with a philosophy of "build it and they will come," but to other hospitals a new era of radical change occurred in healthcare design. Not only did the "space" matter to women who had time to comparison shop before choosing the hospital for the birth, but the "place" mattered as well. The space needed to be a sacred place for new life to emerge, so the birthing centers were designed with many homelike, sacred designs that appealed aesthetically to women and connoted the feeling of home and family, which after all is what birth is about. The family-centered care philosophy and the Planetree philosophy of care were emerging as guiding principles to change the culture of health care (Frampton, Gilpin, & Charmel, 2003; Institute of Family Centered Care, 2008; McKay & Phillips, 1983). The lobbies of the new family-centered birthing centers were often quite similar to nicely appointed homes, with a fireplace, sofas, plump comfortable chairs, lamps, soft music, brightly colored artwork of flowers, children, animals, or nature, and handcrafts such as tapestries, quilts, or framed stitchery. The patients' rooms were similarly appointed, and the surgical tile flooring previously seen in delivery rooms and surgical suites gave way to real wood flooring sealed for protection from fluids or woodlike vinyl applications. A new day had dawned in healthcare facility design, and women were not the only ones to notice the difference. Although maternity centers were not the revenue drivers that cardiovascular, orthopedics, or oncology services were, they were the market drivers for many hospitals. And as patients, their families, and visitors noticed the new look of the birthing centers, there was a new demand that the rest of the hospital look equally hospitable. Soon a new attribute of quality emerged in the eyes of the consumer, and the look of the facility was viewed as a measure of quality (Stichler & Weiss, 2001). Even though reimbursement methods changed over these same decades, consumers still had some choice among healthcare plans, and hospitals that considered the appearance of their physical environment were often viewed by payer and patient as quality hospitals.

The 1990s was a chaotic time in health care, with massive reimbursement changes resulting in major cutbacks in programs and staff. The decisions not only trimmed expenses, but they also nearly eliminated the last shred of trust and confidence that nurses and other providers had in healthcare leadership, resulting in dissatisfaction and turnover. In some organizations these times were referred to as "the medieval ages in health care." Work environments were darkened with a stressed staff, crowded inpatient environments, and failing systems. Healthcare futurists predicted that the sum of reduced lengths of stay, increased numbers of minimally invasive procedures, and the expansion of high-tech diagnostic procedures would result in significant downsizing of inpatient settings and a proliferation of outpatient facilities. Many acute care units were converted to outpatient services, office space, and onsite wellness programs during this time.

Realizing the negative effects of some of the organizational downsizing and deteriorating work environments on staff recruitment and retention, patient outcomes, quality metrics, and performance measures, healthcare leaders began to examine ways to repair the organizational cultures that were completely eroded in the medieval years and to see the hospital environment with a new lens. Many hospitals built with Hill Burton funds in the 1940s and 1950s were no longer able to support new care delivery methods or new diagnostic and interventional technologies. With all the reduction in reimbursement, many not-for-profit hospitals no longer had the money for capital improvements, leaving the facilities to age without repair or renovation. Additionally, new regulations were passed in California requiring all hospitals to meet new seismic requirements, increasing the chances that the hospitals would withstand a major earthquake affecting their area. This regulation alone caused all California hospitals to develop a facility strategic plan that would outline how they would comply with the new regulations by 2015 with either structural renovations or new replacement hospitals. All across the country hospitals began considering the need and cost of renovating or replacing their facilities to meet customer and provider needs, increase capacity (the experiment with downsizing did not work), and accommodate new diagnostic and interventional equipment.

A new interest developed in creating healthcare environments that had a calming and healing effect on both staff and patients. The Center for Health Design (CHD) was instrumental in publishing research findings correlating attributes of the environment on patients' medical outcomes and satisfaction rates (Rubin, Owens, & Golden, 1998). These reports raised awareness that the appearance and design of health facilities were more than marketing tools and that the term "healing environment" was more than a promotional gimmick to draw customers to the hospitals. Ulrich's reports on the effect of patients' views to the outside on their recovery rates and satisfaction levels (Ulrich, 1984) and the positive effects of healing gardens on staff, patient, and family moods and stress levels (Ulrich, 1999) did much to peak interest in the notion that the environment might be important as a healing factor. Although many embraced the concept of the environment as a factor that could enhance healing for patients and families and reduce stress for providers, others were skeptical and demanded evidence to back up the claims that the facility design and appearance improved anything other than market appeal.

Desperately Seeking Evidence

Research on the effect of the built environment on patient and provider outcomes was initiated by the CHD with the leadership of the Research Advisory Committee composed of several luminaries and researchers in design, health care, environmental and organizational psychology, sociology, and the neurosciences. The intent was to seek out existing evidence to guide design decisions, to test the effect of design features on outcomes, to create new knowledge for dissemination, and ultimately to reduce stress for hospitalized patients, their families, and healthcare providers (Cama, 2006a, b). Paralleling the work of CHD, the Coalition for Health Environments Research (CHER) was developed as a nonprofit organization founded by the American Institute of Architects' Academy of Architecture for Health to promote health environments research. Later, the two organizations separated, and CHER formed a 501(c)3 corporation to facilitate collaborative research efforts with other foundations and corporations. With a staff of volunteers and funding from varied sources, CHER produced and disseminated findings from a number of critical research projects that became a part of the foundation for the evidence-based design initiative. Now as a part of CHD, CHER continues as a Research Council of six experienced researchers who direct or conduct research on topics exploring the relationship between environmental design and patient falls, nursing medication errors in an acute care setting, infection control, environmental noise, and safety for patients and providers. CHD has also provided significant leadership in the evidence-based design with the Pebble Project initiative, which provides research consultation to subscribing hospitals interested in using an evidence-based design approach in building projects or in measuring the effect of their new environments on organizational metrics or patient and provider satisfaction (CHD, 2008).

Although the physical environment was not specifically addressed, the publication of the Institute of Medicine's *To Err Is Human* (Kohn, Corrigan, & Donaldson, 2000) transformed facility design from a passing interest to center stage as an important attribute in creating safer environments for patients and staff. The Committee on Quality of Health Care in America and the Institute of Medicine's *Crossing the Quality Chasm* (2001) and its focus on improving safety, quality, and outcomes by analyzing the systems behind inadequate quality of care provided a new framework for healthcare design with the recognition of the interdependence of all changes in a system and the critical need for interdisciplinary groups to collaborate on the redesign of organizational structures and organizational cultures. Although not specifically stated, it is clear that the same mandate has application to the design of healthcare facility structures as well. The facility design as critical component to ensure patient safety was explicitly discussed in *Keeping Patients Safe* (Page, 2004), which recommended improving the patient environment and the nurses' work environment and cited ways to reduce errors with changes in the physical design. With this publication and emphasis from the Institute of Medicine, Agency for Healthcare Research and Quality, Institute of Health Improvement, and The Joint Commission, the notion that the healthcare physical environment made a difference on patient and provider outcomes was finally recognized. Architects, interior designers, engineers, and healthcare executives were challenged to identify innovative designs to address issues that affected the patient and family experience and the providers' work efficiency, stress levels, and total experience. The challenge for innovation was also coupled with the demand for evidence to demonstrate that these new innovative design ideas made a difference as promised in marketing presentations and publications of completed projects.

Dichotomy of Evidence and Innovation

The notion of promoting the use of an evidence-based approach to design is innovative in itself in that most published projects focused on the glossy photos of beautiful new facilities taken before occupancy and accompanied by information related to total square footage, the total construction and project costs, and the names of the designers, consultants, and contractors. The narrative for these projects includes descriptions of the floor plans, specific design features, and the issues and forces that contributed to the design decisions. The merging of innovation and evidence-based design presents an interesting push–pull dichotomy. Evidence-based design combines the findings from previous research that is applicable for a specific project with best practice examples of completed projects, opinions of experts (design and health care), and opinions from the clients (healthcare administrators, providers, and even patients). Conversely, innovative design may not always have directly supporting evidence but provides a fresh, creative look at design challenges coupled with the synergistic thinking of multiple disciplines that cannot be achieved by any other method or approach.

The St. Joseph's Hospital in West Bend, Wisconsin, a member of *Synergy*Health, was one of the first to invite a multidisciplinary team of experts to participate in the design of the new hospital with a goal to improve patient safety through design. The planning group conducted a learning lab conference with local and national experts in safety tapped from the aerospace industry, design, health care, and Six Sigma. The group's findings included safety-driven design principles developed from the top ten design recommendations to enhance safety through design (Reiling, Breckbill, Murphy, McCullough, & Chernos, 2003). This one event and subsequently published findings caught the attention of the Institute for Healthcare Improvement, Agency for Healthcare Research and Quality, and The Joint Commission, who now recommend an interdisciplinary approach to all design projects. To achieve the interdisciplinary approach, all disciplines at the table must have the knowledge and competencies to contribute to a truly collaborative and innovative outcome and be committed to finding the wisdom in the intersections of the disciplines.

MAGIC AT THE INTERSECTION

Is innovation a buzzword or a vision imperative? With so much emphasis on innovation, how can we balance the innovation imperative with an evidence-based design approach built on a foundation of previous research findings, best practice examples, and expert opinion. Can the two coexist? Where do the two concepts intersect?

Innovation has been defined as a new creation (a device, product, service, process, building) that results from in-depth analysis or study of the phenomena or situation (Dictionary.com) or "new ideas plus action or implementation which results in an improvement, a gain, or a profit" (Kelley, 2005, p. 6). Similarly, Carlson and Wilmot (2006) define innovation as "the process of creating and delivering new customer value in the marketplace" (p. 6). The notion that innovation brings new thinking to the table that adds value to the customer and results in an action for change was validated in *The Medici Effect* (Johansson, 2004), but the author states that it is impossible to determine if an idea or vision (design) is truly innovative until society decides whether the idea is both new and valuable. Furthermore, the author posits that real creativity and innovation occur at the intersection where different fields or disciplines meet—the Medici effect—and it is in the connection of different fields where real creative insights occur by connecting concepts from one field with concepts of another. "When you step into the Intersection, you can combine concepts among multiple fields, generating ideas that leap into new directions . . . intersectional ideas . . . . which will make you take a double take" (Johansson, 2004, p. 17).

Differentiating directional innovation from intersectional innovation, Johansson noted that directional innovation creates change in fairly predictable and planned steps, resulting in refinements and adjustments. This type of innovation occurs in health care when we make operational changes to improve quality or efficiency or even minor renovations to update the facility aesthetically. In contrast, intersectional innovations radically change the world and "leaps along in new directions" (Johansson, 2004, p. 19) and can even pave the way for new fields of study. Intersectional innovations can occur for healthcare facility design only when an emphasis is placed on having interdisciplinary teams work together on the design of each department within the healthcare facility to achieve the intersectional innovation. It is hoped that the day when architects design health facilities with a few token administrative people and with minimal input from patients and providers has ended. With an interdisciplinary design process in which nurses, physicians, and other providers are actively engaged in the design, innovative solutions that will be exemplars of the healing environment can finally be realized. "In systems thinking, leaders are aware of the importance of the 'intersections' . . . it is here where much of the work of leadership unfolds" (Porter-O'Grady & Malloch, 2007, p. 30).

Desperately Seeing Synergy

It is a curious notion that architects and healthcare professionals need to work together in the design of a facility, and there are some architects and healthcare executives who still firmly believe that only a chosen few hospitals leaders should interact with the design teams. Their rationale is that including nurses or physicians will drive up project costs because they have too many demands that are not affordable, cause too many costly changes in the drawings, or create unachievable expectations that will result in staff dissatisfaction. Usually, these same executives are not clear about their own vision and goals for the project or cannot articulate the boundaries of the project, such as the design philosophy, budget limits, department priorities, and targeted volumes of patients and/or procedures, which ultimately determines space requirements and costs. Although organizational leaders espouse that they have operational knowledge, often they do not have current understanding of the work at the point of service. Excluding those at the point of service often results in a completed project that is inefficient and inadequate in meeting the needs of the providers or providers. Creating collaborative work groups for the design requires the executive and design teams to trust that the nurses, physicians, and other providers can make the right decisions to achieve the project's goals once they are informed of the critical success factors for the project and then truly engage them in the process. A fine line of distinction exists between asking the providers to participate in the design process in contrast to being fully engaged in the process. Full engagement requires that the members are knowledgeable about the process, possess competencies in articulating and managing abstract concepts, and demonstrate open, active, and respectful communication with other disciplines and stakeholders who may have very competing priorities.

This level of engagement requires truly collaborative relationships that are founded on trust, mutual respect, sharing of information, and a balance of power that is achieved when each participant shares his or her expertise at the table (Kouzes & Posner, 2007; Stichler, 1995). A truly collaborative relationship results in a synergy that cannot be achieved in any other method or process, and most successful design projects were created as a result of interdisciplinary collaborative relationships.

Several factors can ensure a successful collaboration and outcomes that support the initial vision for the project and foster innovative thinking among the team members. These factors are described further below.

Knowledge About the Process

The process of designing and building a new facility follows a predictable process known by the design team but not well understood by most healthcare professionals. Many difficulties can be averted if time is taken to orient those who will be engaged in the design process about the planning, design, and construction process. The project leaders must orient those participating in the design process steps and expand their competencies to engage in each of the following phases:

- Visioning
- Evidence seeking and best practice exploration
- Planning, including space programming, operational planning, and equipment planning
- Conceptual design
- Schematic design
- Design development
- Construction drawings
- Construction administration
- Bidding
- Construction
- Occupancy planning
- Postoccupancy evaluation

A milestone chart where progress can be tracked is helpful to ground assumptions and expectations in reality and to keep the design project on schedule.

Defining Beliefs, Values, and Critical Factors

Often, the most important steps of the project, envisioning the future, is bypassed or rushed to complete the planning stage in which the number and types of spaces within the facility are determined. Too often these practical decisions are made without the context of a desired framework to guide the project. Before the design is initiated, the leadership team and those at the point of service must envision together what the future of patient care will be, how the current realities could be improved or changed, and what features support philosophical notions that are valued and sacred to the organization. Having these discussions during the design phase are important to remind everyone about the critical success factors for the project, but the real innovative thinking must come before the planning and design sessions even begin. As an example, an organization may desire to adopt the Planetree philosophy, which is a healing environment concept that is widely accepted in many hospitals today. The Planetree philosophy has major implications for planning and design, and this philosophy must be articulated to the design team to enable their translation of the philosophy to design concepts that support the philosophy. The philosophy also has major implications for the planning of nursing care delivery that must also be discussed and decided before the design process begins. Adopting a family-centered care model directly influences the design of the patient rooms and the location of waiting and family areas and may include family kitchens where families nurture their loved one with culturally sensitive food choices and preparations.

Other critical issues that must guide design decisions need to be determined before the design process begins, such as patient safety, employee safety, patient-centered care, operational efficiency, or adaptability/flexibility of planned spaces. Patient safety is a critical imperative, and serious consideration and innovative thinking must occur with all disciplines engaged to ensure that all patient care areas are designed to enhance patient safety. Innovative thinkers must work through patient care scenarios and professional functions to identify where possible breaches in safety might occur in the future and design spaces or processes to reduce the probability of occurrence. Some organizations engage in failure mode effectiveness analysis, workflow analysis, or Six Sigma processes for high-risk scenarios to enhance innovative thinking for future process improvements and design solutions. Computer simulation, video enactments, and deep dive experiences can also test the hypotheses that specific design attributes will effectively maximize patient safety and reduce injury or errors.

Evidence from other completed projects can provide insight into the efficacy or cost-to-benefit of specific design attributes or the retrospective study of outcomes resulting from the design (Stone, 2008). The current trend of expanding the size of patient bathroom doors is an example of disciplines coming together to analyze the risk involved of the patient, intravenous pole and pumps, and the nurse moving through the traditionally sized 3- to 4-foot door openings. All three cannot fit at once; this predisposes the patient to a fall or to nurse injury as he or she attempts to prevent the patient's fall. In an attempt to increase the bathroom door size, architects began to use a 2-foot and a 3-foot combination with both doors opening into the bathroom, but most nurses immediately reacted with feedback that trying to keep both doors open while maneuvering the patient and equipment through the door was more hazardous than before. This design option is a real example of design solutions that are adopted without nurses' input. Challenging traditional building guidelines and codes and examining the patient and provider process of moving through the door simultaneously, architects developed a new solution of expanding the doors to 5- or 6-foot openings and using sliding doors to maximize the opening.

Because of architects interacting with nurses, it was determined that another bathroom fall risk resulted from the design of enclosed shower areas where the patient had to step over the lip of the shower, negotiate moving into the shower enclosure, or stand from a wheelchair to step into the shower. An examination of options and innovative thinking resulted in the shower area being an open, integral part of the total bathroom area with sloping flooring and ceiling-mounted shower curtains to contain the water. This bathroom design has decreased the incidence of patient falls in several hospitals. If point-of-service providers were not engaged in the process with the architects, these simple innovations, which have had a significant impact on reducing patient falls and employee injuries, might never have been discovered.

Learning to Communicate and Work Together

The language of architecture, planning, and design is different from healthcare language, and to communicate each discipline must learn the basics of how to communicate in the other's language. Healthcare professionals may have difficulty sharing their knowledge, expertise, and experience in patient care with design professionals who must translate the language of patient care conceptually. The feedback determining if the architect understands the healthcare professional's description of a desired space is often a two-dimensional sketch or a computer-generated drawing that the healthcare provider may not be able to read or understand. How can this gap in communication be closed? How can healthcare professionals grasp how big 100, 250, or 800 square feet is or understand the cost implications of "can we make it bigger"? How can healthcare professionals help architects realize the critical nature of certain design features to ensure patient safety, enhance professional communication, reduce noise, minimize walking distances and other physical stressors, enhance infection control, or ensure immediate access to emergency equipment or diagnostic procedures? These translations of information to the other discipline require innovative ways of communicating about space, place, purpose, and priorities and ways of creating common meaning in the disparate language of differing disciplines.

There is magic and synergy at the intersections of disciplines. Learning to work together, communicate in a common language, articulate innovative solutions, and create shared meanings requires that nurses and other healthcare providers increase their knowledge and competencies in design and designers develop knowledge, competencies, and positive attitudes toward patient care delivery philosophies and processes. Leaders of the design process must engage the participants in the process by enhancing their knowledge of healthcare design process, evidence-based findings, and existing best practice examples. Recognizing the critical importance of the intersection between healthcare practice and the design process, many leaders in both fields are transforming the educational process of nurses, healthcare leaders, and designers.

One innovative group, Nursing in Health Design, has created learning modules about evidence-based design, design phases, healing environments, designing for safety, and other similar topics to enhance nurses' knowledge and competencies in healthcare design (see www.nursingihd.com). Realizing the critical importance of having informed and competent nurses interacting with architects in the creation of patient care environments, the founders created the Web-based self-learning modules, tested the validity of the product with several schools of nursing and hospitals involved in design projects, and created testing methods to measure the effectiveness of the modules on increasing the nurses' attitudes, knowledge, and competence in healthcare design. This innovative and entrepreneurial venture was one of the nation's first examples of nurses learning the language of design to enhance their effectiveness in creating healing environments for patients, families, and providers.

Recognizing that nurses were leading design efforts as consultants in architects' offices, project managers for major building expansions, researchers for evidence-based projects, or educators of nurses at the point of service to enable and empower them to be involved in the design projects, the *Journal of Nursing Administration* initiated a column aimed at advancing the knowledge of nurses about design. Articles disseminating research findings about the effect of design on patient outcomes and staff experiences can be found in most major nursing, medical, and healthcare management journals, whereas before articles of this nature were limited to environmental or design journals, which are not readily assessible to healthcare or design professionals.

In 2007 the interdisciplinary, peer-reviewed *Health Environments Research & Design Journal* was launched with a mission to enhance the knowledge and practice of evidence-based healthcare design by disseminating research findings, discussing issues and trends, and translating research into practice (see www.herdjournal.com). This new scientific journal with an interdisciplinary editorial advisory board creates magic at the intersection of disciplines and has fostered new science focused on healthcare design. With the merging of disciplines around this content knowledge, a new demand for innovative thinking about the education of future healthcare designers has emerged.

EDUCATING LEADERS IN HEALTHCARE DESIGN

Nursing involvement and leadership in healthcare design require an expanded set of competencies from those cited by the American Organization of Nurse Executives (AONE, 2005; Stichler, 2007). Stichler indicated that, in addition to the AONE prescribed skills, nurse leaders in design must master the art of articulating the project's vision to multiple levels of stakeholders and build interdisciplinary teams to work with designers to bring the vision to reality. To ensure the preservation of design features that are critical to the vision and philosophy of care, the nurse leader must have strong financial skills, not only in traditional business and healthcare financing but also in project and construction budgeting and financing, enabling the nurse leader to articulate the cost-to-benefit of specific design features to the board of directors, community leaders, potential donors, and government or grant agencies (Stichler, 2007). Although nurse executives are competent business and financial leaders, the language of construction finance may be new to them and to many healthcare executives. Critical content areas for nurse and other healthcare executives to gain competency include learning the methods to calculate an estimation of probable costs of a project, differentiating between the costs that contribute to the building costs versus the project costs, and capital financing options. Building projects are often the largest capital projects that executives will direct in their careers, and the decisions made will affect patient care delivery for many future decades (Stichler, 2008).

To meet the growing demand for nursing leadership in healthcare design, some schools of nursing are developing courses and/or specialized concentrations in design. Texas Woman's University in Houston, Texas, was one of the nation's first graduate nursing courses focusing on healthcare design for doctoral nursing students. Students examined evidence about design features that promote patient safety, interviewed architects, discussed their own knowledge base and experience as nurses, and created drawings of the "ideal" patient room to enhance patient safety. Partnering with a national vendor specializing in the product research, development, and manufacturing of hospital beds, healthcare furniture, headwalls, and equipment, the entire class was hosted by the company to meet with designers at their corporate offices where the students' "ideal" room was constructed as a mock-up and then evaluated by the students and designers as to its effectiveness in promoting patient safety (Stichler & Cesario, 2007).

Similarly, a collaboration between Emory University's School of Nursing and Georgia Technology School of Design, funded partially by a Robert Wood Johnson grant and under the direction of a nurse researcher and an architect-researcher, developed the *Hospital Room of the Future* course as a prototype for interdisciplinary learning (Lamb, Conner, Ossmann, & Stichler, 2007). Students from multiple disciplines were asked to study specific design problems in health care from their discipline's perspective and then synthesize the multiple perspectives into functional models of innovative solutions. From the students' observations, field notes, discussions, and innovation think tanks, five important lessons about the synergy were realized from the interdisciplinary collaboration:

1. Looking at problems collaboratively challenges past assumptions about how things work or are supposed to work in health care.
2. Discussing how specific design elements could negatively affect patient safety among disciplines motivated the designers to create design solutions to achieve the goals.
3. Learning the language of another discipline and finding a common meaning to frequently used words takes time.
4. Exploiting the diversity in nursing specialties is a major strength that can be used in design.
5. Realizing the importance of what is at stake in getting healthcare design right inspired deeper exploration leading to new innovations in design.

Students reported that ". . . participating in this course was a profoundly rewarding experience . . . in 15 weeks we moved from confusion and frustration to awareness and then awe of the power of the interdisciplinary process and its potential for creativity and innovation" (Lamb et al., 2007, p. 428).

Purdue University's School of Nursing also offers course work toward a Doctorate in Nursing Practice with an emphasis on design of healthcare processes and systems as well as the healthcare environment. The program proposes that graduates of the program work with administrators and design specialists to identify problems in existing designs and use an evidence-based approach in designing future nursing units that are more nurse friendly (Medaris & Novak, 2006).

The magic at the intersection has resulted in a new interdisciplinary approach to healthcare design with an integrated approach to educating future designers with courses of study leading to a doctoral degree by integrating nursing, architecture and design, business, and research. In *A Culture of Improvement Technology and the Western Millennium,* Friedel (cited in Friedman, 2008) stated, "imagine how much better firms and countries could innovate if they could harness the distributed creative potential of all these innovators in waiting . . . in an age of mass innovation, the world may even find profitable ways to deliver solutions to the 21st century's greatest needs . . . the one natural resource that the world has left in infinite quantity is human ingenuity" (Friedman, 2008, p. 166).

INNOVATION IN EDUCATION: CHARTING THE FUTURE OF HEALTHCARE DESIGN AND HEALING ENVIRONMENTS*

Dan is a patient on the medical ward of a small rural hospital. His nurse, Jenny, enters his private room to assess his condition. Dan's wife, Laura, is also in the room sitting in a chair beside his bed. As Jenny approaches Dan, she moves the bedside table out of the way and attempts to push his IV pole closer to the wall to make room for her to take Dan's vital signs. The vital sign cart Jenny has brought in with her gets caught on the corner of the bedside table, as she tries to pull it behind her. This causes the cup of water on the bedside table to spill. Laura jumps out of her chair and tries to squeeze past Jenny in an attempt to be helpful by wiping up the spilled water. As Jenny lowers the side

---

*This section was written by Jamil AlShraiky, MArch, MS, Director of the Healthcare Design Initiative and Assistant Professor in the Department of Interior Design, College of Design at Arizona State University, and Sandra Davidson, RN, MSN, PhD(c), CNE, Director of the Master of Healthcare Innovation Program and Clinical Associate Professor at the College of Nursing and Healthcare Innovation at Arizona State University. These two leaders are transforming the educational experience of healthcare designers by finding the magic of intersecting healthcare and design.

rail of the bed, the power cord of the IV pump gets caught, causing the IV pole to wobble. Jenny reaches out to steady it. Meanwhile, Laura is done wiping the bedside table and apologetically brushes past Jenny again to return to her chair at the bedside. As Jenny applies the blood pressure cuff to Dan's arm, she thinks to herself, "Why is simply getting to the patient so I can provide care such a struggle?"

The scenario above is by no means unusual or unique. Similar interactions play out on a daily basis in hospitals across the country. This single example at the point-of-care is a result of a complex matrix of events and decisions that occurred in the healthcare system (sometimes years in the making) that led to the nature of the interaction between nurse and client at the bedside. The interplay of the built environment, philosophy of care, and hospital systems design is one aspect that combines to influence the quality of the healing environment.

Traditionally, nursing, design, and healthcare management have existed as discrete disciplines, each with its own language, culture, and processes. Each discipline uniquely contributes to the overall quality of care outcomes. Designers of the built environment create the physical context in which care is provided. Nurses enact the processes of assessment, intervention, and ongoing evaluation of client care, whereas health system managers provide the infrastructure (policies, materials, and operations) in which care occurs.

To a large extent the current approach to healing environment design entails each discipline constructing its own version of the environment with a single disciplinary lens. As the planning process progresses, these often disparate disciplinary ideas and views are brought together and through negotiation and rationalization the needs and wishes of each discipline are "retro-fitted" to each other, and the healing environment takes shape. Challenges in the process of amalgamating the needs and desires of each discipline often stem from the lack of awareness and understanding of discipline-specific issues or requirements. For instance, most nurses are not aware of the American Institute of Architects code book regulations that govern hallway widths and placement of fire doors, just as many designers are not aware of time parameters for the administration of thrombolytics in the management of stroke. The point is not for designers to be nurses or nurses to be designers but for each to become better aware of the language, issues, and processes of the other so that shared understanding and true collaboration can occur in the design of healing environments.

The major impetus for the development of Arizona State University's (ASU's) Healthcare Initiative was the collective realization that to truly create optimal healing environments, healthcare-related disciplines need to work together synergistically rather than in isolation of each other. This vision is that no longer will graduate education take place in interdisciplinary silos but that nurses, designers, and health system managers will be educated in the "new discipline" of healthcare design and healing environments.

The Healthcare Initiative represents the formal transdisciplinary collaboration that was launched in the spring of 2008. Partners from the College of Design, College of Nursing & Healthcare Innovation, and the School of Global Management & Leadership came together with industry leaders representing Architecture, Interior Design, Healthcare Systems, and Care Providers to form the Healthcare Initiative Community Advisory Board. This Community Advisory Board meets quarterly to provide input, support, and direction to the growing initiative.

ASU offers the optimal organizational setting for the Healthcare Initiative's innovative new approach to graduate education in healthcare design and healing environments. The Initiative mirrors the aspirations of ASU's vision of the New American University through promoting excellence in specialized research areas of critical importance, increasing access to educational resources for students across many walks of life, and working with the community to impact social development and create positive change. A key vision and focus of the New American University is *intellectual fusion* through cross-discipline collaboration. The Healthcare Initiative fosters intellectual fusion by uniting architecture, interior design, industrial design, landscape architecture, planning, and visual communication design students from within the College of Design and the cross-disciplinary partnerships with the College of Nursing & Healthcare Innovation and School of Global Management & Leadership. Students and faculty of the Healthcare Initiative also engage local hospital/provider partners in reengineering healing environments to create positive patient and nursing outcomes.

This Initiative places ASU at the forefront of emerging educational programs and paradigms. ASU is currently the only university offering a truly transdisciplinary experience in healthcare design and healing environments. The Initiative represents one of the first formal partnerships anywhere in the country between a College of Design and a College of Nursing to address the built environment from a transdisciplinary perspective. This approach provides the opportunity for cutting-edge research and investigation in the healthcare industry. The partnership with the College of Nursing & Healthcare Innovation provides unique insight into clinical research, patient care, and evidence-based practice.

An essential element to the success of this initiative is the engagement of the professional design, healthcare, and business communities to ensure that our graduates are meeting the needs of the marketplace and that the industry has input into how its future leaders are trained. The design, healthcare, and business community leaders are formally involved and invested in the Healthcare Initiative through participation on its Community Advisory Board and informally engaged in providing mentorship and experiential learning opportunities for students.

Upon graduation, it is anticipated that students will be prepared to work in advanced positions such as

- Leadership and decision-making positions in the healthcare industry
- Strategic planners for large healthcare systems and corporations

- Facility programmers for consulting firms
- Innovative collaborators at research centers
- Expert representatives for leading manufacturers and vendors
- Medical planners for planning divisions in architectural and planning firms

Mission of the Healthcare Initiative

The College of Design and the College of Nursing & Healthcare Innovation are moving forward with program/curricular development in healthcare design and healing environments to capitalize on the growing need for implementing patient- and user-centered healthcare environments. The joint effort is envisioned to integrate evidence-based practice, sustainability science, and innovations in the planning, design, and care processes of healthcare facilities. The program is designed to provide a comprehensive, transdisciplinary advanced education. The ultimate mission is to prepare the next generation of healthcare design/practice professionals that will provide leadership for a new vision of healthcare planning, design, and delivery. These graduates will become the industry leaders who will shape the way that healthcare facilities are conceptualized, designed, and experienced. This new generation of healthcare leaders will be poised to fundamentally change how care is provided and how healing environments are designed and built.

The emphasis of the "new discipline" is on understanding the healing experience from the patient's and user's perspectives through facility-related components that cluster into seven curricular themes:

1. Evidence-based design/practice and research
2. Facilities analysis (physical and environmental)
3. Systems planning (systems thinking, programming, and strategic planning)
4. Financial/resources analysis
5. Human factors innovations
6. Regulatory issues (building codes, care policies, accreditation processes)
7. Leadership of innovation and change facilitation

This transdisciplinary approach seeks to integrate and synthesize key principles from architecture and interior design, nursing and healthcare innovation, leadership and management, health and human services, and communication and behavioral sciences.

Nature of the Educational Experience

Throughout the program students are mentored by local healthcare design consultants who have a shared interest with the student or whose expertise relates directly to the student's thesis, capstone, or dissertation topic. Students also team with nurses and clinicians in exploring and vetting their ideas and projects. The program collaborates directly with health system partners and care providers in that topics and design studio projects are put forward by health system partners and are reflective of their real-life challenges and issues. Students also correspond with forward-thinking healthcare researchers to gain insight about their chosen thesis, capstone, and dissertation topics. Several educational experiences of the Healthcare Initiative are highlighted in Boxes 9-1 and 9-2.

The Initiative includes multiple tracks of study in healthcare design and healing environments at the graduate level. Several degree programs are still in the planning/approval phase, with two graduate programs already in existence. Each of these tracks of study is described in Box 9-3.

Finally, an optional study abroad component allows students to explore global trends, issues, and challenges in the creation of healing environments. At present, faculty are working in collaboration with industry partners to plan a trip to Dubai Healthcare City. Albert Einstein is credited with saying, "We can't solve problems by using the same kind of thinking we used when we created them," and the Healthcare Initiative represents a bold step in the direction of creating a new way of thinking about and addressing the challenges facing healthcare. The discipline-specific perspectives used in the past are simply too small to fully grasp the immense challenges we face in health care. Think of viewing a problem from a small submarine portal: There is a limit to what your view will allow you to see and learn about your environment. A transdisciplinary approach creates a different perspective on the problems facing health care. The Healthcare Initiative seeks to design the "skylight view" for the future of healthcare. (See Box 9-4.)

Box 9-1 Healing Experience Studio

At the core, the design studio creates new paradigms in the healthcare industry. The class looks at the patient–nurse environment, how it influences the healing experience, the methodology and flow of nurses' work patterns, and what is required to support a fully positive patient outcome.

A local hospital partner serves as a model for realistic research and impactful issues via the demographics it serves and the powerful mission statement embraced by the staff and administration. A healthcare design studio class in Fall 2009, "The Healing Experience Studio," gives students the task of reengineering acute care environments at this hospital. Students also explore design that improves patient healthcare outcomes, contributes to outstanding care, and reinforces the mission statement of the organization. Proposed benefits to key stakeholder groups include

- Patients
- Hospital staff
- Students
- Industry

Box 9-2 Healthcare Environments Magazine Class

The student-produced healthcare environments magazine is a twofold vehicle for the joint effort. First, the research, writing, design, and production of this magazine, focused on healthcare design from a patient's and a user's perspective, is performed by students from the College of Design, College of Nursing & Healthcare Innovation, and the Walter Cronkite School of Journalism & Mass Communication. Second, this transdisciplinary approach provides an outlet for the dissemination of innovative approaches to healing environments, as well as research and investigation into the creation of optimal healing environments. This publication is differentiated from other healthcare facility or medical healthcare magazines because it strives to combine the user's and patient's perspectives as well as innovative approaches and research on healing environments into the spectrum of articles.

Patient- and user-focused outcomes driven research, in conjunction with evidence-based practice and the leadership of innovations, will form the dominant way of being and operating in the future of healthcare design. When we seek to understand and meet a human's deepest needs, quality of life improves. When quality of life improves, humans can unleash creative thinking and personal power. And when creative power is released: the world changes.

> Dan is sitting in the window seat of Laura's hospital room. He recalls the last time they were both in the hospital was 15 years ago. Laura's room is very different from the room he was a patient in just over a decade ago. Laura's nurse, Terry, enters the room. She stops at the provider-designated sink to wash her hands. Terry continues to the bedside and voice activates in-room vital sign monitoring equipment. Laura's current vital signs are instantly visible on the in-wall smart screen. Terry then tells the voice-activated monitoring system to record the current vitals in Laura's electronic medical record. Dan watches from the comfort of the family-designated zone of the room. He thinks what a great gift is has been for him to be able to stay at Laura's side throughout her recovery and not once has he felt as a family member that he was "in the way."

HARNESSING CREATIVE POTENTIAL TO CREATE TRULY HEALING ENVIRONMENTS

The innovative educational experience described in the previous section will exponentially expand the creative potential in healthcare design because of the intersection of disciplines in creating healing environments for the future. There are direct parallels

Box 9-3 Proposed Graduate Degree Programs

- Master of Healthcare Design and Nursing Innovation (Arizona Board of Regents pending permission/under development). This degree would feature the Healing Experience Studio where design and nursing students would collaborate to solve healthcare design problems and create improved processes and methods aimed at understanding how to design optimal patient and user experiences.
- PhD in Environmental Design and Planning with emphasis in Healthcare Design and Healing Environments Innovation (Arizona Board of Regents pending permission/under development). The doctoral degree is envisioned to require students to synthesize issues in design, health care, and healthcare administration research for a truly comprehensive investigation into evidence-based healthcare design (envisioned to be a partnership with the ASU College of Nursing & Healthcare Innovation and School of Global Management & Leadership).

Graduate Programs Currently Offered

- Master of Science in Design with a concentration in Healthcare and Healing Environments. This degree offers a research-based focus to students from a variety of backgrounds. The MSD implies a strong research orientation while the modifier "in Design" designates professional terminal degree status. The concentration is focused on factors that impact the design and planning of healthcare facilities and healing environments, especially the integration of evidence-based design with the practice of healthcare innovations. Students in this program are mentored by College of Nursing & Healthcare Innovation faculty in addition to faculty from the College of Design. MSD students team with students from other design disciplines and work directly with real clients and healthcare consultants.
- Master of Healthcare Innovation. This interdisciplinary program is offered through the College of Nursing & Healthcare Innovation. The MHI degree focuses on leadership of innovation, transformation management, bioethics, technology, team building, personal development, and evidence-based practice. Major courses include the principles of innovation, systems thinking for innovators, the integration of technology into practice, the individual and innovation, evidence-based innovations, financing for innovation, the challenges of health policy and innovation, and management outcomes resulting from innovation.

Box 9-4 At-a-Glance Healthcare Initiative Highlights

- Transdisciplinary education focus with multiple supporting ASU partners
- Strong support from the design, healthcare, and health administration industries
- Patient/nurse-centered focus in collaboration with actual nurses and patients
- Evidence-based practice and sustainability science are integrated throughout
- Real health system clients and practitioner partners actively participate in the initiative
- Mentorship and outreach opportunities through local and national design firms partners
- Development of a healthcare design research database
- Global perspective through optional study abroad programs

---

with the physiology of wound healing and the creation of a healing environment. Healthcare providers fundamentally know that healing is a very complex process and must occur deep within the wound before the visible wound or disease can be healed. We also know that after the insult or wound occurrence, bleeding occurs with clotting impregnating the wound. Healing is initiated because of an inflammatory process that occurs at the wound site with macrophages and phagocytes dispatched to eliminate bacteria from the site. Secondary healing occurs when granulomatous tissue is formed deep in the wound, knitting the edges of the wound together and creating new epithelial cell growth that closes the wound (Mercandetti, 2008).

This physiological view of wound healing has meaning as we examine the design of healing environments. There are fundamental wounds in healthcare system with resultant hemorrhaging in the *business aspects* (diminishing revenues, escalating expenses, and errors of commission and omission negatively affect patient outcomes), *organizational factors* (negative culture and climate, restrictive and authoritative organizational structures, poor leadership, incivility, workload stress), *professional issues* (concerns about competence, dissatisfaction with the work environment, poor interpersonal relationships, job dissatisfaction, role stress), and the *physical environment insults* (poorly maintained, unsafe, crowded, inefficiently designed) that must be healed.

Healing Environments

Consumers want to be healed when they come to hospitals, and if the body cannot be healed, then there is an important mission to at least address healing of the mind and the spirit. As healthcare professionals we are healers, yet too many providers are too stressed, fatigued, depressed, and oppressed to fulfill the healing role. The literature is replete with evidence about the effect of the work environment on patient and staff outcomes, with work environment defined predominantly as the organization's culture, climate, and leadership milieu (Foley, Kee, Minick, Harvey, & Jennings, 2002; Laschinger & Leiter, 2006; McManis & Monsalve Associates, 2003). What is often missed is considering the physical work environment where health care is delivered as a critical factor in promoting healing of the mind–body–spirit of the patient and the provider. Whereas Hippocrates of Kos, the ancient Greek physician, espoused three factors critical in healing and medicine—the disease itself, the patient, and the physician—Currie stated that there is a silent, often unrecognized fourth factor that subtly influences the whole process of healing—the setting or place or physical environment (Currie, 2007).

The concept of healing environments acknowledges the patients' spirituality and emotional needs as necessary for healing while also valuing the patients' rights to privacy and dignity. Recognizing that illness is a social event, the design team must create healing environments that support the involvement of loved ones and friends in the patients' healing process. Although Hippocrates valued the role of the physician as healer, today we recognize that the "healer" is a multidisciplinary term and all healing professions are influenced by the setting and place where they give care. A true healing environment must "heal the healer" as well.

Healing Places and Spaces

A number of organizations, such as the CHD, Picker Institute, Academy of Neuroscience in Architecture, American College of Healthcare Architecture, Association of Critical Care Nursing, the AONE, Institute of Family Centered Care, Samueli Institute, and Planetree, and numerous individual authors have defined the characteristics of healing environments for patients with such attributes as (1) a connection to nature, (2) safety of patients and providers, (3) patient-centered care, (4) family and social support, (5) self-control and choice in the environment (light, temperature), (6) alternative and complementary healing therapies, (7) healing philosophies, and (8) positive diversions (American Association of Critical Care Nurses, 2005; Center for Health Design & The Picker Institute, 2008; Frampton et al., 2003; Institute of Family Centered Care, 2008; Malloch, 1999; McManis & Monsalve Associates, 2003; Samueli Institute, 2008).

Citing Oldenburg's work that describes a hierarchy of places with home as the first place, work as the second, and gathering places for pleasure as the third place (Oldenburg, 1999), Huelat and Wan (2007) postulated that at the very least we need to create healing environments that provide a positive experience for patients and providers that act as their third place, a place where there is a feeling of well-being. In that sense Huelat and Wan offered eight new attributes to be considered for the healing environment, for which this author has expanded the explanations:

1. *Social immunity* or social neutrality, where the hierarchy of medical care is eliminated and patients, physicians, and providers are all on the same level
2. *Inclusivity,* where there is merging of personalities for an external purpose and where visitors could focus not only on the needs of the sick but also on living well
3. *Conversation* that is engaging, patient focused, and supportive of health and well-being
4. *Accommodating* space, where people feel comfortable and welcomed rather than an intrusion into the care routine
5. *Regular visitors* who come to the designated space for reasons other than to visit the sick but rather to learn, interact, and enjoy the space and place
6. *Simple place* with elements of comfort
7. *Playfulness* with stress-reducing, endorphin-releasing laughter and joy when appropriate
8. *Homelike* with elements of warmth, comfort, and a welcoming sense where a person can feel connected

Huelat and Wan's descriptions of healing environments support the Planetree philosophy, which is gaining wide acceptance in hospitals today. Planetree embraces 10 principles that are considered essential for healing to occur (Frampton et al., 2003):

1. Importance of human interactions and connectedness
2. Importance of family, friends, and social support
3. Empowering patients through information and education
4. Healing designs
5. Nutrition as an integral part of healing
6. Healing arts
7. Spirituality
8. Human touch
9. Complementary therapies
10. Healthy communities

These 10 principles affect the organizational culture and must be considered in the design if the facility is to support the culture of care.

Whatever the philosophy driving the organization's culture or the facility design, the underlying intent of the healing environment is to raise the spirits of patients and providers and all who visit therein. To accomplish this lofty goal, there clearly must be innovative thinking among collaborating disciplines to create healing places and spaces that lift the spirit, rest the mind, and heal the body.

PHILOSOPHY AND CULTURALLY DRIVEN DESIGN

The design and construction of a new building affects everything, including the culture of the organization, and the culture of the organization should drive design decisions about the new facility. There is no more transforming process affecting the culture and operations of a hospital than moving into a new facility. Hamilton, Orr, and Raboin (2008) postulated that "effective transformational change in healthcare organizations is most likely to be sustained when culture change and facility design are jointly optimized" (p. 41). The authors described "cultures" that must be considered to be the philosophical framework for design, including the culture of safety and the culture of patient-, family-, or relationship-centered care. Joint optimization supports the notion of the interdependent relationship between organizational culture and facility design and suggests that the design process provides an opportunity for in-depth cultural and work process assessment, giving the resulting design an opportunity to transform the culture. Initially, the culture and philosophy of care drives the design, but when the facility is completed the built environment influences the culture and care processes. As Churchill (1943) stated in a speech to the House of Lords, "We shape our buildings, and afterwards our buildings shape us."

With this thought in mind, hospitals and healthcare facilities can be transformed to healing environments by adopting healing philosophies that guide design decisions and by the resulting built environment that shapes our lives as patients or providers. A committed vision from leadership must pave the course for all to follow. Transformational leaders inspire others to accomplish what they did not believe they could accomplish (Porter-O'Grady & Malloch, 2007). To create healing environments, all participants need to be inspired by the vision, prepared with the knowledge that it truly makes a difference, and enabled to participate in the transformational process of culture change and facility design. The skeptics and devils advocates, of course, will question if philosophies such as Planetree or Healing Environments really make a difference or if they are just "feel good" initiatives.

New evidence shows that significant differences in outcomes are associated with the cultural and facility transformation resulting from adopting the Planetree philosophy. Stone (2008) reported that patients who were included in the Planetree patient-centered model of care were statistically more satisfied, had shorter lengths of stay, and had reduced costs per case as compared with a matched group who received the traditional care model (869 hospitalized patients undergoing elective total knee or total hip joint replacement surgery).

There are many other examples of the positive effect of jointly optimizing cultural transformation with facility design transformation that are outlined by Hamilton et al. (2008) with outcomes such as reductions in patient transfers, falls, hospital-acquired infections, and medication errors; changes in physician–nurse relationships resulting from decentralized unit design; improved patient satisfaction scores; operational improvements in productivity and cost controls; and improved staff and physician satisfaction scores.

Other researchers have demonstrated the value of decentralized nursing stations as compared with centralized nursing stations when evaluating nursing coordination, consultation, collaboration, and leadership time in the engagement of patient care. All these activities were significantly higher in the decentralized design. Direct care activities were also significantly higher in the decentralized design as compared with the centralized design, whereas the indirect care activities were significantly lower in the decentralized design as compared with the centralized design (Gurascio-Howard & Malloch, 2007). This study is another validation of the effect of the facility design on patient care and the nursing staff's work experience. Evidence is mounting to support decentralized designs for nursing work stations and supply areas to reduce worker fatigue from walking long hallways to gather supplies needed for patient care, to obtain medications, or to document patient assessments and interventions (Hendrich, 2008) and to reduce the scale of nursing units to 32 rooms or less with 20 to 28 rooms being optimal (Ritchey & Stichler, 2008).

Acuity adaptable rooms have also demonstrated their efficacy in reducing the number of patient transfers and hand-offs with the potential to reduce associated errors, reduce employee injuries from physically moving the patients and their belongings from one room to another, and for increasing the flexibility of patient room assignments (Hendrich, Fay, & Sorrells, 2004). These rooms are readily adaptable to any patient type or acuity maximizing rapid patient placement from intake areas such as the emergency department or general admitting.

To ensure employee safety, ceiling-mounted patient lifts have demonstrated cost-to-benefit in reducing employee injury, with some hospitals electing to install them in all patient rooms. Future designs must include space and place near the point of service to store other safe patient mobilization devices such as portable lifts and slide sheets, because evidence supports that immediate access is critical for staff to use these devices.

The ultimate goal of a healing environment is to reduce stress to patients and staff. Mounting evidence demonstrates that facility design can be an important variable in decreasing staff stress and enhancing provider alertness with exterior views from their work stations, particularly when those views were of nature as contrasted to another building (Pati, Harvey, & Barach, 2008), or decreasing levels of stress and improving job satisfaction after moving into a new facility with improved quality of patient rooms and workspaces (Berry & Parish, 2008).

Patients who are transferred from one level of care to another or from one floor to another often experience tremendous anxiety because of the fear of being too far away from the "critical care specialists." From discussions with care providers and patients who had been in the intensive care unit, one design team created a combination intensive care unit and medical surgical (step-down) unit all on one floor rather than "stacking" the intensive care units on a floor above or below the medical surgical units. By having the critical care unit on the same floor as the step-down unit for that specialty, patients and families were less anxious about the transfer. In their minds the critical care personnel were "just steps away" and immediately available if needed (Figure 9-1). Intensive care unit room designs were also quite different from the traditional design, with docking stations and headwalls or power poles with all the medical gases, outlets, and equipment. Figure 9-2 shows an intensive care unit room that was the result of designers and providers working together to answer the question, "what one thing would make the intensive care unit room most efficient?" The result was a headwall-less room with all the medical gases, outlets, and equipment placed on ceiling-mounted articulating arms. This configuration allows the bed to be moved anywhere in the room and still have access to the support boom.

Women in delivery and placed in stirrups in the lithotomy position are always anxious about who is walking in the room while they are in such a compromised and vulnerable position. To address this patient need and to find a more innovative solution,

Figure 9-1 Floor plan of the Critical Care Tower at Arizona Medical Center, in Tucson, AZ.

Integrating the ICU and stepdown units helps to decrease patient transfer anxiety. Although the patients are transferred to a different level of care, the physicians and nurses who cared for them in the ICU are still on the same floor, giving a level of comfort to patients and their families.

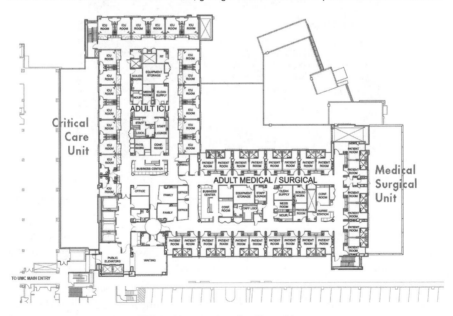

Source: Illustration provided by NTD Architecture, Inc., San Diego, CA.

Figure 9-2 Patient room in the Critical Care Tower of Harris Methodist Medical Center, in Forth Worth, TX.

The ceiling-mounted or wall-mounted articulating power and medical gas booms allow the bed to be moved anywhere in the room. It also allows for 360-degree access to the patient by the interdisciplinary team of providers.

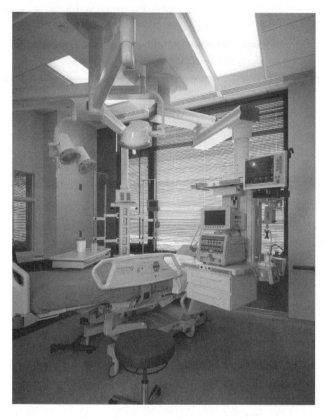

Source: Photo provided by NTD Architecture, Inc., San Diego, CA and Michael Lyon Photography.

a team of architects designed the slanted headwall that angles the patient away from the entry to the room (Figure 9-3). In studying the pros and cons of this design with the providers, some serendipitous advantages were noted. First, the angle created a greater space at the foot of the bed for the delivering doctor or midwife, which solved a recognized problem in rectilinear- or square-shaped rooms with limited space at the footwall. Second, the angle created clearly delineated zones for the patient, the family, and the provider. Third, the designated space for infant resuscitation and stabilization was near the entry door, allowing quick egress to the neonatal intensive care unit for dis-

Figure 9-3 A labor-delivery-recovery-postpartum (LDRP) room in the Women's Pavilion in Scottsdale Healthcare Shea, in Scottsdale, AZ.

An LDRP room with a slanted headwall protects patient privacy during delivery, among other benefits.

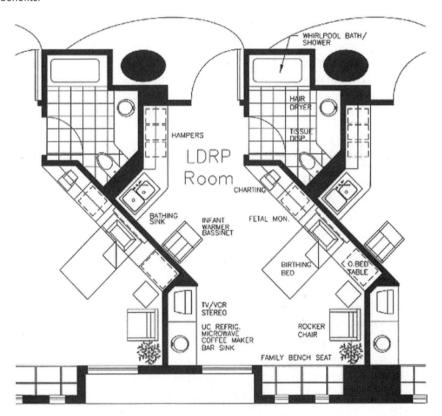

Source: Illustration provided by NTD Architecture, Inc., San Diego, CA.

tressed infants. Finally, patient views to the outside were enhanced because the patient faced the window rather than being parallel to the window. The rooms have been extremely well received by patients, families, and staff.

New innovations in design need to address ways to reduce both patient and provider stress and create emphasis on the healing aspects of care environments. These innovative facilities will likely be the source of competitive advantage and financial growth. To accomplish this leaders must be innovation friendly and challenge what is currently known about healthcare design and traditional construction. To be good community stewards and leaders in all matters pertaining to health, innovative thinkers must focus on transforming the healthcare environment to be sensitive to global warming, climate change crisis, and toxic environmental factors and to redefine design and operations to a sustainable future.

TRENDS AND INNOVATIONS IN FACILITY DESIGN

New studies conducted by nurse, design, and academic researchers are in process to determine the effect of specific design attributes on patient and provider experiences and organization performance metrics. In reviewing the literature and interviewing architects, designers, and nurse executives involved in major building projects, several design trends and new innovations in design were identified.

Patient-Centered Care or Relationship-Based Care Philosophies

- All single-bed room configurations for adults and children (including neonatal intensive care units) to include space and a designated place for families and/or visitors, including comfortable places to sit, sleep, and store personal belongings and space to display family pictures or other personal items
- Designated family retreat areas on the nursing care unit where families can have quiet times to destress from their involvement with patients or support each other when their loved one is dying
- Unit-based family kitchens and eating areas, recognizing that healthy nutrition also feeds the soul
- Way-finding designs that make it easy to navigate to a destination without assistance
- Views of nature in artwork or outside window views (Figure 9-4)
- Diversional activities and options: self-selected artwork or interactive art or complementary therapies such as music, art, aroma, or pet therapies
- Massage, Reiki, healing touch, and guided imagery therapies (Figure 9-5)
- Sacred or quiet spaces such as a chapel or meditation area or Zen garden (Figure 9-6)

Patient Safety Initiatives Supported by Design Decisions

Patient safety should be the first consideration in all design decisions. Designs that support patient safety include the following:

- Wider doors into toilet rooms
- Nonenclosed showers in toilet rooms with sloping floors for water drainage

Figure 9-4 A patient room at Clarian West Medical Center, in Avon, IN.

A patient room with a nature view to the outside. The head wall can provide a handrail for assistance to the bathroom, and space is provided for the paitent's family to stay.

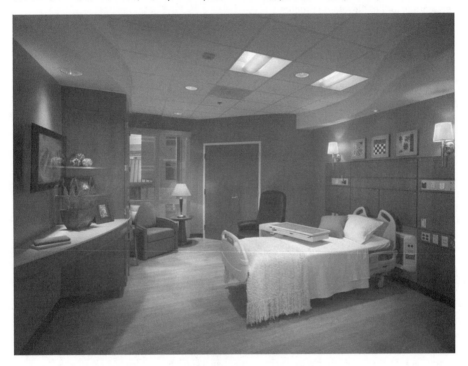

Source: Photo provided by HDS, Inc., Dallas, TX and Ed LaCasse Photography.

- Direct line of sight from the decentralized nursing station to patient from their decentralized or documentation area (Figures 9-7 and 9-8)
- Bathroom located on headwall for continuous hand-rails from the head of the bed to the bathroom
- Automatically controlled lighting when patient leaves the bed at night
- Point-of-service storage for safe patient mobilization equipment and supplies
- Flooring that prevents slippage
- Hand-washing sinks immediately adjacent to the entry door to the room
- Large floor-to-ceiling windows to provide natural lighting in the patient room (Figure 9-9)
- Family and patient respite and informational space and kiosk (Figure 9-10)
- Computerized patient information centers in patient rooms (Figure 9-11)

Figure 9-5 Floor plan of spa areas for Scottsdale Shea's Women's Pavilion, Scottsdale, AZ.

The spa area of hospitals include massage therapies, healing touch, aroma therapies, and retail areas for health-related products.

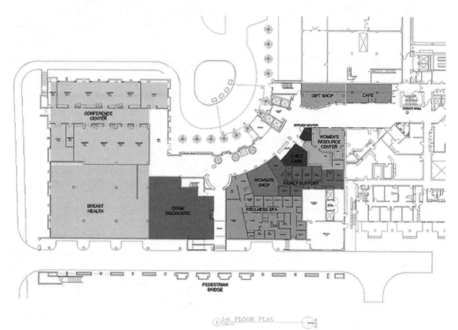

Source: Illustration provided by NTD Architecture, Inc., San Diego, CA.

- Patient discharge lounges
- Antibacterial materials and fabrics
- Acoustical features to minimize noise
- Multiple lighting options with motion sensors and safety guards to prevent patient falls

Design Features to Enhance Employee Safety and Positive Work Experience

- Ceiling-mounted room lifts in all or most rooms; point-of-service storage areas for safe patient mobilization devices (Villeneuve, 2006)
- Decentralized care supplies and equipment storage near point of service

Figure 9-6 The Sletten Cancer Center Chapel, in Great Falls, MT.

The chapel provides patients and families a quiet place for prayer and meditation, and helps meet the spiritual needs of patients, families, staff, and the community.

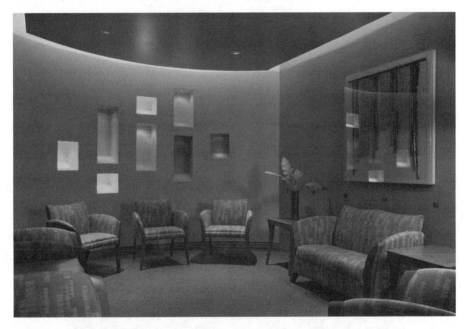

Source: Photo provided by NTD Architecture, Inc., San Diego, CA and J K Lawrence Photography.

- Ergonomically designed work areas for documentation and in patient care areas
- Smaller configurations of nursing care units: either smaller floor plans or room groupings to create smaller care areas (Figure 9-12)
  - Decreases noise due to activity intensity levels
  - Decreases travel distances for nurses
  - Enhances peer-to-peer visibility
  - Maximizes line of sight to all patient rooms
- Respite or quiet room where staff can go for a few minutes of silence to reduce stress of care giving in highly stressful areas
- Designated space for nurse–physician discussions or interactions with other disciplines
- Decentralized nursing documentation stations providing direct line of sight to assigned patients (Figure 9-13)

Clear lines of sight from the nurses' station to the patients' rooms have the potential to decrease patient falls because the nurse can see when the patient is getting out of bed or needs attention.

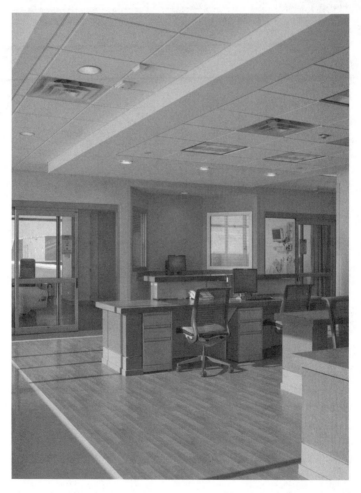

Source: Photo provided by VOA Associates, Inc., Chicago, IL on behalf of the VOA + OWP/P Design Collaborative and Craig Dugan at Hedrich Blessing Photography.

Figure 9-8 A nursing station in Clarian West Medical Center, in Avon, IN.

Decentralized documentation stations provide a clear line of sight into the patient rooms and minimize walking distances for the nurses. The patients' ability to see the nurses has the potential to decrease anxiety.

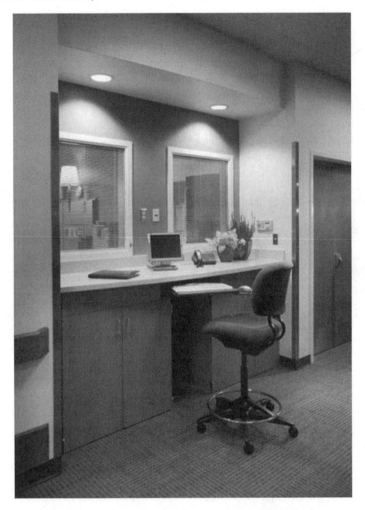

Source: Photo provided by HKS, Inc., Dallas, TX and Ed LaCasse Photography.

Figure 9-9 A patient room in Northwestern Memorial Healthcare's Prentice Women's Hospital, in Chicago, IL.

Patient rooms are zoned to provide space for the patients, their guests and family members, and providers. Large floor-to-ceiling windows provide ample natural lighting.

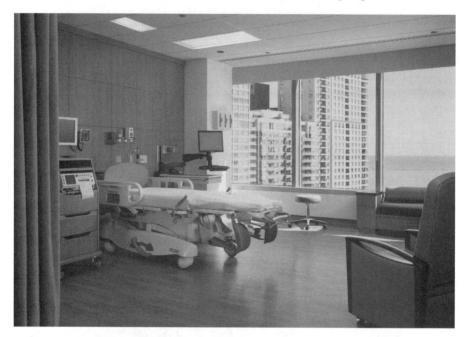

Source: Photo provided by VOA Associates, Inc., Chicago, IL on behalf of the VOA + OWP/P Design Collaborative and Nick Merrick at Hedrich Blessing Photography.

- Hallways that have an aesthetic appeal as contrasted to the long unappealing halls (Figures 9-14 and 9-15)
- Decentralized nursing stations break up the look of the static hallway, decrease walking distances, and create areas where providers can collaborate about the patients' needs (Figure 9-16)
- Multiple documentation sites in and/or near the point of service
- Windows to the outside with views of nature in the centralized communication or business center (formerly known as the nursing station)
- On-stage/off-stage design
- Patient rooms that enhance care and productivity (Figure 9-17)
  - Maximize visibility of patients
  - Maximize usable room space

Figure 9-10 Informational kiosks in Northwestern Memorial Healthcare's Prentice Women's Hospital, in Chicago, IL.

Family waiting rooms offer a diversionary space and information center as a respite for patients' families and guests.

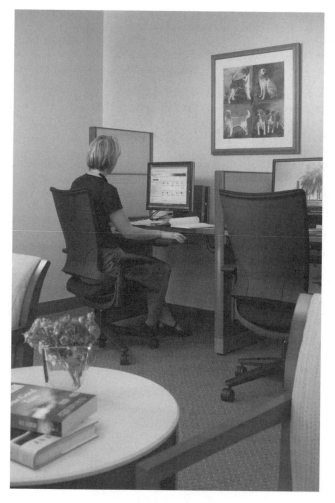

Source: Photo provided by VOA Associates, Inc., Chicago, IL on behalf of the VOA + OWP/P Design Collaborative and Craig Dugan at Hedrich Blessing Photography.

Figure 9-11 A patient room in Northwestern Memorial Healthcare's Prentice Women's Hospital, in Chicago, IL.

Computerized patient information centers in patient rooms provide education, entertainment, and information.

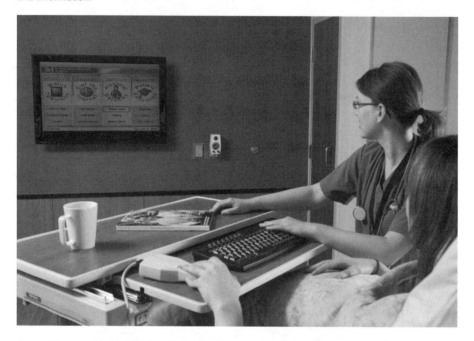

Source: Photo provided by VOA Associates, Inc., Chicago, IL on behalf of the VOA + OWP/P Design Collaborative and Jeff Millies at Hedrich Blessing Photography.

- Widened entry doors into rooms
- Acuity adaptability

Design Features to Enhance Infection Control

- Single-bed patient rooms
- Abundant hand-washing sinks and hand-gel dispensers
- Sharps and contamination boxes in the point of service area
- High efficiency particulate air filters for high-risk areas and laminar flow systems for ultraclean room requirements

Figure 9-12 A floor plan showing smaller patient unit sizes.

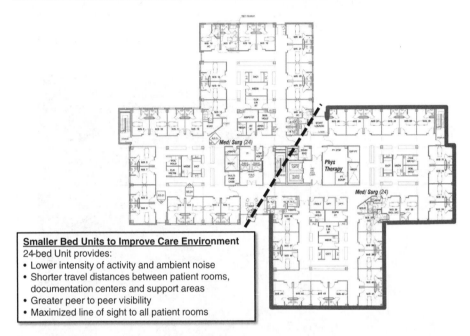

Smaller Bed Units to Improve Care Environment
24-bed Unit provides:
- Lower intensity of activity and ambient noise
- Shorter travel distances between patient rooms, documentation centers and support areas
- Greater peer to peer visibility
- Maximized line of sight to all patient rooms

Source: Illustration provided by HKS, Inc., Dallas, TX.

- Ventilation system cleaning and maintenance to reduce dust and particulate generation; frequent air filter changes
- Antimicrobial materials and fabrics for cubicle curtains and furniture
- Designated enclosed space on each unit for large collection bins for regular and contaminated trash and linen near the service elevator (reduces trash collection in hallways)

Design Implications From Technology Revolutions That Merge Technologies With Interventions

- Surgi-nostic departments with the merge of radiology and surgery where the interventional radiology procedure merges with the operating area
- Emergi-nostic departments with the merge of radiology and the emergency department
- Point-of-service laboratory and pharmacy spaces

Figure 9-13 A distributed documentation station in Penrose Hospital, in Colorado Springs, CO.

Decentralized or distributed nursing stations provide a direct line of sight into the assigned patient rooms.

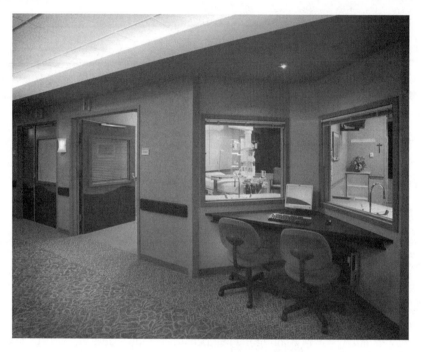

Source: Photo provided by HKS, Inc., Dallas, TX and Ed LaCasse Photography.

- Flexibility and swing use of space (Figure 9-18)
- Bedside documentation with handheld personal digital assistants with docking systems at point of service, hallway decentralized nursing stations, and central nursing station

Community and Education Areas

- Community space such as internal and external gardens (Figure 9-19)
- Community meditative or chapel space
- Education space or resource libraries for the community and staff (Figure 9-20)

Figure 9-14 Static hallways appear to be a "road to nowhere."

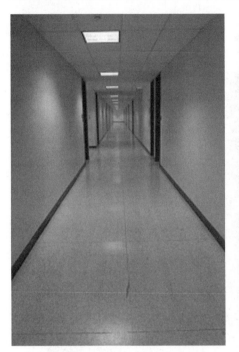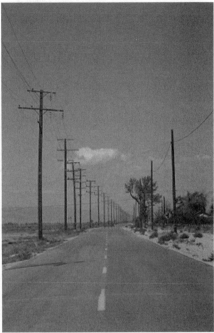

Source: Photos courtesy of NTD Architecture, Inc., San Diego, CA.

- Public spaces with nature integrated into the design with art, water features, plants, fireplaces, and grouped seating with natural lighting (Figures 9-21 and 9-22)
- Lobbies that have multiple functions including
  - Edu-tainment while waiting (Oermann, Webb, & Ashare, 2003)
  - Retail for the convenience of patients, families, and staff (Figures 9-23 and 9-24)
  - Spa areas off of lobby
- Medical concierges that optimize the hospital–community relationship

Innovations to Enhance Patient Flow and Operational Efficiency

- Acuity adaptable or single-bed rooms
- Smaller bed unit size (24 beds optimal) to reduce noise and intensity of activity
- Integration of all invasive procedure activities in one location to maximize staff utilization, material resources, and flexibility of the space for multiple uses

Figure 9-15 Hallway in the Critical Care Tower in Harris Methodist Medical Center, Fort Worth, TX.

Hallways with aesthetic appeal and decentralized nursing stations are both more dynamic and functional.

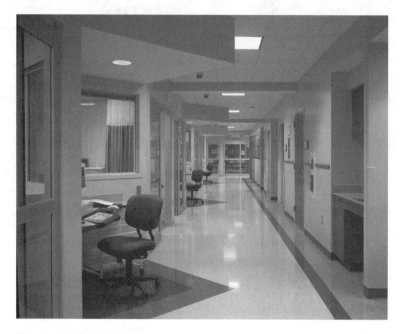

Source: Photo provided by NTD Architecture, Inc., San Diego, CA and Michael Lyon Photography.

These are but a few of the innovations that are transforming the healthcare environment in the creation of healing environments for patients, families, and staff. These innovations create a balance between what is needed to support operations and staff efficiency with what is needed to uplift the mind, body, and spirit in promoting a sense of well-being for all who use and work in the facility.

GOING GREEN: A NEW KEY DESIGN INITIATIVE WITH INNOVATION OPPORTUNITY

"Green Is the New Red, White and Blue" is the title of a chapter in Friedman's *Hot, Flat and Crowded* (2008) in which he describes a series of "great opportunities disguised as insoluble problems" (p. 170). Friedman states that in a flat, Internet-connected world,

Figure 9-16 Hallway in the Holmes Regional Medical Center, in Melbourne, FL.

Decentralized nursing stations break up a static hallway and provide space for interdisciplinary collaboration.

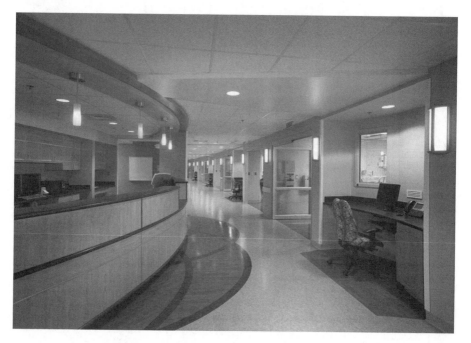

Source: Photo provided by HKS, Inc., Dallas, TX and Ed LaCasse Photography.

what we are doing about resource utilization, environmental pollution, and energy consumption is "becoming more visible, measurable, assessable and inescapable" (p. 171). Although thought to be community beacons for health and caring behaviors, hospitals are major consumers of water, power, and fossil fuel resources and major contributors of all sorts of solid, gaseous, and liquid waste, some of which are toxic to the environment, including a number of greenhouse gases. The medical industry generates more than 2 million tons of waste per year and releases fumes into the environment from incinerators burning medical wastes made of polyvinyl chloride (e.g., flexible intravenous and surgical tubings, syringes, soft plastic bags) that when burnt emit dioxins, mercury, and other toxins known to be carcinogens or are responsible for respiratory ailments and asthma (Minnema, 2008). Indoor air quality is compromised with pollutants from laboratory chemicals, latex, mercury, and a host of other toxic building materials that emit cadmium,

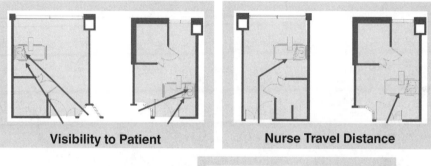

Figure 9-17 Floor plans of patient rooms that enhance care and productivity.

Visibility to Patient

Nurse Travel Distance

Patient Rooms that Enhance Care and Productivity
• Maximize patient visibility
• Shorten travel distances
• Maximize useable room area (entry vestibule)
• Acuity variability and adaptability
• With no lose of patient and family environmental quality

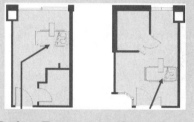

Patient Transport In/Out of Room

Source: Illustrations provided by HKS, Inc., Dallas, TX.

lead, and polychlorinated biphenyls (Roberts & Guenther, 2006). "As the healthcare industry's environmental footprint negatively affects the environment, these environmental impacts may in turn affect human health, and the human health issues further increase the need for healthcare services" (Roberts & Guenther, 2006, p. 82), creating a double loop environmental insult. A number of top executives of large healthcare systems have spoken out about the industry's responsibility to provide leadership in ensuring a healthy global environment as responsible resource consumers and leaders in the sustainability initiative.

The U.S. federal government defines sustainability as "creating new ways for people to live and thrive while keeping the planet's ecosystems and the global social tissue healthy and able to sustain us and future generations" (FedCenter, 2008). More simply put, sustainability is a philosophy and an organizational culture that values meeting the needs of today without compromising the needs of future generations. Sustainability is

Figure 9-18 Floor plan depicting swing space.

Creating flexibility and swing space enhances the adaptability of the facility to patient volume fluctuations and changes in services or care delivery models.

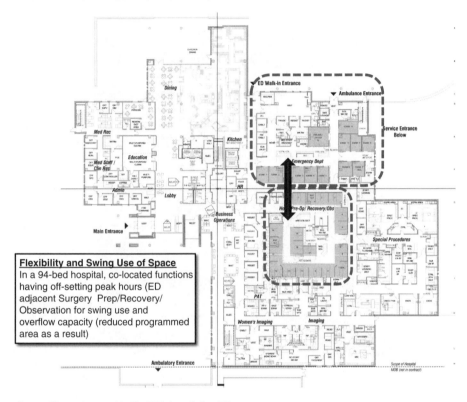

Flexibility and Swing Use of Space
In a 94-bed hospital, co-located functions having off-setting peak hours (ED adjacent Surgery Prep/Recovery/ Observation for swing use and overflow capacity (reduced programmed area as a result)

Source: Illustration provided by HKS, Inc., Dallas, TX.

more than a recycling program; it is all about the four R's: reusing, recycling, reducing the use of fossil fuels and materials that are not biodegradable, and refusing to use materials that emit or degrade into envirotoxins.

Going green can have significant design implications and requires innovative thinking about ways to design and construct buildings that are healthier for the occupants and for the global environment. One innovative solution was to place a green grass roof top that allowed patients to have a view of nature when this would not have been possible without the roof top garden (Figure 9-25). A number of healthcare systems, architects

Figure 9-19 The Internal Gardens-Lobby in Sletten Cancer Center, in Great Falls, MT.

Internal gardens provide a space that can be used for community events in addition to serving as waiting areas for patients and families.

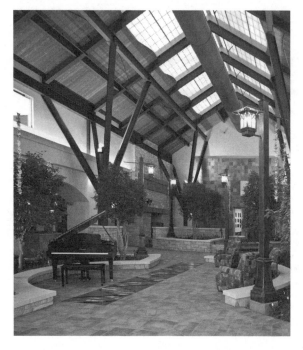

Source: Photo provided by NTD Architecture, Inc., San Diego, CA and J K Lawrence Photography.

and interior designers, professional engineers, and manufacturers of furniture, equipment, and building products have increased their resolve to create sustainable green environments. Accomplishing this goal requires leaders who can inspire everyone in the healthcare setting to value the green initiative by creating a green culture and an environmental mind-set. The first step is to create a green team composed of individuals on the planning, design, and construction team who are certified in leadership in energy and environmental design (LEED) and who have a passion for protecting the environment and ensuring sustainability. Design teams need to create green as a top priority in their design process, and hospital leaders must ensure that green is a major focus of operations as well. New thinking about "going green" is essential to be responsible community leaders in health care.

Figure 9-20 Lobby of Christus Schumpert Medical Center, in Shreveport, LA.

This two-story space for waiting provides a Resource Library on the left and an Education Center on the right, which serve as resources for both community and staff.

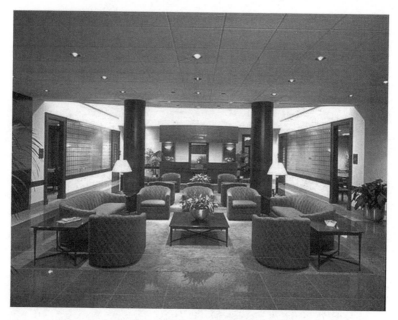

Source: Photo provided by HKS, Inc., Dallas, TX and Smith Photographic Services.

Innovations in Green Design

One of the first hospitals to become LEED certified was Boulder Community Hospital, which used green construction elements such as energy-efficient windows and lighting fixtures, building materials made of recycled or reprocessed materials, water-sparing toilets and urinals, installation of solar panels and wind power turbines, and procurement of furniture and equipment made with environmentally safe material. Other hospitals have followed the "LEED" and have demonstrated significant cost savings and enhanced patient and provider satisfaction and staff retention with sustainable design. Green construction eliminates polyvinyl chloride products and glues and substitutes products such as natural rubber, ceramic or wood flooring, recycled demolition materials, and reconstructed building materials and reduces "sick building syndrome" that often plagued occupants of newly constructed building (Roberts & Guenther, 2006).

Figure 9-21 A lobby in Scottsdale Shea, in Scottsdale, AZ.

A public space featuring natural light, conversation areas for families, and entrances into retail and educational areas.

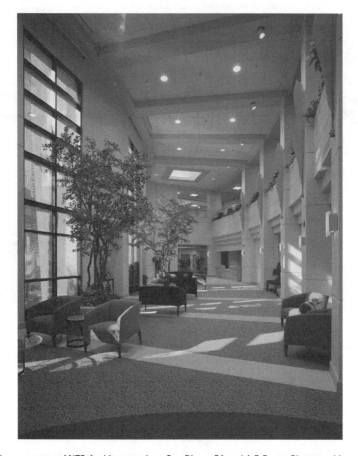

Source: Photo courtesy of NTD Architecture, Inc., San Diego, CA and A.F. Payne Photographic.

There are many opportunities for innovations in going green with sustainable design and "carbon neutral, toxic free, water balanced and zero waste construction" (Guenther, 2008, p. 31). Instead of taking old carpet to the nearest landfill, it can be recycled and reconstructed into new carpet. Use of alternative products instead of vinyl flooring products or vinyl furniture materials can reduce di(2-ethylhexyl) phthalate and its metabolite mono(2-ethylhexyl) phthalate, which are carcinogens. Alternatives for resilient flooring

Figure 9-22 A lobby in Sletten Cancer Center, in Great Falls, MT.

A public space with natural light, water features, and a park-like setting.

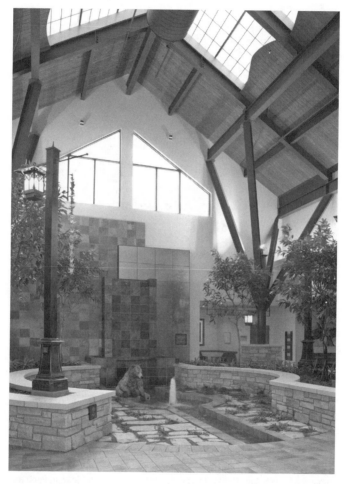

Source: Photo provided by NTD Architecture, Inc., San Diego, CA and J K Lawrence Photography.

and nontoxic wall coverings for health care are outlined by the Toxic Use Reduction Institute. Green alternatives in resilient flooring include the use of natural linoleum, cork, and polyethylene limestone blend and rubber. Enviro-friendly alternatives for wall coverings include biofibers, wool, polyester, wood fibers, and glass woven textiles for wall coverings (Toxic Use Reduction Institute, 2008). Lighting controls can be installed

Figure 9-23 A lobby in Clarian North Medical Center, in Indianapolis, IN.

A multi-story lobby with retail, dining spaces, educational resources, seating, and natural lighting.

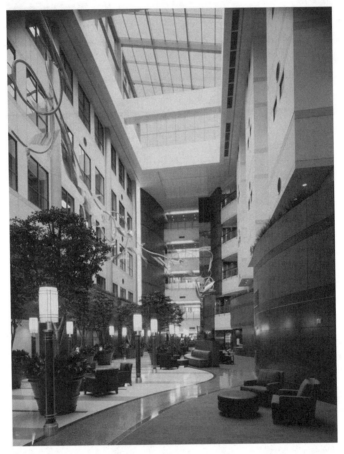

Source: Photo provided by HKS, Inc., Dallas, TX and Jeff Milies at Hedrich Blessing Photography.

in meeting rooms using motion and heat sensors to turn the light on or off, resulting in energy and cost savings. On-site renewable energy sources can be installed such as wind turbines, solar-thermal units, or sun photocells to reduce overall energy and fossil fuel consumption. Shading devices on the exterior of the building can save energy by shading the inside spaces. Use of light shelves in high-volume, windowless spaces can bounce light further into the space, making it appear brighter without additional fixtures, and

Figure 9-24 A lobby in Bassett Army Medical Center, in Fairbanks, AK.

A two-story lobby space combines a waiting area, a convenience store (below) and a Resource Library (above right) with dining, clinic reception, and a children's play area, generating activity and positive distractions.

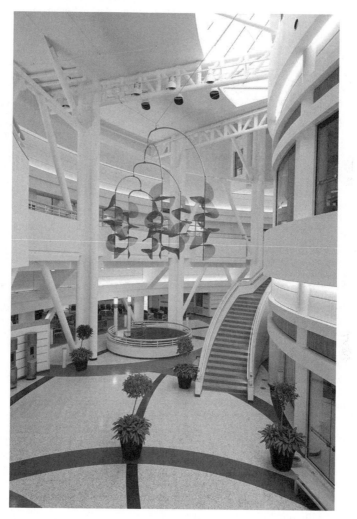

Source: Photo provided by HKS, Inc., Dallas, TX and Blake Marvin Photography.

Figure 9-25 Patient rooms with nature views in Prentice Women's Hospital at Northwestern Memorial Healthcare, in Chicago, IL.

The green roof at Prentice Women's Hospital is one of many efforts to achieve a sustainable facility compatible with Northwestern Memorial Healthcare's standards of excellence. Prentice Women's Hospital was awarded LEED Silver certification in December 2008.

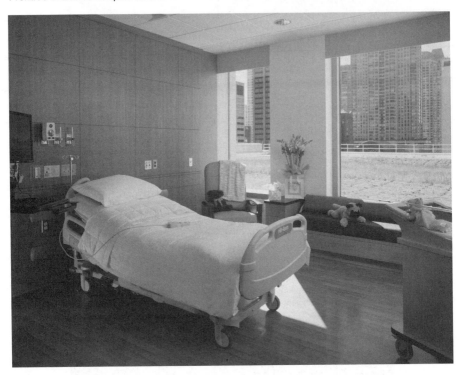

Source: Photo provided by VOA Associates, Inc., Chicago, IL on behalf of the VOA + OWP/P Design Collaborative and Jim Steinkamp at Steinkamp Photography.

florescent lamps without mercury can lower mercury emissions. Selection and procurement of Energy Star equipment and implementing the Green Star Rating System (http://www.gghc.org/links.cfm) ensures more energy efficiency, cost savings, and responsible energy conservation (Energy Star, 2007). Saving water runoff from rainfall in storage tanks can be used for landscape irrigation, conserving clean water.

One innovative architectural firm developed a mock patient room, Green Patient Room, based on evidence of design attributes that enhances healing and the quality of life for patients, families, and providers and materials that were nontoxic and ecofriendly. The prototypical room is being studied to determine its effect on patient outcomes and provider experiences and cost-to-benefit when considering initial costs as compared to life-cycle savings (The Institute for Innovation in Large Organizations, 2008). Another firm has a sustainable "Sites Manager" who directs green construction of projects. Most importantly, going green has to be a conscious choice for daily operations as well as the design and construction of new facilities.

Going green will not happen without transformational leaders who inspire others to value and embrace the importance of enacting green change and move toward a sustainable operation. The new green culture should embrace principles such as (1) creating a healthier workplace, (2) using locally grown food to reduce green gas emissions from trucking food from distant locations, (3) using meditation spaces that preserve local ecosystems in external gardens and using nature and plants indoors to decrease stress, and (4) being a good community neighbor and educating the public on the critical mandate to go green to preserve our planet (Bush, 2008). Transformational leaders must "LEED" the way for water and energy management, environmentally friendly purchasing, and recycling and reusing as much as possible rather than filling up our landfills with reusable materials or creating toxic fumes from incinerating materials that can be cleaned and reused or redistributed for other purposes. Many other positive results from thinking green have also been documented, including energy and water savings; reduced waste/cost; improved indoor air quality; improved patient, provider, and community satisfaction; increased philanthropy and award recognition; and environmental improvements (Serb, 2008). Most importantly, it is simply the right thing to do.

BECOMING AN INNOVATION LEADER IN HEALTHCARE FACILITY DESIGN

"Innovators are those people who know the 99 percent that everybody knows and therefore are able to create the 1 percent that nobody knows. If you don't know the 99 percent, or cannot get access to it, you will not have the foundation to create the new 1 percent. More likely you will just re-create part of the 99 percent that everyone already knows" (Jeff Wacker, cited in Friedman, 2008, p. 166). Imagine if you could just tap into the creativity of the 1% who are going to make a real difference in healthcare design!

In an informal survey this author asked architects, interior designers, and nurse executives (a sample convenient to the author) how they learned about innovations in healthcare design. The designers tended to agree that they learned about new innovations from conferences they attended and talking with design peers, health care providers, and experts in other unrelated fields such as aerospace, education, or business. They indicated that when they had an innovative idea, they would draw it up and test it with others in their own office or in their own discipline (75%), but fewer indicated they would draw it up and test it with healthcare providers (50%). Most agreed they often tried new approaches in design to solve challenges faced in health care, and most held focus groups with patients and families to get their perspective on innovative ideas. It was curious to note that most did not benchmark their project with other completed projects like theirs nor did they search the literature for other similar projects or for evidence that may have addressed a new innovation in health care. All surveyed indicated they talked with healthcare providers about the pros and cons of their new innovative ideas but less with patients and families. Most respondents believed their organization did not promote innovation, and only one respondent reported that his or her organization had a think tank where new innovations were discussed and tested.

Nurse leaders' responses were very similar, and most respondents either directed the project or worked on an interdisciplinary team with designers. All were educated at the graduate level, held executive level positions, and directed multimillion/billion dollar replacement or new hospital projects. Like the designers, most nurses surveyed indicated they learned about new innovations from conferences they attended and by talking with peers in the design field, other healthcare providers, and others in unrelated fields such as aerospace, education, or business. Only 50% indicated that when they had an innovative idea, they would draw it up and test it with others in their own hospital or with those in the design field. All nurse leaders indicated that when they had an innovative idea they would talk about it with those it affected most (75%), but fewer indicated that those discussions would include patients and families (25%). Fifty percent indicated they believed their hospital was known for its innovation.

Overall, nurses and designers reported that "think tank" retreats are needed to develop innovations to address old problems in healthcare design. Expert panels also add a dimension to the think tank approach, and, most importantly, all believed that including past patients and consumer panels in the design process was critical to understanding the facility needs from their perspective. Currie (2007) referred to the physical environment as the fourth factor behind the patient, the disease, and the physician/provider, but the real healing environment is created by the caregivers themselves who find true joy in caring and interaction with patients and their families. The third factor, the provider, is a critical variable in creating healing environments. In response to the question, "what innovations are needed to ensure a safer healing environment for patients and families?", one person summed it up this way: ". . . nurses (physicians too) who remember, every moment during their shift, why they went into nursing! They need to provide sensitivity and caring for the patient and his/her family, no matter what else is going on in their world. The nurse's relationship with the patient is 70–80% of the solution to a healing environment. A caring nurse can overcome all kinds of bad architecture!"

CONCLUSION

Healthcare design is merging the knowledge and science of nursing, medicine, social sciences, architecture, engineering, neurosciences, music, art, and complementary therapies. A new interdiscipline and science is emerging from the magic of these intersections with deep innovative thinking that supports an evidence-based approach to design with an ultimate goal to create healing environments. Healthcare facilities designed today will shape professional practice and care delivery for the next 30 to 50 years as well as our experiences as patients and providers. The design and construction of true healing environments that result in optimal patient outcomes and positive work environments for staff require transformational leaders who use a joint optimization approach merging strong vision, philosophies, and value principles to guide design decisions while simultaneously creating cultural change that inspires staff to higher levels of caring. When it is all said, done, and built, it is still staff members who create the ultimate healing environment for patients and for themselves.

ACKNOWLEDGMENTS

I thank the architects and leaders at the following design firms for their contributions to this chapter with figures, illustrations, personal communication, and survey participation: VOA; NTD Architects, Inc.; HKS Inc.; Jain Malkin Associates; and D. Kirk Hamilton, Associate Professor, Center for Health System Design at Texas A & M. I also thank the nurse executives from Pomerado Palomar Health System and Banner Desert Children's Hospital and Sharp HealthCare System for their contributions of experiences and expertise with large, multimillion dollar hospital projects. Their provider perspective was invaluable. I am also grateful to Sandra Davidson and Jamil AlShraiky who wrote the section on "The Healthcare Initiative: Charting the Future of Healthcare Design and Healing Environments." Their vision for creating magic at the intersection of disciplines will undoubtedly create a better future for healthcare design, and their enthusiasm inspires me.

REFERENCES

American Association of Critical Care Nurses. (2005). AACN standards for establishing and sustaining healthy work environments. Retrieved October 18, 2008, from http://www.aacn.org/WD/HWE/Docs/HWEStandards.pdf

American Organization of Nurse Executives. (2005). AONE nurse executive competencies. *Nurse Leader,* 3(1), 50–56.

Bass, B. M. (1985). *Leadership and performance beyond expectations.* New York: Free Press.

Berry, L. L., & Parish, J. T. (2008). The impact of facility improvements on hospital nurses. *Health Environments Research & Design, 1*(2), 5–13.

Bush, H. (2008). The path to going green. *Hospitals and Health Networks, 38*(8), supplement insert.

Cama, R. (2006a). Linking structure and healing: Building architecture for evidence-based practice. In T. Porter-O'Grady & K. Malloch (Eds.), *Evidence-based practice in nursing and health care.* Sudbury, MA: Jones and Bartlett.

Cama, R. (2006b). The opportunity is now. In S. O. Marberry (Ed.), *Improving healthcare with better building design.* Chicago: Health Administration Press.

Carlson, C. R., & Wilmot, W. W. (2006). *Innovation: The five disciplines for creating what customers want.* New York: Random House.

Center for Health Design [CHD]. (2008). Coalition for Health Environments Research (CHER). Retrieved October 31, 2008, from http://healthdesign.org/CHER/CHER_faqs.php

Center for Health Design & The Picker Institute. (2008). *Consumer perceptions of the healthcare environment: An investigation to determine what matters.* Martinez, CA: Center for Health Design.

Churchill, W. (1943, October 28). Speech to the House of Commons (meeting in the House of Lords). Retrieved June 30, 2009, from http://www.winstonchurchill.org/learn/speeches/quotations

Committee on Quality of Health Care in America & Institute of Medicine (Eds.). (2001). *Crossing the quality chasm: A new health system for the 21st century.* Washington, DC: National Academy Press.

Currie, J. M. (2007). *The fourth factor: A historical perspective on architecture and medicine.* Washington, DC: AIA Press.

Energy Star. (2007). Energy Star for healthcare. Retrieved September 22, 2008, from http://www.energystar.gov/index.cfm?c=healthcare.bus_healthcare

FedCenter. (2008). Sustainability. Retrieved October 15, 2008, from http://www.fedcenter.gov/programs/sustainability

Foley, B. J., Kee, C. C., Minick, P., Harvey, S. S., & Jennings, B. M. (2002). Characteristics of nurses and hospital work environments that foster satisfaction and clinical expertise. *Journal of Nursing Administration, 32*(5), 273–282.

Frampton, S. B., Gilpin, L., & Charmel, P. A. (2003). *Putting patients first.* San Francisco: Jossey-Bass.

Friedman, T. L. (2008). *Hot, flat and crowded.* New York: Farrar, Straus and Giroux.

Guenther, R. (2008). Why should health care bother? *Frontiers of Health Services Management, 25*(1), 25–32.

Gurascio-Howard, L., & Malloch, K. (2007). Centralized and decentralized nurse station design: An examination of caregiver communication, work activities, and technology. *Health Environments Research & Design, 1*(1), 44–57.

Hamilton, D. K., Orr, R. D., & Raboin, W. E. (2008). Organizational transformation: A model of joint optimization of culture change and evidence-based design. *Health Environments Research & Design (HERD) Journal, 1*(3), 40–60.

Hendrich, A. (2008). Unit-related factors that affect nursing time with patients: Spatial analysis of the time and motion study. *Health Environments Research & Design, 2*(2), 5–20.

Hendrich, A., Fay, J., & Sorrells, A. K. (2004). Effects of acuity-adaptable rooms on flow of patients and delivery of care. *American Journal of Critical Care, 13*(1), 35–45.

Huelat, B. J., & Wan, T. T. H. (2007). *Healing environments: What's the proof.* Alexandria, VI: Medezyn.

Institute of Family Centered Care. (2008). Institute of Family Centered Care. Retrieved October 23, 2008, from http://www.familycenteredcare.org/about/index.html

Johansson, F. (2004). *The Medici effect.* Boston: Harvard Business School Press.

Kelley, T. (2005). *The ten faces of innovation.* New York: Doubleday.

Kohn, L. T., Corrigan, J. M., & Donaldson, M. S. (Eds.). (2000). *To err is human.* Washington, DC: National Academy Press.

Kouzes, J. M., & Posner, B. Z. (2007). *The leadership challenge* (4th ed.). San Francisco: Jossey-Bass.

Lamb, G., Conner, J., Ossmann, M., & Stichler, J. F. (2007). Nursing's contributions to innovative hospital design. *JONA, 37*(10), 425–428.

Laschinger, H., & Leiter, M. (2006). The impact of nursing work environments on patient safety outcomes. *JONA, 36*(5), 259–267.

Malloch, K. (1999). A total healing environment: The Yavapai Regional Medical Center Story. *Journal of Healthcare Management, 44*(6), 495–512.

McKay, S., & Phillips, C. R. (1983). *Family-centered maternity care: Implementation strategies.* Rockville, MD: Aspen.

McManis & Monsalve Associates. (2003). *Healthy work environments: Striving for excellence.* Manassas, VA: McManis & Monsalve Associates.

Medaris, K., & Novak, J. C. (2006). New nursing programs seek to improve health-care design, delivery. Retrieved October 23, 2008, from http://www.purdue.edu/UNS/html3month/2006/060126.Novak.dnp.html

Mercandetti, M. (2008, July 22). Wound healing: Healing and repair. *eMedicine Clinical Reference.* Retrieved June 30, 2009, from http://www.emedicine.com/plastic/TOPIC411.HTM

Minnema, L. (2008). Medicine gears up for a code green: Doctors, hospitals put environment on their charts. *The Washington Post,* p. HE05.

Nightingale, F., Barnum, B. (1992). *Notes on nursing: What it is and what it is not, commemorative edition.* Philadelphia: Lippincott Williams & Wilkins.

Oermann, M. H., Webb, S. A., & Ashare, J. A. (2003). Outcomes of videotape instruction in clinic waiting area. *Orthopaedic Nursing, 22*(2), 102–105.

Oldenburg, R. (1999). *The great good place.* New York: Marlowe & Company.

Page, A. (Ed.). (2004). *Keeping patients safe: Transforming the work environment of nurses.* Washington, DC: National Academies Press.

Pati, D., Harvey, T. E., & Barach, P. (2008). Relationships between exterior views and nurse stress: An exploratory examination. *Health Environments Research & Design, 1*(2), 27–38.

Porter-O'Grady, T., & Malloch, K. (2007). *Quantum leadership.* Sudbury, MA: Jones and Bartlett.

Reiling, J., Breckbill, C., Murphy, M., McCullough, S., & Chernos, S. (2003). Facility designing around patient safety and its effect on nursing. *Nursing Economic$, 21*(3), 143.

Ritchey, T., & Stichler, J. F. (2008). Determining the optimal number of patient rooms for an acute care unit. *JONA, 38*(6), 262–266.

Roberts, G., & Guenther, R. (2006). Environmentally responsible hospitals. In S. O. Marberry (Ed.), *Improving healthcare with better building design.* Chicago: Health Administration Press.

Rubin, H. R., Owens, A. J., & Golden, G. (1998). *Status report: An investigation to determine where the built environment affects patients' medical outcomes.* Martinez, CA: Center for Health Design.

Samueli Institute. (2008). *Survey of healing environments in hospitals: Final report.* Alexandria, VA: The Samueli Institute.

Serb, C. (2008). Think green. *Hospitals and Health Networks, 82*(8), 22–26, 35.

Somerville, I., & Mroz, J. E. (1997). New competencies for a new world. In F. Hesselbein, M. Goldsmith, & R. Beckhard (Eds.), *The organization of the future.* San Francisco: Jossey-Bass.

Stichler, J. F. (1995). Professional independence: The art of collaboration. *Advanced Practice Nursing Quarterly, 1*(1), 53–61.

Stichler, J. F. (2007). Nurse executive leadership competencies for health facility design. *JONA, 37*(3), 109–112.

Stichler, J. F. (2008). Calculating the cost of a healthcare project. *JONA, 38*(2), 53–57.

Stichler, J. F., & Cesario, S. (2007). Preparing nurses for a leadership role in designing healthcare facilities. *JONA, 37*(6), 257–260.

Stichler, J. F., & Weiss, M. (2001). Through the eyes of the beholder: Multiple perspective on quality in women's health care. *Journal of Nursing Care Quality, 15*(3), 59–74.

Stone, S. A. (2008). A retrospective evaluation of the impact of the Planetree patient-centered model of care on inpatient quality outcomes. *Health Environments Research & Design, 1*(4), 55–69.

The Institute for Innovation in Large Organizations. (2008). *The business case for green healthcare facilities.* Arlington, VA: Practice Greenhealth.

Toxic Use Reduction Institute. (2008). DEHP. Retrieved November 2, 2008, from http://www.turi.org/library/turi_publications/five_chemicals_study/final_report/chapter_7_dehp#7.1.2

Ulrich, R. S. (1984). View through a window may influence recovery from surgery. *Science, 224*(4647), 420–421.

Ulrich, R. S. (1999). Effects of gardens on health outcomes: theory and research. In C. Marcus & M. M. Barnes (Eds.), *Healing gardens: Therapeutic benefits and design recommendations* (pp. 157–234). New York: Wiley.

Villeneuve, J. (2006). Physical environment for provision of nursing care: Design for safe patient handling. In A. L. Nelson (Ed.), *Safe patient handling and movement: A guide for nurses and other health care providers* (pp. 187–208). New York: Springer.

CHAPTER 10

The Intuitive Leader

Dominique Surel

"The only real valuable thing is intuition."

—Einstein (Cloninger, 2006, p. 16)

The intuitive leader is a novel concept in the realm of leadership. Intuitive thinking and intuitive leadership is the competitive advantage necessary for organizations to succeed in the 21st century. Leaders recognize the critical need to produce innovative organizational systems to accommodate the increasingly complex present and future challenges. However, the traditional repackaging of models continues, and the beneficial effects of implementation are usually short term. New and old issues resurface, and the perpetual motion of introducing the latest repackaged model continues. A new way of thinking and approaching 21st century challenges is necessary to transcend the concept of traditional organizational models and break through into a multidimensional space/time view of reality.

Whereas the 20th century competitive environment focused on developing technology, the critical component to success in the 21st century will be to learn how to develop our most powerful tool, the human brain. Because the source of innovation is the brain, we need to explore how to enhance our thinking processes and develop our brain functions in an innovative manner. Intuitive thinking has become the focus of both the scientific community and the business world. "Landmark studies have found a correlation between business success and intuition. . . . A lot of companies consider intuition a skill and technique they can use to competitive advantage" (Block, 1990, p. 58). Intuitive thinking generates powerful quick insights, clarity of thought, and enhanced forecasting skills. The process of developing one's intuitive thinking has also demonstrated a journey of evolving consciousness.

This chapter explores the meaning and purpose of intuitive thinking, as well as the unique benefits it can deliver, and addresses the following question: Can we expand our brain, our neural pathways, to develop a more precise skill to assess a situation and a feel for future events? Intuitive leadership by definition does not fit into a model because it is a personalized process adapted to each organization's vision, goals, and human potential. This chapter therefore does not deliver a model, and there is not enough space to explore in-depth the techniques to develop intuitive thinking. However, by exposing another view of reality, the chapter challenges the reader to think beyond his or her comfort zone and reveals the instruments necessary for an aspiring intuitive leader to embark on a unique and elevating journey.

INTUITION: QUANTUM INTELLIGENCE

What is intuition? Intuition has been described as a feeling or a knowing. It is that extra knowledge that manifests itself beyond our analysis and sometimes beyond the rational or perceived rational and logical conclusions. It is the question gap between consciously thinking and accessing data and receiving a solution or insight without understanding where it comes from. Intuition is a flash of information that in hindsight was always correct, even if initially it might not have appeared logical from the data we had for analysis.

Because we cannot explain where intuition comes from by using our conventional intellectual skills, the brain, relying on its self-imposed boundaries and filters, often dismisses the intuitive insight as not credible because it cannot authenticate its provenance. Yet scientific research demonstrates compelling evidence that intuitive thinking is linked to clarity of thought, enhanced forecasting skills, and precognition. Most of us use our intuition in all facets of life and decision-making processes whether or not we are aware of it. The difficulty is identifying an intuitive thought and differentiating it from a rational or logical deduction.

Perhaps the most powerful benefit of intuitive thinking is the perceived notion that intuition can provide signals or insights into the future. Scientific research from different labs demonstrates that our physical body responds to stimulus from 4 to 7 seconds before experiencing the stimulus (Bierman, 2000; McCraty, Atkinson, & Bradley, 2004b; Radin, 1997; Spottiswood & May, 2003). Developing this potential skill would obviously have valuable implications to the quality of the forecasting and decision-making process.

> *"We are the architects of our future healthcare system. We are the creators of new realities, and intuition is our major design tool."*
>
> (KAISER, 1987, P. 15)

A study conducted with companies whose profits doubled in 5 years demonstrated that "eighty percent of these organizations were led by CEOs with higher than average intuitive abilities" (Carlson & Kaiser, 1999, p. 50). In the medical field a study conducted with primary care physicians revealed that even evidence-based practitioners "included intuition among the necessary tools for strong clinical decision-making" (Tracy, Dantas, & Upshur, 2003, para. 19, p. 6).

Contrary to popular belief, intuitive thinking is not a sole function of the right brain but rather an interactive process of the whole brain that goes beyond the right brain and left brain concept and involves other organs such as the heart and the gut (McCraty et al., 2004b). Intuitive thinking encompasses knowledge, experience, rational thinking, critical thinking, and emotions.

One of the most articulate papers written on the subject of intuition was by Miller and Ireland (2005, p. 21), who perceived intuition as follows:

> Neither the opposite of rationality nor a random process of guessing, intuition corresponds to thoughts, conclusions, or choices produced largely or in part through subconscious mental processes; a mental tool that is separate from explicit logic and judgment.

Miller and Ireland define intuition as somewhere in the middle of rationality and a somewhat undefined other mental process.

Numerous studies on intuitive thinking agree that there appears to be an unidentified, or yet unexplained, component in the process. Intuition is said to be based on prior knowledge, life experiences, and rational thinking. However, research conducted with children by Carey and Spelke (1996) suggested that intuitive insight and knowledge can manifest itself before it is experienced. Examples are given of children who have theoretical knowledge that has not been learned (Anonymous, 2003), and numerous studies examining the decision-making process continuously demonstrated a yet unexplained factor that intuitive thinkers can identify but not clearly define. McCraty et al. (2004a) pointed out evidence that "there are instances when so-called 'gut feelings' or 'intuitive insights' are found to be valid and related to circumstances so unique that these intuitions do not seem explicable on the basis of prior experience" (p. 133–134).

> *"82 of the 93 winners of the Nobel Prize over a 16 year period*
> *agreed that intuition plays an important role in creative and*
> *scientific discoveries."*
>
> (COOPER & SAWAF, 1997, P. 43)

The growing interest in decoding intuition is a result of the globalizing business environment generating an increasingly complex context, creating scenarios of uncertainty and divergence of value systems in which leaders must make decisions at a much faster pace (Dane & Pratt, 2004; Maani & Maharaj, 2006; Sinclair & Ashkanasy, 2005). The quest for developing decision-making skills to meet the new challenges opens doors to explore the more ephemeral human qualities, such as emotional intelligence, spiritual intelligence, and intuition (Cote & Miners, 2006; Kerfoot, 2005; Zohar & Marshall, 2000). This produces a major shift from the traditional business models whereby emotions in the workplace were devalued and judged as distracting from the bottom line focus. Cote and Miners (2006) noted that "one of the most provocative ideas to emerge from recent discussions of management concerns the possibility that a new form of intelligence pertaining to emotions is related to the performance of organization members" (p. 1).

Hayashi (2001) contended that decision making gets more difficult as an individual moves on from middle management to an executive level in which situations are more complex and quantitative. One executive in Hayashi's research reported individuals who do not use intuition and do not reach senior levels of management have judgment or decision-making skills that falter considerably.

Quantitative and qualitative research demonstrates executive-level decision makers use intuition more often than middle managers (McNaughton, 2003; Sadler-Smith & Shefy, 2004a). Further study by Burke and Miller (1999) suggested that 89% of executives and managers use their intuition in the workplace to make decisions. Sadler-Smith (2004) revealed a correlation between using intuitive decision making and financial performance. Research conducted with real estate decision makers revealed that 100% of participants admitted to using their intuitive thought process in conducting business and 100% declared that their intuitive thinking contributed significant financial value to their business (Surel, 2009).

Patton (2003) posited three types of leaders: those who recognize using intuition, those who understand intuition and try to develop it, and those who do not or cannot access their intuitive skills. Patton further contended that most leaders are probably in between the two extremes, but the key to successfully using intuition is to be aware of the holistic systematic process involved and to notice how much and when rational processing and intuitive processing occur. Patton also agreed with other researchers that intuition happens on the unconscious level, which is why it is important to learn how to discern between an emotional reaction and an intuitive thought.

CREATING 21ST CENTURY COMPETITIVE ADVANTAGE

Need for a New Way of Thinking: Transcending Models

The parameters of interaction in the business world have shifted into an entirely different paradigm that operates in multidimensions of space, time, and events. It is of a holographic and organic nature, and linear thinking no longer suffices to understand and successfully operate in the vastness and with the intricacies involved. Thus a new way of thinking is necessary to generate insightful solutions to rebuild a new organizational order at a higher consciousness level that transcends the concept of current organizational models.

The socioeconomic dynamics in our world have also changed. Business models are defunct. Forcing existing organizational cultures and structures to change to fit into a repackaged conventional model no longer works because models are restricted to their defined boundaries. Carlson and Kaiser (1999) discussed how current management theory is no longer effective and pointed out that nonlinear thinking is already practiced by scientists, inventors, and artists.

The business world now needs to recognize the added value of thinking beyond the traditional linear process and models. Utilizing mostly the left brain is a self-limiting exercise, and executives must "use the more subtle 'winds' of nonlinearity and intuition. Leaders must learn to 'fly', as the stream did, or think differently, if they are to prosper in the future" (Glaser, 1995, p. 51). Glaser (1995) conducted research to evaluate intuition in a research and development environment and found that individuals who were most creative were those who "couldn't seem to conform to the standard ways of thinking, doing research, writing reports, and so forth" (p. 43) compared with those descried as the most educated and intelligent individuals.

This is where intuitive thinking becomes critical. Instead of trying to *change* organizational systems and cultures, leaders must encompass the concept of *transformation* into a system that is multidimensional in time, space, and events and that operates in harmony with the universal, nonlinear, holographic system. Old concepts of, for example, trying to manage and confront chaos must be replaced by new visions of identifying and building on flowing channels within the holographic system. Carlson and Kaiser (1999) noted that "nonlinear intelligence ultimately alters our notions of how reality operates, of the interconnectedness of external and internal words. This ability to shape and interact with reality in a new way is the ultimate innovation" (p. 51).

Forecasting

When risk and uncertainty are present in a decision-making process, the issues of the unknown and prediction arise. Innovation is replete with unknowns at all levels of the process: What are the future trends? Which basic ideas are worth exploring, and how do we develop them? How do we effectively manufacture a product or package a service? What will the market need in the near future, the long-term?

Many of the attempted definitions for intuition contain the concept of prediction. For example, "We conceive of intuition as the ability to make above-chance judgments about properties of a stimulus on the basis of information that is not consciously retrieved" (Bolte, Goschke, & Kuhl, 2003, p. 416). The mention of above chance implies a certain amount of insight or prediction. Furthermore, rigorous scientific studies over the years demonstrated compelling evidence that intuitive thinking does provide knowledge from the future (Bradley, 2006). The missing piece of the puzzle is discovering from where intuition comes and how to harness it. Bradley's discussion points to two factors supported by empirical evidence: The human body is able to sense future events, and the human body uses the physiological structure to capture and process the information. So far, research demonstrates that both the brain and the heart play a major role in the process. Bradley further explained that the process operates on the quantum level of our holographic system.

Anticipating Future Events

Scientific research, using brain wave detectors, demonstrates the brain captures events before the actual activity (McCraty et al., 2004b). Other similar experiments have been conducted as far back as 1975 whereby findings suggest that the brain has the capability of capturing activity signals before they manifest, although the conscious part of the brain does not register the activity until it happens (Levin & Kennedy, 1975). The findings also challenge the popular belief that intuitive thinking is accessing data that have been stored in the brain but not remembered consciously. Research conducted by Don, McDonough, and Warren (1998) discussed event-related potentials and concluded that there is a phenomenon of unconscious precognition whereby part of the brain registers the future activity but does not necessarily transmit it to the awareness part. Further research indicated that skin reacts to future events of about 5 seconds before the stimulus has been activated (Bierman, 2000; Bierman & Radin, 1997; Bierman & Scholte, 2002; Radin, 1997).

These intriguing findings have led to further research exploring the possibility of an internal system in the human body that can capture signals of future events. McCraty and colleagues (2004b) pioneered extensive research into the function of the heart and demonstrated with the use of electrocardiograms that the heart plays a major role in sensing future events: "These data indicate that, on average, the informational input to the heart regarding the future emotional stimulus occurred approximately 4.75 seconds before the stimulus was actually presented" (p. 331).

Although 4.75 seconds may appear to be insignificant, what is significant is demonstration that the human body is capable of receiving future information. Scientific researchers are only at the initial stages of exploring the possibility of a human future-events detection system. The possible explanation is that "some aspect of our perceptual apparatus is continuously scanning the future" (McCraty et al., 2004b). If this concept is true, then it would imply that we could develop our perceptual apparatus and learn how to fine-tune it and develop our sensories to capture future information and send it to our conscious part of the brain. According to McCraty et al. (2004b), there is "strong evidence for the idea that intuitive processes involve the body accessing a field of information that is not limited by the constraints of space and time" (p. 334).

Box 10-1 Outputs of Intuitive Thinking

- Clarity of thought
- Accurate reality map
- Innovative concepts
- Insights: creative solutions
- Accelerated speed of decision making
- Forecasting accuracy (prediction): feeling for trends, future events
- Deeper understanding of the holographic universe
- Higher consciousness (accountability, ethics)
- Knowing
- Wisdom

Quick Decision Making

In today's business environment decision making is preceded by volumes of information with little time for analysis and reflection. Thus clarity of thought is critical. The continuous flow of information is a double-edged sword: More information contributes to a fuller picture, but more information also gives indications that other information is missing. Meanwhile, the decision maker is running out of time. Drury and Kitsopoulos (2005, p. 29) pointed out the following:

> If you need to wait for more information in order to get all the facts—you'll never make a decision. The art of management lies in the ability to make decision in the face of incomplete information. Effective managers of innovation use the minimum amount of information needed for a reasonable and timely decision. One's quick judgment, intuition, and—yes—experience often override the need for data-hoarding and exhaustive analysis. A survey of over 2,000 top executives shows that they rely more on intuition than they admit.

Business leaders are overwhelmed with volumes of information that only add to the complexity of decision making. Sadler-Smith and Shefy (2004b) claimed the human brain has limitations and can execute only so much rational processing at one time. Studies have demonstrated that effective decision makers use both rational and analytical cognitive processes, but they also appear to use skills described as "instinct and intrinsic gifts" (Kopeikina, 2006, p. 19). These special skills are difficult to define and are referred to as intuition and are also linked to sharper forecasting skills (Cartwright, 2004).

In opposite situations, where there is a lack of available information, such as exploring new ventures in unknown environments, intuitive thinking can be critical in making the right decision. A chief executive officer (CEO) of a major energy corporation believes by the time one collected enough information to be 99.9% confident in making the right decision, "that decision has become obsolete" (Sadler-Smith & Shefy, 2004b, p. 77).

Doctors and organizational healthcare executives are faced with increasingly complex decision-making scenarios (Hay et al., 2002; Faugier, 2005). Some of the healthcare industry leaders and practitioners are exploring the concept of innovation in the realm of self-knowledge systems such as evidence-based and intuition-based decision making (Greenhalgh, 2002; Lieberman, Jarcho, & Satpute, 2004; Tracy et al., 2003). Findings in the healthcare industry research demonstrate that intuition, although still not fully comprehended, is accepted as an integral component of making decisions.

Dowie, Professor at the London School of Hygiene & Tropical Medicine (2001), pointed out that decision makers are weighed down by volumes of information and knowledge and new decision systems need to be created that enable practitioners to become more autonomous. He advocated that a deeper and clearer understanding of the decision-making process needs to be studied and mentions the use of intuition.

> I hear people say, there are all these factors and we will consider them all, take them into account, and bear this and that in mind, and bring everything into the equation, giving due weight to this element, and so on. And in the end a decision is made. But no one has any idea about how one has moved from all those bits and pieces to the conclusion. (Kingman, 2002, p. 3)

The following is a typical statement from a nurse referring to a patient: "You start looking for something and you don't know why. Then you start thinking why aren't you happy with him. Sometimes they're feelings of, you can't turn your back on them, apprehension, sort of scared for them" (King & Clark, 2002, p. 328). The nurses described their intuitive thought as a type of apprehension or feeling that there was something they must investigate further, although there was no rational reason to do so. Once they decided to investigate further, they then relied on their knowledge and experience to guide them through their investigation. The specific intuitive thought that triggers the investigation appears to be distinct from any rational analysis.

MAPPING ABSOLUTE REALITY

How Do We Discover What It Is That We Do Not Know?

The ability to map reality in the absolute is a difficult exercise, because it implies no mental filters or boundaries interfering or interpreting the data. Yet mapping the complex reality of the world we live in has become the most critical challenge for leaders. The issue of objective observation has generated enormous volumes of writing over hundreds of years. Is it possible to shut down all our judgments and filters?

How do we discover our blind spots that prevent us from seeing what we cannot even imagine might exist? To incorporate all elements of reality into a map, leaders' breadth of thinking and objective observation need to be extended. Accepting the reality of the new world tends to cause cognitive dissonance, and leaders need to acknowledge this dilemma. This is where intuitive thinking and insights become critical in mapping our reality. Using a model is limiting because it is self-defined and encrypted with conscious and unconscious expectations, assumptions, filters, and human-generated boundaries.

The Holographic Universe

> *"Intuitive managers change the destiny of their organizations*
> *by perceiving pathways not visible to others. I was once explain-*
> *ing an alternative reality to one of my health administration*
> *students. He said, "I don't see it." I replied: "I know you don't*
> *see it, but don't assume because you don't see it, it is not here—*
> most of reality is not within your range of vision."
>
> (KAISER, 1987, P. 16)

The quantum physics theory of our holographic universe is based on the premise that "all objects and entities in the universe are energized in a constant state of oscillation at different energy frequencies" (Bradley, 2006, p. 11). These different frequencies create wave fields that interact with each other and form the holographic system. Thus any and all types of particles are interrelated and communicate at a certain level. These wave fields create flow channels as well as intersections.

The scientific implication is that the human body has the potential of "establishing a bio-energetic means of connection to the energy fields of the external environment through which non-local information can be communicated" (Bradley, 2006, p. 11). The concept of a holographic system is supported by both the physics and neuropsychology communities because it offers a potential explanation for communication phenomena to include nonlocal transfer of information and the reception of intuitive insights and precognition.

To better understand the holographic principle, Bradley (2006) used the analogy of communicating voice information over the telephone. Each event or information is encapsulated in its own type of space–time bubble that retains its entity. However, in a holographic system these information entities sometimes overlap each other and cause an exchange of information that forms and determines future events. The exchange of information occurs when wave fields form harmonic series with synchronized wave peaks and create virtual channels of communication. Tuning into these channels could explain the forecasting characteristic of intuitive thinking. Bradley posited that to tap into these channels, the human being uses both an outgoing wave of energy that is translated into a focused attention to the object or event and an incoming wave field that is captured through the sensory or pyschophysiological system that continuously generates various energy fields. This process enables the individual to capture intuitive insights from the holographic fields.

Today's socioeconomic interactions between complex systems produce waves of increasing unpredictability and friction. For example, values of some cultures are not aligned with our own. The common reaction is to either believe we can change the values of that group or ignore it completely. Either approach is a formula for disaster. Recognizing and integrating these unacceptable components are critical in establishing our reality map, and the intuitive leader will need to seek the flow channels between the opposite groups that would create space for negotiation or mediation.

Thus the issue of knowledge and understanding of how our brain has the potential to interact with the universal hologram becomes critical. If we do not know of this potential, how will we know to use and develop the skill? Because all matter manifests by emitting different wavelengths and frequencies, it is easy to imagine with the proper reception tool, or antenna, the possibility of retrieving the information. Yet it is understandable how this futuristic concept might initially be difficult for the conscious mind to accept. Our brain has been conditioned that unless a concept is proven scientifically or within our rational understanding, the phenomenon probably does not exist.

The following scenario might help place this concept in perspective. Imagine going back in time to the caveman era. We present the caveman with a television and explain that by plugging the wire into the cave wall, not only would a moving, color, and acoustic picture appear, but that by pressing a few buttons on an independent box, a hundred other different channels would appear and that the images could also be in real time from other geographical locations. Impossible? Inconceivable? How many of us can explain how television and other 21st technologies work? How do telephone numbers traverse the ether and reach the right target? If we cannot explain how a technology works, does it mean the technology does not exist? If we cannot explain or understand how some of our brain functions work, does that mean they do not exist or we should not develop them? Perhaps we should first develop these functions and record the results as evidence from which scientific testing can then be conducted, if need be.

Research in quantum physics has demonstrated instant communication of data between particles separated by a huge distance and that particles have the knowledge of the activity before it happens (McCraty et al., 2004b). In 1997 Radin had already demonstrated that human skin could react to an event 5 seconds before it happened. Reiner (2004) suggested that the ability to access future events could be related to the brain function of the unconscious. Furthermore, the process in itself can take the individual to a higher level of consciousness. Do we refuse to explore this concept and close the door to the possibility of transcending our present state of consciousness, or do we have the courage to travel beyond our present mental paradigm and embark on the journey of discovery and higher consciousness?

"For the intuitive manager, the universe is one fabric—an interconnected whole. All parts are joined with subtleties and are affected by the destiny of each part. The manager manages a system that is always more than the sum of its parts. Each system is contained within a larger system and all systems reflect each other."

(KAISER, 1987, P. 16)

Stretching the Brain for Innovative Insight

It might be easy to intellectually understand the workings of the brain, but what may not be as easy is giving up our comfort zone of our current thinking paradigm and apply our newfound knowledge. Acquiring new knowledge stipulates a willingness to accept concepts that do not always make sense in our personal thinking models. This means letting go of some of our suppositions and assumptions and acquiring new knowledge that might challenge our present pylons of belief.

New knowledge can stretch the brain into unknown territory and trigger a myriad of emotions to include resistance and cognitive dissonance. However, recognizing and managing these emotions will open the door to the vast universe of thinking that had been closed off by the old paradigms. This is not to say that one should accept any new concept without critical thinking but rather one should consider a new concept as a possibility until a full spectrum/multidimensional exploration using critical thinking has been effected. The outcome might lead to the conclusion that the concept is not valid, but there will have been two benefits to the exercise: stretching the mind beyond one's conventional paradigm and possibly discovering innovative concepts peripheral to the germane one.

Shifting From Traditional Rational Thinking to Intuitive Thinking

In seeking new decision-making skill sets, Sinclair and Ashkanasy (2005) reported, "Rational decision-making strategies struggle to reach the 50% success mark" (p. 353). The discovery of alternative components to the traditional, rational type of decision-making process would constitute a valuable contribution. Intuition offers another potential characteristic: the ability to have a better feel for the future, therefore enhancing the forecasting ability of decision makers (Radin & Schlitz, 2005).

In attempting to differentiate between normal information processing and intuitive thinking, Bradley (2006) pointed out that information processing occurs in incremental steps and builds up to a conclusion. Intuitive thoughts, however, manifest themselves spontaneously, creating a sense of complete understanding often accompanied by emotions reflecting the characteristics of the thought. This is because the intuitive process appears to encompass the entire physiological human system and would explain why individuals can sometimes feel goose bumps, a gut feeling, a sound, image, or other sensorial feelings.

Cole (2006), in researching intuition and consciousness development, noted the importance of recognizing sensory signals: "Sensory raw material—what we see, taste, hear or smell—the experience of existence, is the 'raw data' through which social life is understood" (p. 343). Identifying and recognizing the relationship between a sensory signal and a specific cognitive process or thought could be instrumental in defining intuition.

Sadler-Smith and Shefy (2004b), in attempting to explain descriptors, identified intuition on two levels: a knowing that occurs on the intellectual level and a feeling that manifests through the body or through the senses. The two may manifest at the same time, which is why it may be difficult for an individual to describe. Conventional language in this case is very limiting because it is a rational process and words are, in themselves, illustrations of concepts. Through training, an individual can develop a separate type of language to interpret the meaning of the sensory feelings.

Intuition manifests itself differently for each individual. It can be a physical feeling, a vision, picture, an emotional feeling, or a mental feeling full of information that is difficult to translate into conventional language (Sadler-Smith & Shefy, 2004b). Jeter (2003) indicated physical manifestation of intuition might be either pleasant, such as warm feelings, or unpleasant, such as headaches or stomachaches. It is therefore important to be able to identify any correlation of intuitive thought with physical or emotional manifestations.

SHIFT INTO INTUITIVE LEADERSHIP

Because intuitive leaders operate in the holographic dimension, they need to shift their traditional thinking from trying to manage change and chaos to identifying flow channels and synchronicity. Managing change and chaos stipulates that the attention is on the disturbing energy. Disturbing energy is a reality that must be expected in any system, but intuitive leaders need to go beyond the initial reaction of wanting to control or confront the disturbance and look at the entire system to discover flow channels. Intuitive thinking offers the potential to travel beyond our boundaries by sensing resonance, identifying flow channels, and scanning the horizon and identifying areas of nonresistance. The intuitive leader therefore needs to have the ability to understand resonance, synchronicity, to generate fresh insights. The areas of nonresistance are opportunities for synergies, partnerships, a new direction, or innovation.

The focus on confronting change must be replaced by developing a clearer mind and sharper skills to anticipate future events that foster innovation. The singular characteristic of intuitive thinking is that the process is not constrained by boundaries or models. It transcends all parameters and boundaries and incorporates the entire spectrum of the brain functions from the extreme right brain to the extreme left brain qualities, to include an unknown functional component that makes intuitive thinking unique. In research conducted with real estate professionals, participants referred to an unknown piece in the process of intuitive thinking that is related to a higher force that cannot be specifically described but in general terms was referred to as "law of the universe" (Surel, 2009, p. 211). It is this ethereal component that is linked to enhanced forecasting skills.

Intuitive-based organizational systems need to be created from the essence and souls of the individual employees. Leaders therefore need to use their brain differently to create truly functional systems that can inspire followers to operate at their highest potential. Organizational cultures and systems are only as good as the individuals. True change for corporate culture can happen only by addressing the souls of the individuals. Intuitive leaders need to understand the reality map, set the example by learning and evolving, and provide the means and inspiration for employees to do the same.

Intuitive thinking is the catalyst and generator of innovation, creativity, and artistic inspiration. There is also agreement that intuition is a critical strategic decision-making factor for corporations operating in fast-cycle markets. The corporations must be dynamic to sustain their competitive advantage and continue to be high-performance businesses (Miller & Ireland, 2005; Ramphal, 2003; Sadler-Smith & Shefy, 2004a). Corporations in the fast-cycle markets tend to be in technical sectors where innovation is critical for sustaining a competitive advantage.

Although aspects of the process of intuitive thinking are still not demystified, successful entrepreneurs and global corporations are not afraid to capitalize on this skill to develop their competitive advantage and maintain successful strategies. Intuitive thinking is gaining recognition. Schulz (1998, p. 26) noted the following:

> Numerous studies have shown that the use of intuition in any number of
> fields is often what separates the men from the boys—that is, the experts from
> the amateurs. It's the quantum quality that gives an individual an edge over
> others in this field and boosts him into the "expert" stratosphere.

Sundgren and Styhre (2004) conducted a study on the role of intuition in the research and development of new drugs in one of the biggest pharmaceutical companies, AstraZeneca. In 2003 AstraZeneca employed over 10,000 people in its research and development department, with a budget of $2.7 billion. Creating new drugs is the life force of a pharmaceutical company. The qualitative research methodology, based on interviews, focused on the specific concept of intuition defined as a type of thinking that is used under time pressure, is not rational, and is identified as a gut feeling. The definition also took into consideration that although science did not identify intuition in scientific terms, it generates valuable knowledge.

The researchers summarized their findings as follows: "This study suggests that intuition is an intrinsic part of the creative process in drug discovery and thus an important organizational resource" (Sundgren & Styhre, 2004, p. 279). They identified three distinct roles intuition can play in new drug development: First, intuition widens the breadth of thinking and opens the creative channels; second, it opens channels of communications between different scientific sectors; and third, it allows early identification of ideas that lead to scientific breakthroughs. In essence, the research implied intuition is the precursor to innovative thinking.

Although rational thinking is still a valuable, if not critical, element of decision making, it appears necessary to develop a complementary approach in making decisions more effectively. Using one's intuition could be a quick and accurate solution. As Miller and Ireland (2005) indicated, "A framework focused on strategic planning suggests intuition as a hunch is important when planning for ambiguous futures" (p. 24). Miller and other researchers also contended this is true in situations where the leader chooses to deviate from the perceived norm or to experiment with innovative methods, creating a complex situation (Jeter, 2003; Patton, 2003).

Alchemical Process

An individual does not spontaneously become an intuitive leader after attending a few seminars, learning a technique, or following a model. Learning to become an intuitive leader is a highly personalized and continuous transformational process. It is a commitment that stipulates an intellectual and spiritual opening to concepts that are not integrated into most traditional business models. The process is an alchemical mastering and transmutation of the intellect, the soul, the heart, and the sensories. The critical components of transmuting into intuitive leadership include knowledge, life experience, rational and logical analysis, emotional intelligence, critical thinking, and spiritual intelligence combined with a yearning to discover new horizons and a higher consciousness.

"Like lucid dreaming, intuition comes to those who seek the experience. Resolve to develop this capacity and it will begin to appear."

(KAISER, 1987, P. 16)

Box 10-2 Alchemy: The Process

Alchemy, the precursor to modern science, offers protocols to transmute elementary material into higher-level material. What has eluded scientists is the expectation that the results would materialize on the physical level. Those who have practiced alchemy discovered that the process of understanding the principles of combining different energies, both physical and mental, generates a higher and more powerful understanding of how our world functions and how to *plug into* the multidimensional holographic system.

The original concept of alchemy is to reach perfection through the physical and spiritual realms. Alchemists tried to transmute metals into higher matter such as gold by using a rigorous process that included the spirit and the intellect. What has been retained in our modern world is the personal transformational journey that alchemists experienced while conducting their experiments and acquiring wisdom. Alchemists were very strong individuals who worked alone and developed a philosophy of the cosmos that reflected our modern holographic concept and incorporated some of the quantum physics principles.

References to alchemy and the concept of transmutation are found as far back as the 3rd century B.C. in China. Alchemy then migrated to the Western world during the 3rd and 4th centuries A.D. to Greco-Roman Egypt. Evidence of alchemical work can be found in most civilizations throughout the ages to include the Arab countries, which also made significant contributions. Because the alchemical process is based on the individual's personal transformation, the concept of alchemy was thus generally misunderstood and created cognitive dissonance among the general populations. This drove alchemists to operate in isolation and in secret. Their knowledge and wisdom were passed on by word of mouth to only a select few.

Elements of Transmutation

Learning
The intuitive leader's learning process is similar to that of the alchemist. Although alchemists studied written works, they did not rely on books only to advance in the field. What fueled the process of personal transformation was the continuous thirst to investigate and think outside of their and others' paradigms. Alchemists learned the laws of resonance and developed their sense of observation and sensitivity. They trained themselves to tune into both external and internal environmental changes and nuances. As their intellect broadened beyond their own and others' belief systems, they broke through their boundaries and self-doubt and thus entered the cosmic world of multidimensions.

In modern times Cloninger (2006) discussed how to foster intuitive thinking within the educational system and suggested that the traditional methods of teaching that focus on learning without reflection stifle intuition: "We need to make room in analytic activities for synthesis, reflection, and meditation on what is being studied" (p. 26). The intuitive leader must provide learning opportunities within the organizational structure to foster the same transformational process to the employees. The learning environment in an intuitive organizational culture offers periodical forums between departments to create cross-pollination and exchange current thoughts and knowledge about innovation. These forums, or meetings, act as a catalyst to identify valid innovative concepts and push the development into a realistic and successful direction. It is the intuitive leader's responsibility to monitor the exchanges and manage these relationships.

Reflection, Meditation, Contemplation, and Meaning

Reflection time is an important component of the alchemical process. During this time the brain integrates and transmutes all information, data, and experience to create insights at a higher level of consciousness. True reflection creates an empty space in which we can recognize what we do not know, identify more effective actions, and build our intuitive skills to scan the horizon.

Reflection creates a space that generates intuitive thinking by creating a decompression chamber whereby the intuitive leader can consciously disconnect the mental control mechanisms of rational analysis and open the portal to insightful intuitive thoughts. It is not a question of shutting off the rational brain function but rather to surrender control. Let the natural forces flow as they may and let them free associate with experiences, rational thought, and other mental functions such as intuitive thought process. As Wheatley (1992/1999) pointed out: "If we want to influence any change, anywhere, we need to work *with* this powerful process rather than deny its existence" (p. 147). From this process meaning will emerge. Reflection enables the individual's mind and sensories to feel the experiences, integrate the information, and identify the holographic interconnections that lead to intuitive insights. The discipline of making time for reflection also tempers emotional characteristics and fosters tolerance and patience.

Reflection space therefore creates the ideal environment for innovative and creative thinking. Dr. Melanie Polkosky, a social-cognitive psychologist, recommended that innovators "envision a unique, interesting auditory environment and realize it much in the way of a soundtrack or sound effects might be developed for a movie" (2008, p. 7) to elicit creativity.

Intuitive insights generated from reflection lend structure to formulating strategies and solutions. This is not to say that the existing organizational structure and processes are to be ignored. On the contrary, they represent the infrastructure and roots, but the intuitive leader operates his or her leadership function from a higher level that is globally and universally connected. Insights either fit into the organization's adaptive and organic structure or change processes and some structure to foster flow channels internally and with the external environment.

Listening

An important component of reflection is the art of listening. Without listening, there is no true exchange, no lessons learned. Without listening, there is nothing for reflection and no opportunity to develop wisdom. Daniel Goleman (2000), the pioneer of emotional intelligence, described listening as an art that includes multiple functions such as "asking astute questions, being open-minded and understanding, not interrupting, seeking suggestions" (p. 176). In researching the emotional intelligence factor among executives, Cooper and Sawaf (1997) stated, "listening is a matter of paying deep, genuine attention—with eyes open and seeing, mind open and learning, heart open and feeling. This is how we pay fundamental respect to our conversation partner and to the dialogue itself. It may be the most significant step some managers can take to increase productivity and innovation" (p. 73).

Listening is a critical factor in scanning the horizon for signals of potential change. The intuitive leader must be vigilant at all times to minimize the elements of surprise that can emerge from the future horizon. Corporations that work largely with contractors and suppliers around the world and operate within different models and value systems need to be extremely vigilant in scanning their horizon for signals. Boeing's research and development department, concerned about establishing a strong competitive advantage in innovation, recognized the value of listening and established "listening posts" throughout the world (Swain, 2007, p. 60). Boeing's Phantom Works, whose business is mostly with suppliers and partnerships around the world, sought to "connect all the right people together" (p. 62) to maximize the flow of information exchange through their listening posts. David Swain, Boeing's retired chief technical officer, stated clearly that "You have to have these listening posts or you'll waste way too much money doing stuff that's been done" (p. 65).

Synchronicity and the Principle of Similars

Carl Jung defined synchronicity as "a meaningful coincidence of two or more events, where something other than the probability of chance is involved" (Senge, Scharmer, Jaworski, & Flowers, 2004, p. 159). Synchronicity manifests, or rather is recognized, when an individual is intuitively in tune with the holographic system. Synchronicity does not happen because someone is intuitive, but it is the intuitive skill that enables the individual who is operating within the flow channels to notice synchronous events. Synchronicity is visible to those who know it exists and who learn how to recognize the signals. The phenomenon of synchronicity is enhanced when an intuitive leader is flowing within the holographic channels rather than fighting blockages. Operating at the same level of flow in the hologram are other individuals with similar goals and vision and the interconnectedness grows among them. Modern quantum physics supports this phenomenon by explaining that particles that were once together continue to react similarly, faster than the speed of light, when they are miles apart (Phillips, 2006). Another example of synchronicity would be individuals who think and operate on a specific flow-path of the holographic system meeting others of the same nature.

It is therefore important for the intuitive leader to be aware of these laws of physics so that he or she can be more attentive and conscious while scanning the horizon and building relationships for events that are generated by these laws. Manifesting synchronicity stipulates clarity of thought and a focus of the intention to project a clear energetic signal into the holographic system that can be received by others who are traveling on that pathway.

INSTRUMENTS AND RECEPTORS OF INTUITIVE THINKING

The HeartMath research group conducted extensive neuroscience research on intuition and posited three major neural networks: the brain, the heart, and the intestinal track, which would explain how intuitive thoughts appear to be felt in the gut (McCraty et al., 2004b). However, results of the research demonstrated that "the heart is involved in the processing and decoding of intuitive information" (McCraty et al., 2004a, p. 133) and that furthermore, "the heart appears to receive intuitive information before the brain" (McCraty et al., 2004b, p. 325) and that "intuitive perception is a system-wide process in which the heart and brain (and possibly other bodily systems) are involved together in responding to intuitive information" (McCraty et al., 2004b, p. 327).

Other research in the realm of intuition demonstrates that although the conscious mind might not differentiate a logical or rational thought from an intuitive one, the human sensories such as the skin or stomach appear to immediately react. Furthermore, compelling evidence demonstrates that both the brain and the heart react emotionally before a stimulus is physically received by the participants (McCraty et al., 2004b). The heart has an interesting literary link throughout the times and in different cultures by being associated with meaning and knowing. Interestingly enough, the oldest Chinese symbol that represents the mind is that of a heart (Senge et al., 2005).

Cognition and the Brain

The most powerful yet most underused instrument we possess is our brain. In recent years the field of neuroscience has made exceptional findings with state-of-the-art equipment such as functional magnetic resonance imaging (fMRI). Scientists demonstrated that if we use our brain in specific areas, new neural pathways grow to accommodate an increase in that particular function or to accommodate an increase in volume of information. The field of neuroscience is expanding its boundaries and forging ahead to explore links between cognitive functions and brain wave activities with highly sophisticated imaging technology (Farah & Wolpe, 2004). fMRI technology, for example, is so precise it can determine that a person can have a knowing about oneself without having to retrieve information from the part of the brain that stores autobiographical data (Lieberman et al., 2004).

Similar research reveals the brain may consist of multiple self-knowledge systems such as "evidence-based and intuition based self-knowledge" (Lieberman et al., 2004, p. 421), specifically identifying intuitive thought versus evidence-based knowledge, which retrieves information from the memory of experience or learned knowledge. Other research indicates each life experience triggers growth of new neural connections that in turn affect the way the brain treats new material it receives (Murray, 2004). By practicing intuitive thought processes, one might be able to develop the brain in that area, thus further developing the intuitive process.

Extensive research in cognitive psychology and theoretical reasoning has generated different approaches as to how the rational interplays with intuition, but the common thread is that intuitive thinking "involves a complex interplay of cognitive, affective and somatic elements" (Hodgkinson, Langan-Fox, & Sadler-Smith, 2008, p. 11). The consensus is that the brain uses a combination of life experience, knowledge, rational and logical analysis, and pattern recognition. Intuitive thinking is not a function of its own but an amalgamation of all brain functions and physical sensories that incorporates a yet undefined element that specifically generates insight and forecasting capabilities.

The essence of intuitive thinking uses the whole brain to integrate space, time, and action events into one holographic picture. Our first reaction might be to question if it is possible. Initially, we encounter our cultural and mental blockages and biases. Cognitive dissonance erupts. But how do we know it is impossible? Is it because we have not experienced it yet? How do we know for sure that the limitations to the intuition concept are real and not just a limitation in our programmed mental framework? How do we know what we do not know? Are we trapped by our fear of the unknown?

Sensors

Intuitive thoughts are received in different ways depending on the individual. The reception can be intellectual by visualizing a picture, by physical feelings detected by our sensors such as goose bumps or warmth through the skin, by emotions such as elation or fear, or even by an impulse from the gut or from the heart. George Soros, for example, who made millions in currency speculation, explained he receives reliable intuitive signals by a specific backache, always followed by an important market change. Soros changed his monetary positions whenever the backache manifested (as cited in Stewart, 2002).

McNaughton's (2003) research demonstrated that each individual has his or her own way of accessing the intuitive process, and some use more than one technique. In his research 65% of interviewees listened to what they called their internal voice, whereas 45% received the intuition in a visual form and 23% practiced some form of physical exercise to trigger their intuitive thought process.

At first it is difficult to grasp the intuitive signal because "The flash of insight—intuition—comes and goes like quicksilver and it takes a bold step and imagination to use the form or idea to create meaning . . . . effective workers utilize this practice wisdom instinctively, artfully and, possibly, unconsciously" (Milner, 2006, p. 66). The intuitive leader therefore needs to heighten his or her mental and physical awareness in learning to identify intuitive signals.

> *"If the senses don't actually perceive the world, if they are instead participating parts of the mind-world as a whole, a radical re-understanding of perception is necessary."*
>
> (ELEANOR ROSCH, COGNITIVE SCIENTIST, BERKELEY, AS CITED IN SENGE ET AL., 2005, P. 209)

The Heart

In a unique study of the heart, McCraty et al. (2004a) reported there are instances when so-called intuitive thoughts cannot be related to prior experience or knowledge and "the psychophysiologic systems receive and process information about a future event before the event actually happens" (p. 134). Their findings indicate the brain does not hold the major role in processing information because the heart plays a direct role in processing data before the body senses the event. The findings further demonstrate a correlation between intuitive process and specific heartbeats.

The findings relate to discoveries in quantum physics and demonstrate that either instant communication of data occurs between particles separated by a huge distance or that particles have knowledge of the activity before it happens (McCraty et al., 2004a, p. 134). The findings relate to quantum physics findings regarding nonlocal communication (Dunne & Jahn, 2003), and further research by Radin (1997) demonstrated that skin reacts to an event 5 seconds before it happens.

The study by McCraty et al. (2004a) on intuition supported Radin's findings. Using an electroencephalogram to measure cardiac changes and relating them to specific cortical activity, findings demonstrated not only that the body does respond to intuitive stimulus but also that it does so many seconds before the individual registers the activity. The electroencephalographic measurements demonstrate it is the heart that triggers the reaction, not the brain. According to the researchers, the study proves the body "is continuously scanning the future" (p. 133). They explain the heart processes the stimulus, which in turn creates a signal that the sensors, such as the skin, can detect.

Other research using the electroencephalogram to measure skin conductance and the electrocardiogram to measure cardiac accelerations and decelerations demonstrated that the heart is involved in the processing and decoding of intuitive information. Once the prestimulus information is received in the psychophysiologic systems, it appears to be processed in the same way as conventional sensory input (McCraty et al., 2004a). The findings present compelling evidence that the body's perceptual apparatus is continuously scanning the future. It is important for the aspiring intuitive leader to have this knowledge so that he or she can become aware of these functions, gain a better understanding of how the human system works, and therefore develop these powerful skills.

Emotions

The root of the word emotion comes from the Latin *motere* or to move. Daniel Goleman, a pioneer in emotional intelligence, states that emotions "fuel our motivations, and our motives in turn drive our perceptions and shape our actions. Great work starts with great feeling" (2000, p. 106). Emotions have only recently been accepted in the business world as significant influencers in decision making.

However, there is another aspect to emotions. Research revealed that some emotions are actually impulses triggered by the reception of intuitive thoughts. Bradley (2006) reported that "intuitive foreknowledge involves perception of implicit information about non-local objects and/or events by the body's psychophysiological systems" (p. 1) and "intuitive perception of a future event is related to the degree of emotional significance of that event" (p. 1). Emotions, if understood and managed, can therefore be used as an intuitive detection and connection tool. Bradley implied that if an individual focuses emotionally to the target object or event, he or she could tune into the holographic channels, connect to the target, and obtain implicit information about future possibilities of the target.

Breuer (2004), in an article published in *Scientific American,* conducted fMRI experiments demonstrating emotions are definitely detectable and attributable to specific brain functions. The research implied fMRI studies may lead to major discoveries in brain function, including the demystification of intuition. LeDoux (2003) and Ekstrom (2004) contended that neural synapses can develop and new ones be created if the individual uses them more often and in a different way. The more one uses intuition, the more the neural synapses might develop, which implies that one can develop intuitive skills without truly understanding the actual process. The aspiring intuitive leader should therefore learn about the meaning of emotions and monitor his or her emotional impulses to identify which ones are actually responses to intuitive information versus a personal reaction to a situation or to another person's behavior.

"Emotions are a "signal system" and source of information and energy."

(COOPER & SAWAF, 1997, P. 36)

Passion and Positive Thinking

Passion is a personal energy that fuels one's direction and drive. Passion is the ultimate cruising speed of one's motivational drive. Because emotions and energy are an integral part of intuitive thinking, passion plays a central role in the development of intuitive leadership. Emotions are communicated energetically, and the intuitive leader communicates his or her visions and goals not just through strategic planning and language, but by his or her own emanation of that thought.

Bradley (2006) described the entrepreneur's passionate attention as "the biological energy activated in his emotional connection to the object of interest (e.g., the quest for future opportunities in a certain field of business)" (p. 15). In our holographic system, passion is a highly intensive attention projected onto a target that can be a future idea, innovation, or event. This human-generated energy travels the spectrum of the holographic system until it resonates harmonically with a similar frequency and/or wavelength of the target. The resonance establishes a communications conduit from which a well-trained intuitive brain can receive the information.

Bradley's (2006) research demonstrated that having a positive feeling versus a negative one plays an important part in scanning the horizon. The "adoption of positive emotional interest involved in the act of 'paying attention to' distant locales or nonlocal objects, establishes a relationship of phase-conjugated-adaptive-resonance with the quantum level of an object at the distant location" (p. 14). Bradley concluded that this process "enables the body to receive and process quantum-holographic information about nonlocal objects and events spectrally encoded in the movement of energy" (p. 14). A positive attitude or feeling can be compared to the *on* position and a negative feeling as the *off* position in terms of being able to connect into the hologram.

ISSUE OF EXPERIENCE

Experience is only one of the components in the formula of intuitive thinking. Lessons are drawn from experience and contribute to the knowledge base that is accessed by the intuitive process. For innovation to break out into truly creative modes, however, alternative thinking processes are needed. Contemporary views caution that experience is not the only crucial factor: "While experience is obviously valuable, it can also lead to fossilization, resistance to change, and stifling of the imagination. . . . In order to invent and innovate, we must break with experience and let our imaginations soar. Relying solely on experience to gain wisdom inhibits creativity" (Drury & Kitsopoulos, 2005, p. 28).

If the innovative thought process relies only on known data and experience, then there is little space, if any, to explore possibilities beyond these defined databases. What emerges are repackaged ideas based on already known information. Creative thought process, in order to discover novel and seminal concepts, can use experience and information databases as a springboard to leap outside this defined space and into the holographic system where the unknown and truly innovative concepts can be discovered. Drury and Kitsopoulos (2005) pointed out that "Relying solely on experience to gain wisdom inhibits creativity" (p. 28). Yet many decision makers prefer to stay in that comfort zone of experience, whereas others who do transcend their known experience boundaries and achieve true innovation are reluctant to put forth their new concepts for fear of rejection from those who cannot see beyond their self-defined paradigms.

As past experiences accumulate, they tend to mold our mindset. Before we realize it, our mindset is based on not only events from our past but on our own personal experience of them, which creates a rather self-limited paradigm. The individual falls into a routine mode that lessens sensitivity to unusual signals that might be flagging an upcoming crisis or an innovative solution. Another issue to think about is how we have experienced a specific event or concept in the past could be different if we reexperienced the event in today's timeframe and context with our new knowledge and information. Equipped with new knowledge and perhaps a way of thinking that has evolved, we may not gain the same insights that we did in the past.

INSEAD Professors Sengupta, Abdel-Hamid, and Van Wassenhove (2008), in researching the role of experience in leadership, stated that "in big complex projects, managers tend to draw on experience that doesn't help, or actually hurts the project" (para. 4). The researchers specified that "Managers tend to learn the wrong lessons and apply them again and again in a way that's fundamentally counter-productive" (para. 6). Simulations were run as part of the research, and managers continuously repeated the same errors even with feedback between each simulation.

More specifically, a study in clinical decision making exploring the utilization of evidence-based medicine by physicians and the role of intuition concluded that "primary care physicians see no opposition between research evidence and clinical intuition" (Tracy et al., 2003, para. 24). Greenhalgh (2002), in researching the issue of evidence-based decision making, stated that the false dichotomy between evidence and intuition should be recognized and that it is not a zero-sum relationship. According to Greenhalgh, "it is now time to raise the status of intuition as a component of expert decision-making" (p. 399).

Studies using fMRI posited that experience functions as a modifier of neural connections, thus making information processing more efficient by enabling the brain to build shortcuts (Berns, 2008). This process, however, creates an unconscious dependency on past experience, and a vicious circle is created in terms of continuously operating within the constraints of previous experience and not being able to see beyond one's own thought model defined by those personal experiences.

Berns (2008) pointed out that if an individual imagines something never seen before, then the brain cannot find a previous experience link and creates novel perceptions and ideas and, more importantly, "reconfigure neural networks so that you can see things that you didn't see before" (p. 53). A new stimulus or a jolt from something unknown triggers the thinking function beyond the constraints of past experience: "The more radical the change, the greater the likelihood of fresh insights" (p. 53).

The brain reorganizes its perception field only if it receives a stimulus that is unknown, especially if it is precipitated from an environment outside one's expertise or comfort zone. This is why analogy exercises conducted in creativity sessions usually generate repackaged concepts and not true innovation. Berns (2008) suggested one way of breaking the brain from automatically using these shortcuts is to pay attention to intuition and "allow yourself the freedom to write down gut feelings, even if they're vague or visceral . . . only when you consciously confront your brain's shortcuts will you be able to imagine outside of its boundaries" (p. 55).

Bern's (2008) findings would explain the experiment conducted by Sengupta et al. (2008) whereby after repeated simulations and getting feedback from each one, the managers repeated their mistakes. The quality of the feedback could also be tainted by the individual's brain that is operating in the closed thinking loop based on past experience. Thus the intuitive leader needs to be aware of this trap and be responsible for communicating this knowledge throughout the organization so that others can benefit and enhance their own intuitive thinking process.

Creating the Intuitive Organizational Environment

Shifting an organization's culture and processes into an intuitive environment is a course of action that must be done harmoniously. There is no model to impose. An intuitive organizational system is a dissipative structure, as explained by Ilya Prigogine in Gilstrap (2007). A dissipative system is one that can reorganize itself to a higher level to accommodate additional volumes of data or increasingly complex functions. Dissipative, or self-renewing, systems are stable over time. As the intuitive leader conducts the shift from a more traditional organizational structure into an intuitive one, the existing system and its subsystems will reach a point of saturation. The intuitive thinkers in the organization who are knowledgeable about dissipative structures will notice first the fluctuations caused by the impending saturation and thus be able to anticipate the needs for the higher level restructuring and derive the insights to formulate the new processes and functions.

From a traditional viewpoint, the intuitive organizational structure and culture is an organic, adaptive, and self-organizing system that operates in a nonlinear holographic paradigm. The intuitive leader needs to provide the necessary structure to coach employees in shifting out of a linear mode of thinking and to anticipate new concepts that initially might not resonate with their traditional mental paradigms.

> *"The more I read about self-renewing systems, the more I marvel at the images of freedom and possibility they evoke. This is a domain of independence and interdependence, of processes that support forces we've placed in opposition—change and stability, continuity and newness, autonomy and control—and all in an environment that tests and teases and disturbs and, ultimately responds to changes it creates by changing itself."*
>
> (WHEATLEY, 1992/1999, P. 98)

More specifically, in team building individual strengths and fortes need to be identified and developed. The intuitive leadership identifies and incorporates employees' aspirations to formulate appropriate incentives that go beyond the basic Maslow's hierarchy of needs. As financial and other basic needs are met, the intuitive organization provides the cultural fabric for employees to find meaning in their work and strive for self-actualization.

Intuitive leadership focuses on inspiring individuals to reach their potential by building on their strengths and identifying other emergent skills. In some ways intuitive leadership reflects the basic philosophy of appreciative inquiry whereby organizational change is based on identifying an organization's and employees' strengths instead of battling with the weaknesses and negatives (Sekerka, Brumbaugh, Rosa, & Cooperrider, 2006). In building organizational structure, intuitive leaders work with positive flow channels and elicit employees' strengths.

The shift into an intuitive environment must be done organically. The intuitive leader can start the process by first communicating knowledge and understanding about the values and benefits of functioning in an intuitive environment. Then, communication channels between departments need to be opened and discussion forums need to be scheduled. Transparency is key, and the intuitive leader is accessible and actively implicated in the organizational transformation.

The intuitive leader in coaching the executive team and managers wants to foster the same philosophy of being actively implicated with and being accessible to employees and other teams. Standard Chartered Bank ensures that its executives are actively integrated with various departments by maximizing face-to-face interactions even if it means extensive travel (Gratton & Erickson, 2007). Standard Chartered Bank perceives this effort as an investment in generating a true collaborative culture that increases efficiency. In launching a new program, for example, employees "had an almost uncanny ability to understand who the key stakeholders at each branch were and how best to approach them" (p. 104). This was attributed to the relationships that were previously nurtured during the face-to-face interactions.

It is therefore the intuitive leader's responsibility to create an organizational environment that is open and fluid to ensure harmonious and constructive flows in the organizational structure. The intuitive leader should be in tune with the group's ethos, incorporating the goals and objectives of employees, to help create meaning. The traditional policies of forcing and breaking through are replaced by the concept of identifying flow channels, synchronicity, and synergies to create integration both internally between departments and externally with the environment.

Well-known healthcare advisor Leland Kaiser, a strong advocate of intuitive leadership, stresses the importance of understanding the concept of how elements of reality are interrelated. Kaiser (1987) pointed out that when thinking about an ideal hospital system "you are attempting to come into resonance with its larger order or pattern of being. If you are successful in your linking, you will become a conscious agent of evolution in the American healthcare system" (p. 16).

PERSONAL INTUITIVE LEADERSHIP ATTRIBUTES

"To have a conscience is to be in touch with the hidden, inner truth of the soul."

(ZOHAR & MARSHALL, 2000, P. 209)

The intuitive leader is open to discovering the unknown, courageously willing to look beyond the conventional paradigms and pioneer an alchemical path for others to follow. The intuitive leader values the rational and logical thought processes and seeks the equilibrium point with the more ethereal concepts of intuitive thinking. As a pioneer, the intuitive leader anticipates resistance but knows how to communicate wisdom and knowledge through inspiration and example by traveling the positive flow channels of the organizational structure and interfacing harmoniously within the universal holographic system. In times when society follows set models, trendy thoughts, and other formulated solutions that appeal to the quick applications mindset, the intuitive leader must have the audacity to think for him- or herself and the stamina of believing in the higher consciousness.

Intuitive leadership style is inspirational and demonstrated through example. Intuitive leadership is similar to a calling whereby the individual is personally compelled to lead through the values of intuitive thinking. Humility and empathy are key in communicating and coaching others in the art and science of intuitive thinking. The intuitive leader needs to surrender his or her ego and manage emotional impulses. The characteristics of intuitive leadership describe an individual who is transparent, daring, and capable of letting go of ego-fueled behavior. Facing resistance and criticism, the intuitive leader must demonstrate a delicate balance between tenacity in effecting the shift and empathy toward those who do not understand or who will not embark on the transformational journey.

> *"Consciousness is far more than intellect: it gives us a capacity for relationship, a potential for a direct and profound intimacy with life."*
>
> (MOSS, 2007, P. 65)

Shift Agent

The intuitive leader acts as a shift agent in implementing intuitive thinking to specific organizational functions and processes. The intuitive leader needs to set the example for the employees by being transparent with his or her personal transformational process, thus communicating the knowledge acquired. The implications include giving employees time and space to discover and exercise their own intuitive thinking and to offer their insights. The focus is on the individuals and on building the organizational system by identifying and developing positive traits and strengths. Providing coaching to help employees identify their fortes, emergent skills, and motivational criteria provides the intuitive leader with the basic values to create an organizational culture that has meaning to the employees.

Because events and issues are all at some level interrelated, when faced with resistance the intuitive leader seeks interconnections, resonance, and flow channels instead of battling head-on with chaos. By letting go of the need to control the destabilizing forces, the intuitive leader finds *pockets of calm* within the chaos that leads to the flow channels. When faced with resistance, instead of imposing change the intuitive leader should choose to fuel or encourage the pockets of calm to develop and grow and thus create a positive critical mass of energy that entrains those who resist or gives them the option to leave because their values and motivations are not in resonance with the organization's culture and mission.

Kaiser (1987) stated that an intuitive leader encounters resistance because he or she advocates to create an imagined reality rather than fight with the difficulties. Abandoning the comfort zone of battling against change or problematic issues can appear threatening as individuals believe they are losing control. Kaiser posits the root of the problem is "we do not teach our healthcare professionals to manage uncertainty or view ambiguity as a desirable precondition of creativity. Their security is vested in the status quo and the "old ways" not in themselves or their vision" (p. 15). As a shift agent the intuitive leader must take this into consideration and provide learning and coaching opportunities to elicit individuals' intuitive potential and help build their self-confidence of their potential in creative thinking.

> *"The more evolved you are, the more of the universe is in your view."*
>
> (YASUHIKO KIMURA, CITED IN PHILLIPS, 2006, P. 49)

Improvisation

In managing day-to-day operations, the intuitive leader must continuously stay in tune with the big picture of reality, the holographic system. Instead of relying on a model or formula, the intuitive leader's reference points are rooted in the concepts and real-time dynamics of the holographic design, utilizing the intuitive tools such as scanning the horizon for signals and recognizing synchronous events. Addressing the critical issues of operating in complex adaptive systems, McDaniel (2007) recommended that leaders use improvisation: "It is improvisation that will enable organizations to generate productive responses to changing conditions" (p. 32). Improvisation entails exploring and testing scenarios without any expectations of where it might lead. Because this process can be risky, intuitive thinking becomes critical.

Plans, processes, and procedures are inescapable and valuable, but it is important to provide space and time for employees to think and live outside those parameters. Balance and equilibrium are key. Plans tend to rule the daily tasks and schedules and can hypnotize employees into routines operating strictly inside the confines of the plans. When a critical issue emerges, decision makers react within those same boundaries without mining into the larger holographic system for insights.

An example of improvisation in a critical situation is on 9/11 when the Saint Vincent Catholic Medical Center's phones went down. Technicians had the insight to improvise telephone communications by making technical changes to their computer system. Many other facilities whose phone systems were down were able to connect into Saint Vincent's improvised communication system and tend to the disaster (McDaniel, 2007). The success of this improvisation was due to the relationships that had been built both internally and with the external environment as well as the leadership that enabled the time and space for improvisation.

> *"While it is tempting to want to defeat uncertainty and surprise with control and planning, it is improvisation that will enable organizations to generate productive responses to changing conditions."*
>
> (MCDANIEL, 2007, P. 32)

Personal Attention and Energy

Because scanning the horizon for signals of change or for emerging trends is an important function for the intuitive leader, sharpening attention skills and fueling passion enhances the accuracy of the exercise. Bradley (2006) commented that "it is also clear from recent research that nonlocal perception is related to the percipient's degree of emotional arousal generated by an object. It is the individual's passion or 'rapt attention'— biological energy activated in his emotional connection to the object of his interest—that generates the outgoing attentional wave directed to the object" (p. 12).

Bradley (2006), in discussing the importance of emitting outgoing waves through the emotion of passion to tune into the holographic system, explained that calming other emotions and attention to other events intensifies the outgoing wave of passion and thus strengthens the communication path within the holographic system. Freeing the brain of extraneous thoughts and emotions fuels the outgoing waves that capture information and receive it through the heart. The heart then sends a signal to the brain to notify the consciousness of incoming information.

Interpersonal Relationships

Good relationships and conviviality are crucial conditions in creating a healthy intuitive environment. In alignment with the holographic concept of organic and adaptive systems, the intuitive leader also needs to develop relationships outside the organization to create the necessary holographic connections and flows that link and generate synchronous events. It is through these relationships that potential collaborations and partnerships can be discovered in areas that would otherwise not have been discussed or explored.

For example, Adidas AG manufactures the soles of some of their sports shoes with tread designed by Goodyear Tire & Rubber Co. (Balasubramanian & Bhardwaj, 2008). The reputation of Goodyear and the perception of robust tires gripping the road are transferred to Adidas' sports shoes. The alliance, however, went beyond the design stage and into marketing the product. The shoes display the Goodyear brand name on the outsoles. This creative alliance between a tire manufacturer and a sports clothing manufacturer is an example of how intuitive thought process and good relationships generate true innovative thinking that is not necessarily based on past experience.

> *"I don't think of leadership as a position. I don't think of leadership as a skill. I think of leadership as a relationship."*
>
> (PHIL QUIGLEY, EX-CEO OF PACIFIC BELL, AS CITED IN COOPER & SAWAF, 1997, P. 51)

COACHING

In an intuitive organization where communication of knowledge and encouraging individuals to reach their potential are key factors, the issue of coaching takes a central role. The intuitive leader must be accountable and have a direct participative role rather than hire outside consultants who are not leaders and will teach theory with case studies that are only generic examples and do not represent the soul of the client organization.

PepsiCo's past CEO, Roger Enrico, who was known to be brilliant in marketing and who acted upon his instinct (Benezra, 1996), realized the importance of being personally implicated in cultivating the organization's culture and vision. "The two years before he became CEO, Enrico devoted more than 120 days exclusively to coaching and mentoring the next generation of PepsiCo leaders. He personally designed a program called Building the Business, and over 18 months he ran the program 10 times, with classes of nine participants each time" (Klein, 2003, p. 208).

Intuitive thinking is not easy to teach because it is an experiential process that needs to be elicited from the individual. It is important to understand that knowledge about the principles of intuition can be communicated but the actual intuitive thinking process must be elicited and experienced by the learner. In this case, "All of Peter Senge's materials extolling the virtues of a learning organization or a teaching organization aren't enough if you don't have the tools to improve the intuition of others" (Klein, 2003, p. 209).

Therefore the personal implication of the intuitive leader in coaching is critical because it gives employees the opportunity to interact directly with a successful intuitive leader. The coaching process also develops internal relationships that are a critical attribute of the intuitive organizational fabric. There is a major difference between learning the theory and living the experience. With the basic theory of intuition, one can learn intuitive thinking by interacting with intuitive peers. Intuitive thinking is a process and a way of life and cannot be learned only by theory and case studies. The element of life, experience, relationship with peers, and soul are the critical elements.

APPLICATIONS OF INTUITIVE LEADERSHIP

Maximizing Team Dynamics

In building an intuitive organizational structure, the intuitive leader understands that the structure of processes must be flexible to enable fluid communications and exchange of knowledge. As Carlson and Kaiser (1999) pointed out, innovative ideas can be suffocated when the downstream organizational channels operate in a closed system.

At a branch of the Max Planck Institute in Germany, Cooper and Sawaf (1997) described "the feeling of incredible excitement in that lab. It was contagious. I realized that what was taking place was innovative collaboration of the highest order. Times of intuitive flow: From one discovery to the next" (p. 211). The director of the lab attributed this intuitive flow to the fact that the lab had selected true innovators—individuals who thrived in the process of creation and whose job was to do only what they do best: come up with innovative ideas. They "were told that each study must hold the promise of providing something of value to humanity or to the healthy future of our planet" (p. 212). This gave meaning to their work and a *raison d'être*. The effectiveness was striking: "every year they were publishing hundreds of studies on their findings" (p. 212).

The communications structure of an intuitive organization is unique to each corporation because it is tailored to the organization's specific industry characteristics and the organization's goals, vision, employees' values, and collective style and culture. For example, in a study on leadership in the nursing environment, Michaels (2002) described the formation of circle communication that "is a form of group exchange that builds a network of relationships, a sense community. Through practices of active listening, intentional speaking, and conscious self-monitoring circle communication emphasizes individual contribution while building consensus to fulfill the purpose of the group" (p. 1). Michaels also specified that these meetings are not mandatory but by invitation, which changes the tone and creates a more convivial atmosphere.

One of the differentiating characteristics of an intuitive thinking environment is it provides an innovation time/space from which creativity can emerge independently from past experience. An intuitive environment fosters thinking and reflection beyond the traditional boundaries of our thought models and encourages employees to communicate insights that might at first appear out of the ordinary and may not fit into conventional thought models. This is true intuitive innovation, even though the raw insight might be delivered in a form that initially is not apparently implementable. It is the responsibility of the intuitive leader to encourage and provide the environment for employees to take the raw insight and play with it until an application with purpose emerges.

BP, in an effort to create effective executive teams, instituted a policy of rotating executives from acquired firms into different positions across the corporation. BP believed that changing roles frequently "forces executives to become very good at meeting new people and building relationships with them" (Gratton & Erickson, 2007, p. 103). As another example of fostering a collaborative environment, in 2005 Fred Goodwin, CEO of the Royal Bank of Scotland, built a 350-million-pound building designed especially to encourage the exchange of ideas. The building features an atrium with an open layout so that employees have a better chance of running into each other (Gratton & Erickson, 2007). The physical transparency in design may subliminally foster a more open-minded and transparent mentality and behavior.

Power of Collective Intuitive Thinking

Research on collective thinking demonstrates that there can be significant value created in the quality of ideas (Eisenhardt, 1999; Surowiecki, 2004). Eisenhardt conducted decision-making research with executives and concluded that "The most effective strategic decision makers made choices that were fast, high quality, and widely supported and did so by building collective intuition" (p. 65). The general concept of collective thinking posits that given a group of intelligent individuals, their aggregate information or knowledge can be at a higher level than on an individual basis (Surowiecki, 2004). Surowiecki commented that the process of creating collective thinking identifies upfront critical differences in ideas and immediately discards those with the less probability of success.

Not all groups of thinkers are automatically wise, and the possibility of groupthink is always present. Poor decisions can be made if groupthink is allowed and the lowest common denominator ideas are taken. It is therefore imperative that the intuitive leader be intellectually sharp, understands the dynamics of collective intuition, and knows how to guide the group to the highest level of decision making.

Some corporations realize the importance of fostering collective thinking and that individuals need to develop interpersonal and intellectual skills to understand the dynamics of collaboration that in turn generates collective thinking. In a study on collaborative teams, "PricewaterhouseCoopers emerged as having one of the strongest capabilities in productive collaboration" (Gratton & Erickson, 2007, p. 106). At the time of the research, PricewaterhouseCoopers counted 140,000 employees in 150 countries. The corporation's training program includes "modules that address teamwork, emotional intelligence, networking, holding difficult conversations, coaching, corporate social responsibility, and communicating the firm's strategy and shared values" (p. 106). Once a collaborative esprit is created, the interpersonal and intellectual dynamics are in place to generate productive collective thinking forums.

When building teams, the intuitive leader must take into consideration employees' preferences about working individually or in teams. The literature on creativity and team building reveals that some individuals are more creative on their own, whereas for others team interaction can also trigger creativity. The intuitive leader respects the need of individual workers and provides them with the environment they need to help them reach their potential. In exchange, these individuals will be asked to participate and interact in teams to share their insights. Fostering a safe team atmosphere where no contribution is judged or ridiculed encourages intuitive insights and promotes collective intuitive thinking.

Strategic Decision Making

Decision makers operate in an environment of continuous change in which even reference points weaken or disappear, whereas others emerge and present new challenges. Yet grounded and focused strategic decision making is what carries the organization through turbulence to meet the goals and remain successful. In a study about strategic decision making in high velocity markets, Eisenhardt (1999) concluded that "Building collective intuition . . . enhances the ability of a top-management team to see threats and opportunities sooner and more accurately" (p. 67). The research demonstrates that successful intuitive decision makers use as much information and data as the less successful ones. The differentiating factor appears to be the reflection time that is provided for generating intuitive insights and regular meetings to foster collective intuitive thinking.

Eisenhardt (1999) gave the example of a successful computer company that "is known for its ability to reposition the firm adroitly as opportunities shift" (p. 67). The organization "measures everything. They examine an array of key operating performance metrics that they collectively track monthly, weekly, and sometimes daily: inventory speed, multiple cash-flow measures, average selling price of products, performance against sales goals, manufacturing yields, customer-acquisition costs, and gross margins by product and geographic region . . . they also pay attention to innovation-related metrics" (p. 67). The list goes on and covers similar intricate measurements of the external marketplace about competitors, including industry gossip. The company attributes its success to its collective intuitive culture. At regular meetings individuals pool their real-time information and generate collective insights to map a more accurate picture of reality and future trends. In a more traditional organization, strategic decisions might be made using parts of the information, with in-depth accounting-based analysis, and independently by different vice presidents with few, if any, regular meetings.

Companies that do not hold regular meetings do not establish a bond among individuals that creates a safe environment to brainstorm or express a view that might not initially appear viable until it is processed further and properly contextualized by others in the meeting. The added value of this type of established familiarity creates a faster paced decision-making process. Individuals recognize each others' fortes or specialty of thinking and learn how to best rely on each other. Eisenhardt (1999) commented that "when intense interaction focuses on the operating metrics of today's businesses, a deep intuition, or 'gut feeling' is created, giving managers a superior grasp of changing competitive dynamics" (p. 69).

Predictive Decision Making

The issues of risk and uncertainty in decision making bring up the concepts of unknown and prediction. Many of the attempted definitions for intuition contain the concept of prediction. For example, "We conceive of intuition as the ability to make above-chance judgments about properties of a stimulus on the basis of information that is not consciously retrieved" (Bolte et al., 2003, p. 416). The mention of above chance implies a certain amount of insight or prediction.

Radin (2004), the renowned psychologist and researcher of intuition, stated that intuitive thoughts can provide correct information about the future, without using inference, as well as information about emotions and intentions of other individuals. Wackermann, Seiter, Keibel, and Walach (2003) conducted an experiment using electroencephalographic technology to test two individuals in two separate electromagnetically insulated rooms. One individual sent a mental signal, whereas the other was the recipient. The findings demonstrated a correlation of brain activity in terms of the recipient registering brain activity as the other person sends the message.

The medical care environment particularly focuses on the use of intuition to enhance predictive decision making. Nursing examples abound, for example, such as the nurse who, by trusting her intuitive thought, saved a 3-year-old boy's life. Although logically nothing should have led her to check on the boy, she listened to her inner voice and discovered he was experiencing respiratory problems and she was able to save his life (Leonard & Sensiper, 1998). Doctors attribute this type of predictive insight to intuition because the individuals have no laboratory information or the formal knowledge to back up their decisions.

Kerfoot (2005) described some emergency room nurses who could codify the condition of a patient entering the room before any other data were available. Kerfoot described the skill as intuitive thought process and agreed with Faugier (2005) that this type of thinking focuses first on the brain by recognizing certain patterns and then using intuitive thought process but that it is a combination of both functions.

Crisis Decision Making

The intuitive leader averts crises and chaos by scanning the horizon of the holographic reality and synchronizing the sensors to capture and understand the signals. Mitroff

(2004) was adamant that "Far in advance of their occurrence, all crises send out a trail of early warning signals" (p. 82). If signals are picked up and processed into the organization's internal and external reality map, then crises can be mitigated or even avoided.

Mitroff (2004), a specialist in crisis leadership, cautions about the nature and definition of a crisis. An event that does not have a major impact on the entire organization might not be a crisis but an emotional over-reaction from a leader who is not centered or connected to the whole picture of the event. Naglewski (2006) guards us against emotional and ego-driven reactions: "Nothing hurts effective decision-making more than allowing ego or insecurity to drive a crisis decision" (p. 49). Part of the intuitive leader's training is to learn to let go of the ego and learn how to use emotions as sensors rather than a channel for personally invested interests and goals.

Mitroff (2004) suggested "A crisis is something that cannot be contained completely within the walls of an organization" (p. 63). It is therefore important for the intuitive leader to be able to reflect if an event is truly a crisis or not by using intuitive thinking and rational analysis. More importantly, the intuitive leader's skills in scanning the horizon for signals of change become a critical attribute in being able to judge the scope of the potential crisis event.

Patton (2003) posited that intuition has a stronger role during a crisis because of the lack of time available for the decision-making process. Many sectors such as the military, police officers, paramedics, and fire fighters operate under constant stress and develop their intuitive skills. Because intuitive thinking accelerates decision-making time by providing clarity, it would enable leaders to avoid potential crisis situations and immediately start focusing on the next issues.

The demise of both Enron and Arthur Andersen resulted in thousands of layoffs for Enron as well as billions in shareholder losses, disastrous impact on the pensions of thousands of former employees, and produced the biggest corporate bankruptcy in U.S. history. In analyzing the decisions that were made during the crisis, Naglewski (2006) stated that these individuals "were certainly intelligent, educated, and business savvy people, and they had the benefit of hindsight into the failure of similar critical decision-making situations to provide some guidance" (p. 46). In reviewing the attributes of the decision maker, one word or concept is absent: intuitive thinking. Could Arthur Andersen employees have made more appropriate decisions had they been trained in intuitive thinking? Naglewski's view is that "Decision makers at Andersen appear to have denied reality, to have lost control of the situation, and not to have learned from the mistakes of others in similar circumstances" (p. 46).

Although it is impossible to judge whether or not intuitive thinking would have saved the situation, it is obvious that intuitive thinking addresses the weaknesses pointed out in the crisis decision-making scenario, especially in terms accepting reality and seeing the potential impact and repercussions the decisions would have had in the holographic picture of reality.

LEADERSHIP AND THE FUTURE

"Intuition is the last frontier of the mind, since it is an aspect of cognition that knows no boundaries."

(CLONINGER, 2006, P. 15)

Scientific evidence supporting the existence and value of intuitive thinking is compelling. Yet the question remains, why is the phenomenon stigmatized? Why is it that those who use and experience intuitive thinking in the workplace hesitate to share their experience with others in fear of being mocked? Cloninger (2006) attempted to answer these questions by stating that intuition "puts us in touch with an immensity that is frightening to individuals who seek to assure measurable objectives" (p. 26).

Are we prisoners of our own consciousness? This chapter puts forth a challenge to those who can or wish to visualize a higher level of consciousness within themselves and society. Believing is like listening. If we do not listen, we will not hear. If we do not believe in intuition, we will not access it. The portal to the cosmic multidimensional universe is open to each of us. We now have the knowledge of how to operate in the fields of resonance and the holographic universe. The question to the aspiring intuitive leader is this: Do I have the courage to walk through the portal of the future and higher consciousness?

REFERENCES

Anonymous. (2003). A Mozart with numbers. *Strategic Finance, 84*(11), 64.

Balasubramanian, S., & Bhardwaj, P. (2008, October 20). Notice me: Cutting through the marketing clutter. *Wall Street Journal*, p. R8. Retrieved July 1, 2009, from http://online.wsj.com/article/SB12242710967 9945225.html

Benezra, K. (1996). Roger Enrico. *Adweek Western Edition, 46*(41), 56–60.

Berns, G. (2008). Rewiring the creative mind. *Fast Company, 129*, 51–56.

Bierman, D. J. (2000, September). Anomalous baseline effects in mainstream emotion research using psychophysiological variables. *Journal of Parapsychology.*

Bierman, D. J., & Radin, D. I. (1997). Anomalous anticipatory response on randomized future conditions. *Perception and Motor Skills, 84*, 689–690.

Bierman, D. J., & Scholte, H. S. (2002). Anomalous anticipatory brain activation preceding exposure of emotional and neutral pictures. Paper presented at Toward a Science of Consciousness IV, Tucson, Arizona.

Block, B. (1990). Intuition creeps out of the closet and into the boardroom. *Management Review, 79*(5), 58–60.

Bolte, A., Goschke, T., & Kuhl, J. (2003). Emotion and intuition: Effects of positive and negative mood on implicit judgments of semantic coherence. *American Psychological Society, 14*, 416–421.

Bradley, R. T. (2006, February 8–10). The psychophysiology of entrepreneurial intuition: a quantum-holographic theory. Proceedings of the Third AGSE International Entrepreneurship Research Exchange, Auckland, New Zealand.

Breuer, H. (2004). Anguish and ethics. *Scientific American, Special Edition, 14*(10), 10–12.

Burke, L. A., & Miller, M. K. (1999). Taking the mystery out of intuitive decision making. *Academy of Management Executive, 13*(4), 91–100.

Carey, S., & Spelke, E. (1996). Science and core knowledge. *Journal of Philosophy of Science, 63,* 515–533.

Carlson, L. K., & Kaiser, K. (1999). Intuitive intelligence. *Health Forum Journal, 42*(5), 50–54.

Cartwright, T. (2004). Feeling your way: Enhancing leadership through intuition. *Leadership in Action, 24*(2), 8–11.

Cloninger, K. (2006). *Curriculum and teaching dialogue.* Charlotte, NC: Information Age Publishing.

Cole, K. (2006). The last putting *themselves* first III: Progress, intuition and development studies. *Progress in Development Studies, 6,* 343–349.

Cooper, R. K., & Sawaf, A. (1997). *Executive EQ: Emotional intelligence in leadership and organizations.* New York: Perigee Books.

Cote, S., & Miners, C. T. H. (2006, March). Emotional intelligence, cognitive intelligence, and job performance. *Administrative Science Quarterly, 51,* 1–28.

Dane, E., & Pratt, M. (2004). Intuition: Its boundaries and role in organizational decision-making. *Academy of Management Best Conference Paper.* MOC, A1–A6.

Don, N. S., McDonough, B. E., & Warren, C. A. (1998). Event-related brain potential (ERP) indicators of unconscious psi: A replication using subjects unselected for psi. *Journal of Parapsychology, 62,* 127–145.

Dowie, J. (2001). Decision technologies and the independent professional: the future's challenge to learning and leadership. *Quality in Health Care, 10*(Suppl II), ii59–ii63.

Drury, M. L., & Kitsopoulos, S. C. (2005). Do you still believe in the seven deadly myths? *Consulting to Management, 16*(1), 28–31.

Dunne, B. J., & Jahn, R. G. (2003). Information and uncertainty in remote perception research. *Journal of Scientific Exploration, 17*(2), 207–241.

Eisenhardt, K. M. (1999). Strategy as strategic decision making. *Sloan Management Review, 40*(3), 65–72.

Ekstrom, S. R. (2004). The mind beyond our immediate awareness: Freudian, Jungian, and cognitive models of the unconscious. *Journal of Analytical Psychology, 49*(5), 657–682.

Farah, M. J., & Wolpe, P. R. (2004). Monitoring and manipulating brain function: New neuroscience technologies and their ethical implications. *The Hastings Center Report, 34*(3), 35–45.

Faugier, J. (2005). Basic instincts. *Nursing Standard, 23*(19), 14–15.

Gilstrap, D. L. (2007). Dissipative structures in educational change: Prigogine and the academy. *International Journal of Leadership in Education, 10*(1), 49–69.

Glaser, M. (1995). Measuring intuition. *Research Technology Management, 38*(2), 43–46.

Goleman, D. (2000). *Working with emotional intelligence.* New York: Bantam Books.

Gratton, L., & Erickson, T. J. (2007). 8 ways to build collaborative teams. *Harvard Business Review, 85*(11), 100–109.

Greenhalgh, T. (2002). Intuition and evidence—uneasy bedfellows? *British Journal of General Practice, 52*(478), 395–400.

Hay, J., LaBree, L., Luo, R., Clark, F., Carlson, M., Mandel, D., et al. (2002). Cost-effectiveness of preventive occupational therapy for independent-living older adults. *Journal of the American Geriatrics Society, 50*(8), 1381–1388.

Hayashi, A. M. (2001). When to trust your gut. *Harvard Business Review, 79*(2), 59–65.

Hodgkinson, G. P., Langan-Fox, J., & Sadler-Smith, E. (2008). Intuition: A fundamental bridging construct in the behavioural sciences. *British Journal of Psychology, 99,* 1–27.

Jeter, T. R. (2003). Knowing without knowing: Urban public middle school administrators' perceptions of intuition in decision-making (Doctoral dissertation, University of Hartford, 2003). *Dissertation Abstracts International, 63*(12), 4168.

Kaiser, L. R. (1987). The intuitive manager and innovation. *Healthcare Forum Journal, 30*(6), 15–17.

Kerfoot, K. (2005). Learning intuition—less college and more kindergarten: The leader's challenge. *Urologic Nursing, 25,* 404–406.

King, L., & Clark, J. M. (2002). Intuition and the development of expertise in surgical ward and intensive care nurses. *Journal of Advanced Nursing, 37*(4), 322–329.

Kingman, S. (2002). Intuition versus analysis: The benefits of modeling health care decisions. Department of Public Health & Policy, London School of Hygiene & Tropical Medicine 7. Retrieved July 1, 2009, from http://www.lshtm.ac.uk/php/publications/briefing7.pdf

Klein, G. A. (2003). *Intuition at work.* New York: Currency Books.

Kopeikina, L. (2006). The elements of a clear decision. *MIT Sloan Management Review, 47*(2), 19–34.

LeDoux, J. (2003). *Synaptic self: How our brains become who we are.* New York: Viking Adult.

Leonard, D., & Sensiper, S. (1998). The role of tacit knowledge in group innovation. *California Management Review, 40*(3), 112–133.

Levin, J., & Kennedy, J. (1975). The relationship of slow cortical potentials to psi information in man. *Journal of Parapsychology, 39,* 25–26.

Lieberman, M. D., Jarcho, J. M., & Satpute, A. B. (2004). Evidence-based and intuition-based self-knowledge: An fMRI study. *Journal of Personality & Social Psychology, 87*(4), 421–435.

Maani, K. E., & Maharaj, V. (2006). Links between systems thinking and complex decision making. *System Dynamics Review, 20,* 21–48.

McCraty, R., Atkinson, M., & Bradley, R. T. (2004a). Electrophysiological evidence of intuition: Part 1. A system-wide process? *Journal of Alternative and Complementary Medicine, 10*(1), 133–143.

McCraty, R., Atkinson, M., & Bradley, R. T. (2004b). Electrophysiological evidence of intuition: Part 2. A system-wide process? *Journal of Alternative and Complementary Medicine, 10*(2), 325–336.

McDaniel, R. T., Jr. (2007). Management strategies for complex adaptive systems. *Performance Improvement, 20*(2), 21–42.

McNaughton, R. D. (2003). The use of meditation and intuition in decision-making: Reports from executive meditators (Doctoral dissertation, Fielding Graduate Institute, 2003). *Dissertation Abstracts International, 64*(05), 1750.

Michaels, C. L. (2002). Circle communication: An old form of communication useful for 21st century leadership. *Nursing Administration, 26*(5), 1–10.

Miller, C., & Ireland, D. H. (2005). Intuition in strategic decision making: Friend or foe in the fast-paced 21st century? *Academy of Management Executive, 19,* 19–30.

Milner, V. (2006). Uncommonly sensible social work practice: Using depths of conventional wisdom and spirituality to match what we know with what we sense. *Social Work Review, 18*(3), 61–68.

Mitroff, I. I. (2004). *Crisis leadership: Planning for the unthinkable.* Hoboken, NJ: Wiley.

Moss, R. (2007). *The mandala of being: Discovering the power of awareness.* Novato, CA: New World Library.

Murray, E. (2004). Intuitive coaching. *Industrial and Commercial Training, 36*(5), 203–206.

Naglewski, K. (2006, Spring). Are you ready to make effective decisions when disaster strikes? *Journal of Private Equity, Special Turnaround Management Issue, 9*(2), 45–51.

Patton, J. R. (2003). Intuition in decisions. *Management Decision, 41,* 989–996.

Phillips, J. (2006). *The art of original thinking: The making of a thought leader.* San Diego: 9th Element Press.

Polkosky, M. (2008). Intuiting design. *Speech Technology Magazine.* Retrieved July 1, 2009, from http://www.speechtechmag.com/Articles/Column/Interact/Intuiting-Design-49902.aspx

Radin, D. I. (1997). Unconscious perception of future emotions: An experiment in presentiment. *Journal of Scientific Exploration, 11,*163–180.

Radin, D. I. (2004). The future is now. *Shift: At the Frontiers of Consciousness,* 38–39.

Radin, D. I., & Schlitz, M. J. (2005). Gut feelings, intuition, and emotions: An exploratory study. *The Journal of Alternative and Complementary Medicine, 11,* 85–91.

Ramphal, S. (2003). Global governance or a new imperium: Which is it to be? *The Round Table, 369,* 213–219.

Reiner, A. (2004). Psychic phenomena and early emotional states. *Journal of Analytical Psychology, 49,* 313–336.

Sadler-Smith, E. (2004). Cognitive style and the management of small and medium-sized enterprises. *Organization Studies, 25*(2), 155.

Sadler-Smith, E., & Shefy, E. (2004a). Developing intuition: Becoming smarter by thinking less. *Academy of Management Proceedings*, PC1.

Sadler-Smith, E., & Shefy, E. (2004b). The intuitive executive: Understanding and applying "gut feel" in decision-making. *Academy of Management Executive, 18*(4), 76–91.

Schulz, M. L. (1998). *Awakening intuition: Using your mind-body network for insight and healing.* New York: Harmony Books.

Sekerka, L. E., Brumbaugh, A. M., Rosa, J. A., & Cooperrider, D. (2006). Comparing appreciative inquiry to a diagnostic technique in organizational change: the moderating effects of gender. *International Journal of Organization Theory and Behavior, 9*(4), 449–489.

Senge, P., Scharmer, C. O., Jaworski, J., & Flowers, B. S. (2005). *Presence: An exploration of profound change in people, organizations, and society.* New York: Currency Books.

Sengupta, K., Abdel-Hamid, T. K., & Van Wassenhove, L. N. (2008). The experience trap. *Harvard Business Review, 86*(2), 94–101.

Sinclair, M., & Ashkanasy, N. M. (2005). Intuition: Myth or a decision-making tool? *Management Learning, 36,* 353–371.

Spottiswood, J., & May, E. (2003). Skin conductance prestimulus response: Analyses, artifacts and a pilot study. *Journal of Scientific Exploration, 17,* 617–641.

Stewart, T. (2002). How to think with your gut. *Business, 2.0,3*(11), 98–104.

Sundgren, M., & Styhre, A. (2004). Intuition and pharmaceutical research: The case of AstraZeneca. *European Journal of Innovation Management, 7*(4), 267–279.

Surel, D. (2009). Identifying intuition in the decision-making process: A phenomenological research study. (Doctoral dissertation, University of Phoenix, 2007). *Dissertation Abstracts International, 69*(10).

Surowiecki, J. (2004). *The wisdom of crowds.* New York: Random House.

Swain, D. O. (2007, January). Achieving R&D leadership. *Research Technology Management,* 60–65.

Tracy, C. S., Dantas, G. C., & Upshur, R. E. G. (2003). Evidence-based medicine in primary care: Qualitative study of family physicians. *BMC Family Practice, 4,* 6.

Wackermann, J., Seiter, C., Keibel, H., & Walach, H. (2003). Correlations between brain electrical activities of two spatially separated human subjects. *Neuroscience Letters, 336,* 60–64.

Wheatley, M. J. (1992/1999). *Leadership and the new science.* San Francisco: Berrett-Koehler Publishers.

Zohar, D., & Marshall, I. (2000). *SQ: Spiritual intelligence the ultimate intelligence.* New York: Bloomsbury Publishing.

Index

Page numbers followed by *b, f,* or *t* indicate boxes, figures, or tables, respectively.